Beyond Biomechanics

Psychosocial Aspects of Musculoskeletal Disorders in Office Work

About the editors

Sam Moon, MD, MPH, is on the Duke University faculty in Occupational and Environmental Medicine. He is Board certified in occupational medicine, a Fellow of the American Academy of Family Physicians, and a Diplomate of the American Board of Pain Medicine. He lectures and writes on various topics, including pain disorders as they relate to work. His consulting practice emphasizes individual and corporate strategies for health, prevention, and productivity. Sam Moon consults nationally, and serves as Corporate Physician for several companies in the Research Triangle Park and in Southeast USA.

Steven L. Sauter received his PhD in Industrial Psychology from the University of Wisconsin, and later headed the Behavioral Science Program in the University's Department of Preventative Medicine. He currently serves as Chief of the Applied Psychology and Ergonomics Branch at the National Institute for Occupational Safety & Health (NIOSH), and as Adjunct Professor of Human Factors Engineering at the University of Cincinnati's Department of Mechanical, Nuclear, and Industrial Engineering. His research interests focus on occupational stress and ergonomics, with a special emphasis on office and computer work. He is an Associate Editor of the *Journal of Occupational Health Psychology*, and has authored and edited several books and articles on the psychosocial aspects of occupational health, including *Promoting Health and Productivity in the Computerized Office* (with Marvin Dainoff and Michael Smith, Taylor & Francis, 1990).

Beyond Biomechanics

Psychosocial Aspects of Musculoskeletal Disorders in Office Work

EDITED BY

S. D. MOON

Duke University Medical Center, Division of Occupational and Environmental Medicine, Durham, North Carolina, USA

AND

S. L. SAUTER

National Institute for Occupational Safety and Health, Taft Laboratory, Cincinnati, Ohio, USA

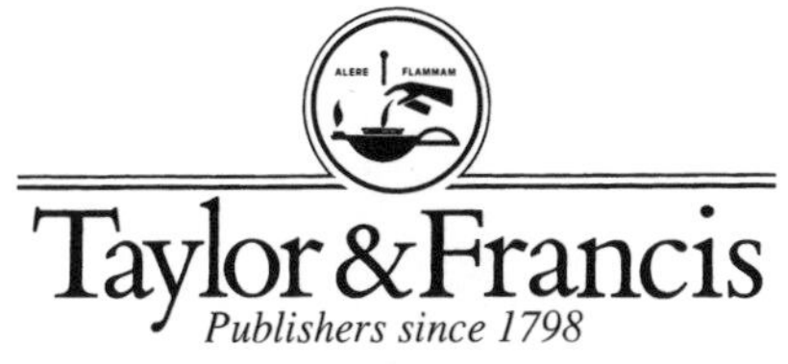

UK Taylor & Francis Ltd, 1 Gunpowder Square, London EC4 3DE
USA Taylor & Francis Inc., 1900 Frost Road, Suite 101, Bristol, PA 19007

The opinions, findings, and conclusions expressed in this volume are those of the individual authors, not of the editors nor of the National Institute for Occupational Safety and Health (NIOSH). The editors cannot assume responsibility for the validity of all materials or for the consequences of their use. Mention of company names or products does not constitute endorsement by the editors or by NIOSH.

British Library Cataloguing in Publication Data

A catalogue record for this book is available from the British Library.
ISBN 07484 0321 3 (cased)
ISBN 07484 0322 1 (paperback)

Library of Congress Cataloging in Publication Data are available

Cover design by Amanda Barragry

Typeset in Times 10/12 pt by Santype International Limited, Salisbury, Wilts., England
Printed in Great Britain by T J Press (Padstow) Ltd

To Robin and Ezra, with gratitude for patience and support

SDM

Contents

Contributors

BEN AMICK
Yale University School of Medicine, New Haven, Connecticut, USA

BRUCE BERNARD
National Institute for Occupational Safety and Health, Cincinnati, Ohio, USA

SIDNEY BLAIR
Loyola University Medical Center, Maywood, Illinois, USA

LESLIE BODEN
Boston University, Boston, Massachusetts, USA

RICHARD BUTLER
University of Minnesota, Minneapolis, Minnesota, USA

PASCALE CARAYON
University of Wisconsin, Madison, Wisconsin, USA

DELIA CIOFFI
Dartmouth College, Hanover, New Hampshire, USA

E. N. CORLETT
University of Nottingham, United Kingdom

JENNIFER R. EGERT
Duke University Medical Center, Durham, North Carolina, USA

MICHAEL FEUERSTEIN
Uniformed University of the Health Sciences, Bethesda, Maryland, USA

LAWRENCE J. FINE
National Institute for Occupational Safety and Health, Cincinnati, Ohio, USA

WILBERT E. FORDYCE
University of Washington School of Medicine, Seattle, Washington, USA

LINDA FRAZIER
Duke University Medical Center, Durham, North Carolina, USA

HAROLD GARDNER
Options & Choices, Inc., Cheyenne, Wyoming, USA

TOM HALES
National Institute for Occupational Safety and Health, Cincinnati, Ohio, USA

JAY S. HIMMELSTEIN
University of Massachusetts Medical School, Worcester, Massachusetts, USA

BRUCE HOCKING
Telstra, Melbourne, Australia

E. HOEKSTRA
National Institute for Occupational Safety and Health, Cincinnati, Ohio, USA

JOE HURRELL
National Institute for Occupational Safety and Health, Cincinnati, Ohio, USA

STANISLAV KASL
Yale University, New Haven, Connecticut, USA

FRANCIS J. KEEFE
Duke University Medical Center, Durham, North Carolina, USA

SAMUEL D. MOON
Duke University Medical Center, Durham, North Carolina, USA

GLENN PRANSKY
University of Massachusetts Medical School, Worcester, Massachusetts, USA

STEVEN L. SAUTER
National Institute for Occupational Safety and Health, Cincinnati, Ohio, USA

JAMES A. SKELTON
Dickinson College, Carlisle, Pennsylvania, USA

MICHAEL J. SMITH
University of Wisconsin, Madison, Wisconsin, USA

TERRY B. SNYDER
University of Massachusetts Medical School, Worcester, Massachusetts, USA

CRAIG STENBERG
Duke University Medical Center, Durham, North Carolina, USA

NAOMI G. SWANSON
National Institute for Occupational Safety and Health, Cincinnati, Ohio, USA

TORES THEORELL
Karolinska Institute, Stockholm, Sweden

R. H. WESTGAARD
The Norwegian Institute of Technology, Trondheim, Norway

Foreword

This set of papers, bringing together material concerning the interaction between psychosocial and physical factors in the occurrence of musculoskeletal diseases in the office, is timely. Evidence in this field from the working world outside the office environment has been discussed by researchers for many years, but until now the office has not had major attention in this respect.

While office work has major differences in the activities undertaken when compared with, for example, construction work or hospital nursing, the pressures on individuals arising from organizational pressures and social interactions and norms can be equally influential. In the first of these areas we have recognized the influence on safety of peer pressure to take risks arising from a concept of masculinity. In the nursing profession a caring intention can foster the belief that a patient should be moved from the floor, after falling, as quickly as possible. This can put the caregiver at serious, and often unnecessary, risk. More generally, management pressure for output will sometimes cause them to turn a blind eye to unsafe practices in spite of their own promulgated rules. In each of these cases there is a mismatch between appropriate activities and cultural norms which influences the probability of safe behavior.

But recognizing a possible set of influences is a long way from defining its contribution in terms that can be applied to injury reduction. While much work continues, as it must, on the nature of the responses of the muscles and joints to loading, the broadening of the research area to see injury in the full ecological context of people in their total environment is an important advance in the struggle to improve work and work safety.

This broader perspective is one that ergonomists have sought to adopt, recognizing that there are interactions between the various factors that influence human performance apart from their direct effects. Matching these many factors to the capabilities and other requirements of people has always been more than anthropometry and biomechanics, although it needed a lot of work in these basic areas before we could usefully turn our attention to the wider field.

An industrial study illustrating this point is that of the Saab-Scania engine assemblers (Edgren, 1985). Objective measures of the physical work capacity of the assemblers demonstrated a range of strengths, while ratings of perceived exertion for their work showed a low rating – very weak – for all of them. Yet musculoskeletal upper limb injuries in this group were very high.

A 12-month prospective study was run, with 25 assemblers. Physical work capacity with an arm ergometer was measured before and after study, as was a measure of preferred work rate. Although their work capacity revealed a range of abilities, the preferred work rates were very similar, being positioned in the middle of the range of the objective measures. It was proposed that for the 13 whose preferred rate was above their capacity, they were at risk. For those in the reverse situation, no risk existed.

At the end of the study the musculoskeletal condition of 10 of the 13 who were at risk had deteriorated, as had that of two in the other category. The 'motivation' to work at a particular rate, arising from their experience of assembly, had encouraged them to work beyond their capacity. To paraphrase Edgren's concluding comment, non-risk individuals are physically strong compared to the chosen work rate, whereas the at-risk ones are physically weak in relation to the demands but ambitious to achieve the norm, emphasizing the effects in this case of social expectations for common levels of performance on injury causation.

While cases such as this are not rare in the literature, progress towards a full understanding is slow. Even where the knowledge is relatively strong, modifying the social norms is a long process. Nursing is the leading profession that experiences back disorders. In the United Kingdom the Royal College of Nursing has, since 1979, steadily advanced the quality of patient handling, and produced the definitive treatise on the subject (Corlett *et al.*, 1992). But it was 15 years before hospital managements could begin to institute 'no-lifting' policies. Three are already in evidence in UK hospitals and many are under development. The clear reduction in risk and the changes in injury levels are not the product of good training and good handling practice only, but equally importantly, of changes in both management and nurses' perceptions of the nurse's role and work. These last have been the key factors in enabling the necessary changes to be instituted, and in achieving the subsequent improvements (Tracy, 1994).

In the half century since the recognition of the interactions in the workplace which gave rise to the term 'sociotechnical system', we have moved steadily towards the study of work from an increasingly holistic viewpoint. These studies have allowed many developments in practice which have demonstrated the validity of the approach. Increasingly we are looking beyond the task, to the work and the system in which the work is done. Good work performance and safe work are products of good system design, and better understanding of that system at the crucial interface between the tasks and the individual is the contribution of this book.

E. N. CORLETT

REFERENCES

CORLETT, E. N., LLOYD, P. V., TARLING, C., TROUP, J. D. G. and WRIGHT, B. 1992 *Guide to the Handling of Patients*, London: National Back Pain Association.

EDGREN, B., 1985, *Perceived Exertion, Motivation and Health: An Industrial Experience*, Stockholm: Dept of Work Sciences, The Royal Institute of Technology.

TRACY, M., 1994, personal communication.

Preface

This book explores, but does not systematically chart, a large and sometimes controversial subject with indefinite boundaries. It is the outgrowth of a multidisciplinary conference convened at Duke University in the fall of 1993 to address non-biomechanical influences on musculoskeletal disorders in office work. Such disorders, particularly in association with the use of video display terminals (VDTs), have been a problem of concern internationally for over a decade. Biomechanical stressors such as awkward postures in keyboard operation have long been suspected as a primary source of these problems. But in recent years, an impressive body of literature has accumulated which also implicates so-called 'psychosocial factors' in the causal path. In the domain of VDT work, well over a dozen studies can now be identified that link factors such as low social support at work or low worker autonomy to an increased prevalence of musculoskeletal disorders. However, important aspects of this relationship await clarification. For example, there is little consensus on precisely which features of the psychosocial environment represent key risks for musculoskeletal disorders. (Indeed, the concept of psychosocial factors is itself somewhat abstract.) Additionally, the relative influence or effect size of psychosocial factors on musculoskeletal disorders in office work is uncertain, and there is little consensus on biological or other mediating mechanisms. The aim of the workshop was to address these areas of uncertainty, with the goal of better understanding prevention measures for musculoskeletal disorders in office work.

To ensure effective coverage of this subject, a multidisciplinary group of scientists representing the areas of social and organizational psychology, medical anthropology, occupational medicine and rehabilitation, office ergonomics, job stress, and health-care economics was invited to contribute to the workshop. Thus, although workshop topics were framed roughly as 'psychosocial', the discussion was far reaching and ranged from behavioral, to economic, to sociopolitical issues. Further, the emphasis on musculoskeletal disorders in the office environment was repeatedly blurred through reference and extension to other work environments and demands. The contents of the present volume reflect this breadth.

The core chapters in this volume are presented in Parts One and Two, followed by a third section of commentary on selected issues raised in the core chapters. The volume begins with discussions and supportive evidence of theoretical models and mechanisms linking psychosocial factors and musculoskeletal disorders in office work. The presentations range from very broad treatment of this subject, such as efforts to integrate psychosocial and ergonomic stressors in a comprehensive causal model (e.g. Chapters 1 and 2), to papers that more narrowly probe suspected effects of psychological demands on musculoskeletal response (e.g. Chapter 5). Of special significance, an entire body of social psychological literature on symptom perception is introduced for the first time into the discussion of musculoskeletal disorders in office work (Chapter 3).

To some extent, Part Two of the volume continues with the discussion of efforts to explain the relationship between psychosocial factors and musculoskeletal disorders. But interwoven with the discussion in a more explicit way are implications and direction for management and prevention of musculoskeletal disorders, as well as for further research on both etiology and prevention. These implications cut across the entire spectrum of prevention: from organizational and workstyle interventions focused on primary prevention (Chapters 11 and 15), to tertiary prevention via symptom management (Chapter 10).

Although the chapters in this volume illuminate potential paths between psychosocial factors and musculoskeletal disorders and, by extrapolation, suggest avenues for intervention, we should not lose sight of the fact that knowledge in this area is still quite rudimentary. Many of the viewpoints expressed in this volume await confirmation, and some of the findings are subject to multiple interpretations. Additional perspectives, as contained in Part Three, were sought for some of the issues and material that seemed especially challenging. Because current knowledge is far from complete, uncritical or narrow conclusions drawn by the reader regarding the way that psychosocial factors influence musculoskeletal disorders in office work are, at best, likely to be unproductive.

With regard to intervention, the complex etiologic picture argues for a comprehensive approach which addresses biomechanical, organizational and, where feasible, individual and societal factors. However, there is concern that an etiologic focus on psychosocial factors may serve to personalize the cause and reduce the credibility of musculoskeletal disorders in office work (e.g. Chapter 13). In this regard, some of the papers (e.g. Chapters 12 and 14) seem highly skeptical of the importance of biomedical/biomechanical explanations of musculoskeletal disorders in office work. Such interpretation could inappropriately detract from a public health prevention approach wherein the front line of defense is primary prevention at the workplace (i.e. work redesign in contrast to worker-focused strategies such as stress management).

On the other hand, several papers argue that the psychosocial perspective is not incompatible with the public health or biomedical tradition. Chapters 1, 2 and 8 all suggest ways to enlarge the biomedical/biomechanical framework to accommodate a variety of psychosocial effects. Additionally, some authors who highlight the role of psychological and cultural influences on musculoskeletal disorders, in contrast to biomechanical mechanisms, are still strong proponents of organizational interventions (e.g. Cioffi in Chapter 3, Hocking in Chapter 9). In our view, there is no theoretical basis or practical reward for tension between the biomedical or public health tradition and the reality of psychosocial influences on musculoskeletal disorders in office work. However, broader acceptance of this perspective and a fuller understanding of the causes and control of musculoskeletal disorders in office work depends on closer dialogue between occupational medicine and social science such as that initiated at the Duke workshop.

Finally, we wish to acknowledge and thank the individuals and organizations who helped to make the Duke workshop and this publication possible. We are grateful to the Duke University Division of Occupational and Environmental Medicine and the Office Ergonomics Research Committee for their sponsorship of the workshop; to the workshop participants and representatives from industry and labor for their insightful and lively discussion; to Donald Elisburg, Gary Greenberg, and the many other reviewers for their editorial assistance in preparing this volume; and especially to the individual authors for their thoughtful contributions and patience during the editorial process.

STEVEN SAUTER and SAM MOON

PART ONE

Evidence, Models, and Mechanisms

CHAPTER ONE

An ecological model of musculoskeletal disorders in office work†

STEVEN L. SAUTER and NAOMI G. SWANSON

INTRODUCTION

There is increasing recognition that so-called 'psychosocial' factors in the workplace are somehow involved in the etiology of work-related musculoskeletal disorders, especially in the context of office work involving video display terminals (VDTs). In an expansive review of the epidemiologic literature on psychosocial factors and musculoskeletal disorders, Bongers and de Winter (1992) concluded that monotonous work, high perceived workload, time pressure, and low control and social support were all related to musculoskeletal symptoms among workers. This relationship is captured in a metaphor by Hocking (1990) which likens work-related disease to an iceberg floating in a social sea (workplace psychosocial environment). Disease is more or less manifest as the iceberg floats higher or lower as a function of conditions in the psychosocial sea.

Despite the mounting evidence, the notion that psychosocial factors affect musculoskeletal disorders has met with some uncertainty. As we see it, the problem is twofold, having to do with (1) confusion regarding the concept of psychosocial factors, and (2) questions regarding possible causal mechanisms linking psychosocial factors and musculoskeletal disorders. These uncertainties are elaborated further as follows.

The expression 'psychosocial factors' is a nonspecific term and involves a vernacular that is unfamiliar outside the stress arena. In its general usage in occupational health, the term has served as catch-all in reference to nonphysical elements of the job/work environment, including organizational climate or culture, aspects of work organization such as the complexity of tasks, and even psychological attributes of workers such as job attitudes (e.g. job satisfaction) and personality traits. Such breadth is not inappropriate (International Labour Office, 1986; Chapter 4 of this

† The views expressed here are those of the authors, and not necessarily those of the National Institute for Occupational Safety and Health.

volume), but it likely contributes to confusion in interpreting what is meant when we speak of psychosocial factors in relation to health problems.

A related issue is that psychosocial factors, such as organizational climate, can be difficult to measure as objectively as many physical workplace hazards such as lifting requirements or the presence of toxic agents. Information on workplace psychosocial factors is usually subjective and obtained through surveys or other self-report techniques. Further, some theorists place greater emphasis on individual appraisals (perceptions) of the environment, in contrast to the objective environment, in determining health risks (e.g. Lazarus, 1966) of psychosocial factors. This subjectivity can create uncertainty in interpreting whether self-reports of workplace psychosocial conditions represent attributes of the environment or whether they are highly individualized perceptions, which leads to uncertainty in ascribing risks associated with workplace psychosocial factors to the job or to the individual.

Uncertainty results also from the absence of a satisfactory or widely accepted framework for explaining causal linkages between psychosocial factors and musculoskeletal disorders. Concepts of disease in Western culture are dominated by the biomedical model, involving biological determinism or mediation of disease processes. Some investigators have proposed that muscle tension secondary to stress may account, in part, for the relationship between psychosocial factors and musculoskeletal disorders (Ursin *et al.*, 1993; Ursin *et al.*, 1988; Waersted *et al.*, 1991; Westgaard and Bjorklund, 1987). But, with this exception, there has been limited discussion or evidence of biological mediation between psychosocial factors and musculoskeletal disorders.

In the wake of the repetition strain injury (RSI) epidemic which engulfed Australia during the 1980s (see Hocking, 1987a, for an overview), mechanisms involving psychological mediation of the relationship between psychosocial factors and musculoskeletal disorders have been proposed. However, this type of explanation has had mixed reception. Within a biomedical paradigm, the implication of psychological processes in the etiology of disease may create the impression that the disease is not 'real' (see Chapter 13 of this volume for a broader discussion of this issue). Various Australian explanations for RSI have emphasized psychiatric mechanisms or other abnormalistic processes (see Bammer and Martin, 1988; Mullaly and Grigg, 1988; Spillane and Deves, 1987), which probably serves to exacerbate this effect. Further, implication of psychological mechanisms may be seen by some as 'victim blaming,' in that it appears to shift the etiologic focus toward the worker and away from the job.

The present discussion attempts to address some of these areas of uncertainty. The primary goal is to suggest ways in which workplace psychosocial factors can influence musculoskeletal disorders. The intent is not to diminish the importance of physical ergonomic factors and biomechanical mechanisms in the etiology of work-related musculoskeletal disorders but, rather, to suggest a more holistic framework which incorporates both psychosocial and physical ergonomic components.

We begin with an attempt to shed further light on the concept of psychosocial factors. Then a hypothetical model of workplace psychosocial factors and musculoskeletal disorders is presented. An important feature of the model is that psychological mediation of musculoskeletal disorders is discussed in terms of normal psychological processes which are fairly well understood in social and health psychology. Finally, research supporting constituent pathways in the model is presented with an emphasis on studies of VDT work.

PSYCHOSOCIAL FACTORS

Few explicit definitions of the expression 'psychosocial factors' can be found in the literature. In the context of work, definition is often by reference to specific conditions such as lack of autonomy, increased work pressure, difficult interpersonal relationships at work (e.g. see National Occupational Health and Safety Commission, 1986). Other definitions simply distinguish physical and nonphysical aspects of the job. Evans *et al.* (1994, p. 2) define the psychosocial environment at work as 'the way production of goods and services is organized and . . . the social climate of the setting produced by the activities of the organization and the people in it,' in contrast to 'physical' factors which refer to 'inanimate components of the work setting.' A similar distinction is made by the World Health Organization (WHO), European Office, in a 1989 report on psychosocial and health aspects of VDT work (WHO, 1989).

Embedded in these approaches to psychosocial factors is the notion of psychological salience; i.e. psychosocial factors have some kind of psychological representation, meaning or valence within the individual. For example, in defining psychosocial stressors, Van Harrison (1983) emphasizes the 'symbolic meaning' of actions and conditions in the workplace.

The International Labour Office (ILO) and WHO carry this concept a step further. In a joint report, ILO/WHO define psychosocial factors as aspects of the work environment, of the extra-work environment, and of the individual which interact to affect well-being (and performance), with an emphasis on psychological effects (ILO, 1986). In effect, this is a simple expression of an occupational stress model or process. In this approach, psychosocial factors can be understood as any factor or condition, whether individual or work related, that contributes to the stress process.

Although it is a significant overgeneralization, it can be said that all theories of stress/occupational stress (e.g. Caplan *et al.*, 1975; Hurrell and Murphy, 1992; Kagan and Levi, 1971; Karasek and Theorell, 1990; Matteson and Ivancevich, 1989; McGrath, 1970; Smith and Carayon-Sainfort, 1989) can be reduced to a common theme: psychological stress is understood as a *process* involving the interaction of environmental demands with individual attributes (needs, expectations, resources, etc.), which leads to acute psychological, behavioral, and physiological reactions and ultimately affects physical health. This core feature is illustrated in Figure 1.1, which shows a generic or simplified version of the Kagan and Levi (1971) and other (e.g. Cooper and Marshall, 1976; Hurrell and Murphy, 1992) psychosocial stress models. In this type of model, individual factors are usually considered as intervening variables which serve to modify the relationship between environmental demands (stressors) and stress responses (strains/ill health); i.e. the model gives primacy to environmental factors in determining health outcomes. (Other models such as Caplan *et al.* (1975) posit more direct effects of individual factors, placing stronger emphasis on the actual fit or balance between environmental demands and individual resources as a determinant of stress.)

Not shown in this model is the appraisal process postulated by Lazarus (1966) which occurs at the intersection of environmental demands and individual variables. As described by Lazarus, appraisal is a multistage cognitive process in which the individual first evaluates the threat potential of the environmental stimulus, and then the availability of individual coping resources. In this schema, stress is regarded

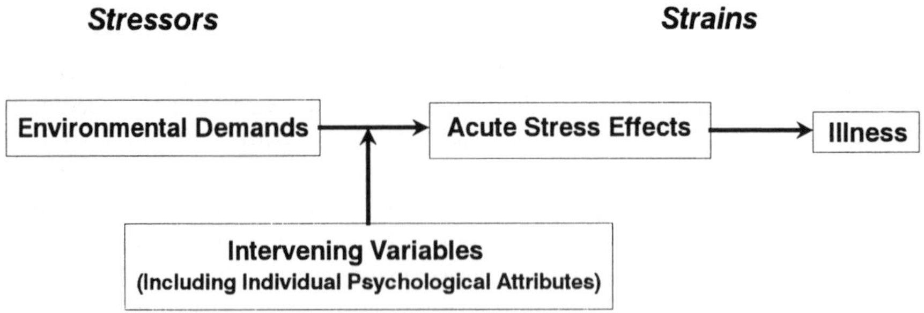

Figure 1.1 The psychosocial stress model.

as a highly individualized and subjective or intrapsychic phenomenon and, thus, the etiological and prevention focus shifts away from environmental conditions toward individual factors. While not denying individual variability in appraisal, critics of Lazarus assert that there are certain environment/job conditions which most workers appraise as threatening most of the time, which argues more for an environmental emphasis (see Brief and George, 1991).

Reviews and studies of job stress provide insight to specific individual factors and working conditions that feed the stress process, and help to provide a more concrete understanding of psychosocial factors. With regard to individual factors, Payne (1988) identified three classes of variables corresponding to (1) genetic factors (e.g. intelligence), (2) acquired aspects (e.g. social class, culture, educational attainment), and (3) dispositional factors (e.g. personality characteristics or attitudes such as job satisfaction). The latter two classes of variables are of special significance to the present discussion. Cultural factors are seen as potent psychosocial determinants of musculoskeletal and other occupational health disorders (Hocking, 1987a, 1987b; Mechanic, 1972). Also, negative affectivity, a dispositional factor characterized by undifferentiated subjective distress, is increasingly associated with elevated levels of somatic complaints (Cohen *et al.*, 1995; Watson and Pennebaker, 1989). Bergquist *et al.* (1995a), for example, have shown that negative affectivity is associated with increased neck–shoulder discomfort in VDT users.[1]

The stress literature also suggests specific classes of psychosocial factors pertaining to working conditions (Cooper and Marshall, 1976; Evans *et al.*, 1994; ILO, 1986; Matteson and Ivancevitch, 1989). The ILO/WHO taxonomy (ILO, 1986), for example, categorized work-related psychosocial factors into (1) physical environmental conditions, (2) factors intrinsic to the job (e.g. workload and design of tasks), (3) arrangement of work time (e.g. hours of work and shift schedule), (4) management/operating practices (e.g. workers' roles, participative management, relationships at work), and (5) technological change.

Kasl (1992) has attempted to dimensionalize working conditions as risk factors for mental health in a way that may also prove useful for understanding work-related psychosocial factors. Elements in the Kasl (1992) taxonomy are summarized as follows:

- Physical aspects of work: physical environmental conditions at work (e.g. heat or chemical exposure) including physical ergonomic demands such as lifting requirements.

- Temporal aspects of the job: hours of work and work–rest schedule, work shift, work pace, etc.
- Job content: scope and repetitiveness of tasks, use of skills, vigilance/mental workload demands, participation in decision-making, clarity of demands, etc.
- Interpersonal relationships: group cohesion, supportiveness of peers and supervisors, availability of feedback, etc.
- Organizational aspects: tall/flat organizational structure and associated bureaucratic characteristics.
- Financial/economic aspects: pay methods, benefits, etc.
- Community/societal aspects: status/prestige associated with the job.

Like ILO (1986), Kasl also adds 'change in the work setting' as a separate psychosocial dimension, particularly in regard to potential for promotion, demotion, job loss, etc. Additional dimensions, which might be considered for this list based on their prominence in prior and current stress research, include work roles (clarity, conflict, and number), human resource systems (training, career development opportunities, etc.), and organizational climate (values, communications styles, etc., in the organization). However, there is a considerable degree of arbitrariness here, and there is no single classification scheme that predominates in the organizational psychology or stress literature.

Both ILO (1986) and Kasl (1992) include physical environmental conditions as a psychosocial hazard. However, although it may be a fine point, the following distinction can be made. Unlike other dimensions, the immediate or direct effect of physical environmental conditions (except for aesthetic aspects of the environment) are somatic, not psychological. Psychological effects occur only as a secondary phenomenon following from the experience of somatic symptoms or disorders resulting from the physical exposure. This argues against the inclusion of physical environmental factors as primary psychosocial factors.

As a group, these dimensions of work are often referred to as job design or work organization factors because, to a large extent, they derive from the way that work systems are designed or organized. In subsequent discussion, the expression 'work organization' is used broadly in reference to any work-related risk factor for job stress, whereas the expression 'psychosocial factors' refers to attributes of both the job *and* the individual that contribute to job stress.

PSYCHOSOCIAL PATHWAYS TO MUSCULOSKELETAL DISORDERS

Three types of explanations for the association between work-related psychosocial factors and musculoskeletal disorders seem especially plausible. In a report on VDT work and musculoskeletal disorders in news editors, the National Institute for Occupational Safety and Health (NIOSH) postulated that (1) psychosocial demands and job stress may produce increased muscle tension and exacerbate task-related biomechanical strain, (2) psychosocial demands may affect awareness and reporting of musculoskeletal symptoms, or affect perceptions of their cause, or (3) the association may be related to a causal or correlational relationship between psychosocial and physical demands (NIOSH, 1993). These types of mechanism have been suggested by several investigators (Bergquist, 1984; Bongers and de Winter, 1992; Bongers *et al.*, 1993; Sauter *et al.*, 1983a; Sauter *et al.*, 1983b; Ursin *et al.*, 1988).

This chapter incorporates all of these pathways into a formal causal model, which builds on earlier efforts by the authors to model the relationship between psychosocial factors and musculoskeletal disorders in office work (Sauter, 1991; Sauter and Swanson, 1993; Sauter *et al.*, 1983a; Sauter *et al.*, 1983b). This model, shown in Figure 1.2, represents an integration of the generic psychosocial stress process illustrated in Figure 1.1 into the traditional biomechanical model of musculoskeletal disorders. This integration can be seen in Figure 1.3, which decomposes the present model into biomechanical, psychosocial and cognitive components.

Recently, researchers from the TNO Institute of Preventive Health Care in the Netherlands have described a generic model of workplace psychosocial factors and musculoskeletal disease with pathways similar to those depicted in Figures 1.2 and 1.3 (Bongers and de Winter, 1992; Bongers *et al.*, 1993).[2] However, an important distinguishing feature of the present model is the attention to cognitive processes, described below, which mediate between biomechanical strain and the development of musculoskeletal disorders (i.e. the shaded area in Figure 1.2 and the 'cognitive' component in Figure 1.3).

According to the present model (Figure 1.2), musculoskeletal disorders can be traced ultimately to the nature of work technology, which includes both the nature of tools and work systems. In the case of office or VDT work the chief tool is the VDT/computer, and the nature of work can be defined as mechanized or automated information work. As shown in the model, work technology has a direct path to physical demands, as defined by the physical coupling between the worker and the tool (i.e. workstation ergonomics), and also a direct path to work organization. The influence of industrialization/mechanization on the specialization of job tasks, recognized since Adam Smith (1976), is an example of the latter. The pathway from work organization to physical demands suggests that the physical demands of work are exacerbated by organizational demands; for example, increased specialization leads to increased repetition.

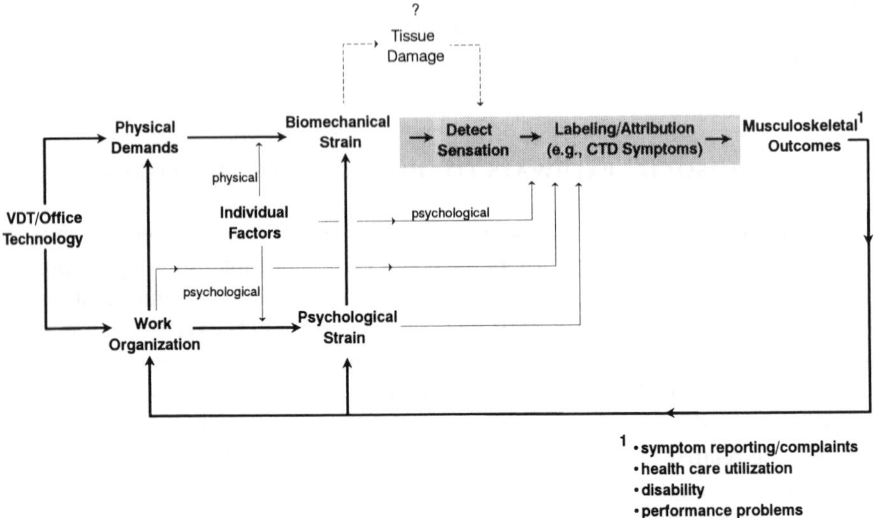

Figure 1.2 An ecological model of musculoskeletal disorders in VDT work.

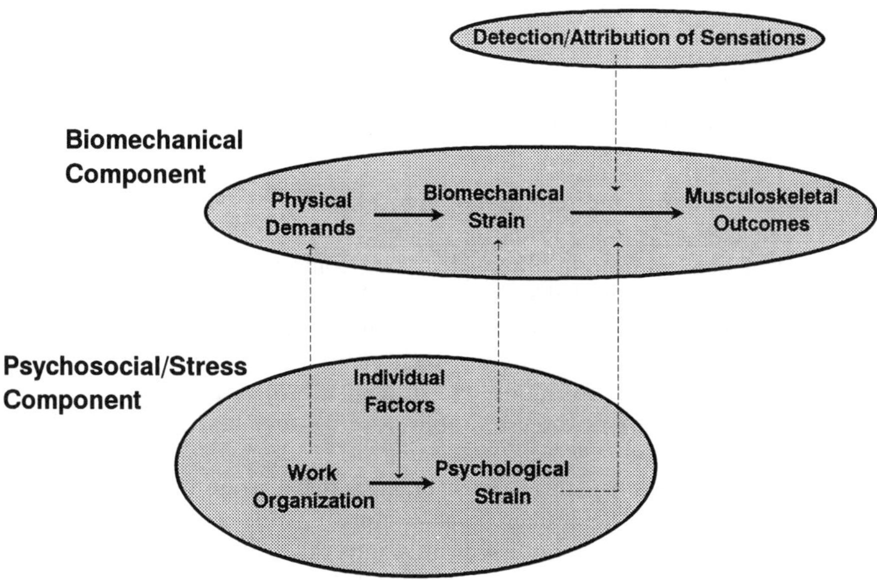

Figure 1.3 Components of the ecological model.

The present model also shows a direct path between work organization and psychosocial strain (stress) which, in turn, influences musculoskeletal outcomes via two routes. First, psychological strain is hypothesized to produce muscle tension, and possibly other autonomic effects, which compound biomechanical strain induced by task-related physical demands. This effect is depicted by the arrow between psychological strain and biomechanical strain in Figure 1.2. Second, psychological stain is hypothesized to moderate the relationship between biomechanical strain and the appearance of symptoms. (Moderating effects are denoted by faint arrows in Figure 1.2.)

The model also suggests that the relationship between biomechanical strains (i.e. internal physiological events) and the development of musculoskeletal symptoms is mediated by a complex of cognitive processes (denoted by the shaded area in Figure 1.2), which involves the detection and labeling/attribution of somatic information (symptoms). As discussed by Cioffi (Chapter 3), development of symptoms is not a direct or predetermined response to some internal physiological event. Rather, it is a highly malleable, interpretive process which is subject to influence by contextual and experiential factors. Unfortunately, however, the rather extensive psychological literature on the perception and attribution of symptoms (see Chapter 3; Cioffi, 1991; Pennebaker and Hall, 1982) has received little or no attention in ergonomics and occupational health.

With regard to the perception of symptoms, Figure 1.2 shows that the connection between biomechanical strain and musculoskeletal outcomes is influenced not only by psychological strain, but also by individual and work organization factors apart from the contribution of these factors to psychological strain. Factors such as organizational safety climate, for example, may have a direct influence on how

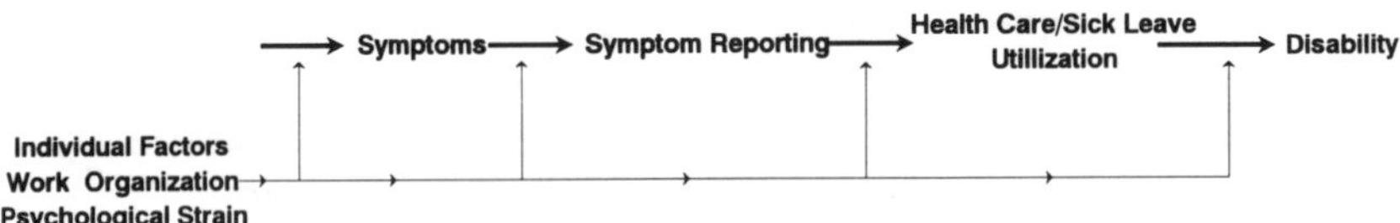

Figure 1.4 Moderating effects of psychosocial factors on musculoskeletal outcomes.

workers detect, interpret and respond to physical (somatic) sensations, regardless of whether safety climate actually results in stress.

For ease of presentation, multiple effects are combined in Figures 1.2 and 1.3 under the rubric of 'musculoskeletal outcomes.' As shown in Figure 1.4, it would be more appropriate to describe these effects in terms of a continuum of events involving first the development of symptoms, then symptom reporting and health-care utilization, then sick-leave utilization and disability, etc., and it can be postulated that psychological factors as discussed above are instrumental in the evolution of each stage.

Figure 1.2 also shows a pathway from biomechanical strain to tissue damage to somatic interpretation. The broken lines comprising this pathway indicate that physical damage or disease is not necessarily integral to the model; i.e. all that is essential are conditions that give rise to musculoskeletal symptoms.

Finally, the model suggests that the experience of musculoskeletal disorders feeds back to influence stress at work (this is the pathway between physical environmental factors and stress mentioned in the preceding discussion of psychosocial factors), and it is likely that these disorders also prompt work redesign. It is because of these closed system properties, as well as the fact that the model incorporates inputs from both the physical and psychosocial work environment, that we refer to the model as an 'ecological' model of musculoskeletal disorders.

EVIDENCE FOR THE MODEL

There are insufficient data to fully substantiate the pathways between work organization and musculoskeletal disorders illustrated in Figure 1.2. Key problems in the extant literature, as pointed out by Bongers and de Winter (1992), include inadequate exposure assessment for the physical or psychosocial factors, and failure to disentangle effectively the effects of these two sets of variables. Further, while many studies link work organization and musculoskeletal outcomes, the effect sizes are often quite small. Also, few studies establish intermediary effects, which is essential to identify specific pathways. Finally, most of the pertinent studies are characterized by cross-sectional designs which limit causal inferences, including direction of causation between psychosocial and musculoskeletal measures. These deficiencies notwithstanding, we believe that select studies offer circumstantial support for several of the pathways in Figure 1.2. These studies are discussed below, with the emphasis on investigations of musculoskeletal disorders in office/VDT workers.

The Path from Office Technology to Work Organization

The mechanization of office work, which was associated with the introduction of the typewriter at the turn of the century, produced changes in the organization of office work not unlike the effects of mechanization in manufacturing processes. As described by Giuliano (1982), the mechanized or 'industrial' office resulted in the standardization of office jobs and fragmentation of tasks and responsibilities characteristic of assembly-line work. VDT (computer) technology offers promise for reversal of these effects through enlargement of tasks and skills in office work (e.g. see Johansson and Aronsson, 1984). However, the indication is that some types of VDT work are still stuck in the industrial age (Stellman *et al.*, 1987), or may even exacerbate the adverse organizational aspects of office mechanization. For example, a 1981 NIOSH investigation of clerical workers who used VDTs and their counterparts who did not work with VDTs found that VDT users reported significantly less autonomy and role clarity, and greater work pressure and management control over work processes (Smith *et al.*, 1981). Identical findings were obtained in a subsequent NIOSH investigation of VDT users and non-users in Wisconsin (Sauter *et al.*, 1983a, 1983b). A much larger 1987 study at Columbia University (Stellman *et al.*, 1987) compared all-day VDT users with part-time users and several groups of typists and clerical workers. In contrast to all other study participants, the all-day VDT users reported significantly higher levels of workload demand and repetition, and lower levels of decision latitude, ability to learn new things on the job, and understanding of the overall work process.

Many additional studies have investigated organizational aspects of VDT work, but strict comparisons with non-computerized workplaces has been difficult in recent years because VDTs have become ubiquitous and suitable comparison groups are therefore unavailable. Still, review of this work suggests a pattern of effects consistent with the reduction of tasks, skills, and autonomy, etc., as discussed above (see WHO, 1989).

Pathways from Work Organization to Musculoskeletal Outcomes

An impressive number of studies in the last decade have linked workplace organizational factors to upper extremity musculoskeletal signs and symptoms among VDT/keyboard users (Bergquist *et al.*, 1995, a and b; Gomer *et al.*, 1987; Canadian Labour Congress, 1982; Green and Briggs, 1990; Hales *et al.*, 1994; Hopkins, 1990; Lim and Carayon, 1993; Linton and Kamwendo, 1989; NIOSH, 1992; NIOSH, 1993; Pot *et al.*, 1986; Ryan and Bampton, 1988; Sauter *et al.*, 1983a, 1983b; Spillane and Deves, 1988; Westgaard *et al.*, 1993). Factors predictive of musculoskeletal outcomes in these studies include limited rest pauses, routine tasks, uncertain job future, highly variable workload, time pressure and heavy workload demands, high mental workload, low co-worker and supervisory support, low worker autonomy, and low peer-group cohesion. Several of these factors (e.g. heavy workload demands and low autonomy, low supervisory support, and low peer-group cohesion) were predictive of musculoskeletal problems in multiple studies.

Figure 1.2 shows two principal pathways from work organization factors to musculoskeletal disease, one mediated by psychological strain and one mediated by increased physical demand. With regard to the latter, it is evident that the VDT itself imposes musculoskeletal demands relating to the posture required to view the display and operate the keyboard, etc. However, it is intuitive that extent of exposure to these demands, as well as exposure to other generic risk factors such as repetitive motion (e.g. excessive keying), is influenced by work organization factors such as the complexity of tasks (which would affect cycle time). At least two studies have shown a relationship between organizational and physical stressors in VDT work (Sauter *et al.*, 1983a; Stellman *et al.*, 1987), with correlations as high as 0.38 reported between these two classes of variables (Sauter *et al.*, 1983b). Although an artifactual relationship (resulting from the effect of technology on both work organization and physical demands) cannot be ruled out, data by Lim and Carayon (1993) argue for a causal link. Using path analysis to explore the relationship between organizational factors, ergonomic demands and psychological stress, these authors reported a direct path from organizational factors to ergonomic (physical) demands.

Research support for linkages in the pathway between work organization and musculoskeletal disorders which is mediated by psychological strain is also available. Using structural analysis methods, Sauter *et al.* (1983b) found that factors such as job future uncertainty, social support and workload demands influenced somatic symptoms in VDT users by way of an intermediary effect on mood disturbances. A study of keyboard operators performing postal letter-sorting tasks (Gomer *et al.*, 1987) linked every element in the pathway mediated by psychological strain in Figure 1.2. Specifically, tasks involving increased visual search and memory demand were associated with reports of increased mental demand, spectral changes in the forearm electromyogram (EMG) and increased forearm tremor, and increased musculoskeletal discomfort. Similar multilink associations were reported by investigators from the Karolinska Institute (Theorell *et al.*, 1991), although the study population did not include office workers. Increased psychological demands at work were associated with increased worry, fatigue and sleep problems which, in turn, were associated with behavioural indicators of muscle tension, which were associated with increased back, neck, and shoulder discomfort.

Other studies address specific links within the psychologically mediated pathway. Lim and Carayon (1993) and Bergquist *et al.* (1995a) reported associations between indicators of psychological strain (fatigue and stomach reactions, respectively) and upper-extremity musculoskeletal symptoms (Lim and Carayon, 1993; Bergquist *et al.* (1995a) and diagnosed disorders of the upper extremities (Bergquist *et al.*, 1995b).

As early as 1951, Lundervold (1951) demonstrated effects of psychological demands on muscle tension in keyboard operators, supporting the link between psychological strain and biomechanical strain in the present model. More recently, Waersted *et al.* (1987, 1991) investigated static muscle loading as a possible mechanism linking work organization, psychological strain, and musculoskeletal disorders among VDT users. Consistent with extensive prior research showing effects of psychological demands on muscle tension (see Ursin *et al.*, 1988, and Waersted *et al.*, 1991 for a review), increases in low-level muscle tension in the trapezius were induced by increasing the complexity and attentional requirements in VDT tasks. Although the overall group effects were modest, averaging about 0.5–1.0 per cent of maximum voluntary contraction (MVC), considerable interindividual variability was seen, with some subjects producing sustained loads up to 6.0 per cent MVC. The latter level is within the range thought by Jonsson (1978) to pose risk for musculoskeletal disease with chronic exposure. In this regard, it is notable that Kogi (1982) reported Japanese research showing sustained muscle loads in the range of 20–30 per cent in the forearm extensors among office machine operators (although a possible linkage to psychosocial demands was not discussed).

It is plausible that the direct, neurogenic effects of psychological demand on muscle tension and ensuing biomechanical strain are complemented by stress-related endocrine effects on musculoskeletal function; for example, an effect of catecholamines on the vigor of keying action (Lim and Carayon, 1993; Theorell *et al.*, 1991). However, there has been little empirical study of such mechanisms.

Despite the evidence supporting the bold pathway in Figure 1.2 from organizational factors to musculoskeletal outcomes via psychological strain, it is difficult to rule out a competing pathway involving direct effects of organizational factors or psychological strain on the perception and attribution of symptoms (i.e. the pathway denoted by the faint arrows from work organization and psychological strain in Figure 1.2). (This effect is examined in the discussion on somatic interpretation below.) But a more fundamental issue is whether effects attributed to the pathway from work organization through psychological strain are possibly confounded by physical effects related to (1) the path from work organization through physical demands, or (2) the covariation of physical and organizational demands resulting from the effects of technology on both of these classes of variables.

Two lines of evidence can be raised against the confounding hypothesis. First, for several types of factors found to predict musculoskeletal outcomes among VDT users, a significant effect on physical demand would seem unlikely. Examples of these types of factors include low group cohesion, work clarity, and staff support, which were predictive of RSI cases in the study by Ryan and Bampton (1988), or uncertainty regarding job future and reduced supervisory support which were predictive of musculoskeletal symptoms in a NIOSH study of telecommunications workers (NIOSH, 1992). Unlike organizational factors such as time pressure or repetitive work, it is difficult to see how changes in these conditions could elicit changes in physical workload demands (i.e. the pathway from organizational demands to physical demands would not seem to be operative).

More compelling are the results of studies that statistically separated effects relating to physical and psychosocial factors and, thus, are able to demonstrate effects unique to the psychological pathway.[3] Using multiple regression methods, Sauter *et al.* (1983a, 1983b) reported a significant association between worker autonomy and musculoskeletal symptoms in VDT users after adjusting for a wide variety of variables denoting physical stressors. Similarly, NIOSH (1993) found an association between supervisory support and hand/wrist symptoms in news editors after adjusting for the amount of time spent typing. Additionally, Bergquist *et al.* (1995), Lim and Carayon (1993) and Ryan and Bampton (1988) all were able to separate, to some extent, the effects of physical and organizational factors in predicting musculoskeletal problems in VDT users.

Similar evidence of effects uniquely attributable to psychosocial factors comes from Arndt (1987), Linton (1990), and Theorell *et al.* (1991), although none of these studies employed VDT users. The Arndt (1987) and Theorell *et al.* (1991) studies are of particular interest. Arndt found increased electromyographic activity in assembly workers who were implored to speed up, but who were unable to respond with increased work speed (virtually eliminating any possibility of a confound with physical factors). Like several VDT studies, Theorell *et al.* (1991) found effects of psychological demands on back, neck and shoulder symptoms after adjusting for physical demands (lifting demands, awkward postures, etc.). Similar to Gomer *et al.* (1987), the Theorell *et al.* (1991) study was also able to demonstrate intermediate linkages of psychosocial demands to psychological strain, muscle tension (self-reported only), and ultimately to musculoskeletal discomfort.

Finally, inherent limitations of cross-sectional studies, which is the predominant methodology in VDT health research, pose a potential problem. The cited associations between organizational factors and musculoskeletal disorders might result from an influence of symptoms on job perceptions, not the reverse. Two studies, however, tend to discount this possibility. Hopkins (1990) studied the organizational environment in workplaces with high and low prevalences of RSI. However, ratings of organizational factors were obtained from asymptomatic workers only (thereby eliminating the possibility of a symptom influence on job perceptions). Almost without exception, ratings of organizational factors were more negative in the high (RSI) prevalence workplaces. Similar findings are reported by Hales *et al.* (1994) who observed an association between fear of job loss and neck, shoulder, and elbow symptoms in directory assistance operators. Fear of job loss ratings within job sites were rescored based on values obtained from asymptomatic workers, and then associations with musculoskeletal symptoms were re-examined. The results showed that symptoms levels were still positively associated with fear ratings; i.e. higher in units with higher fear ratings.

Psychological Mediation of the Path from Biomechanical Strain to Musculoskeletal Outcomes

Thus far, it has been suggested that psychosocial factors might contribute to musculoskeletal disorders via two paths: one involving effects on physical workplace demands, and a second involving stress-related effects on muscle function. A third possible mechanism bears some similarity to what has been referred to as an 'iatrogenic' process (deriving from the Greek *iatros*, meaning physician, and *genesis*).

The iatrogenic hypothesis has been heavily promoted as a partial explanation for the surge in upper-extremity musculoskeletal disorders witnessed internationally in the last decade. According to this hypothesis, musculoskeletal discomfort and fatigue are endemic in VDT work. Environmental forces, including not only medical practitioners, but also social and cultural factors, legal-compensation systems, and workplace industrial relations then encourage the interpretation of discomfort as signals of underlying injury and promote the development of sick roles and disability (Bell, 1989; Cleland, 1987; Hadler, 1986, 1990). Although the iatrogenic hypothesis has not been empirically tested in the context of VDT work, this type of explanation finds support in the medical anthropologic and sociologic literature which identifies significant cultural variations in response to somatic symptoms (see, for example, Hocking, 1987b; Mechanic, 1972).

The iatrogenic hypothesis converges to some extent with an extensive area of investigation in psychology which offers a theoretically deeper and richer formulation for explaining iatrogenic-like effects on musculoskeletal disorders. Extensive research in social and cognitive psychology in the last two decades has sought to explain how people interpret internal somatic information such as sensations associated with emotional response or illness. Space does not permit more than the briefest summary of this work (see Chapter 3 of this volume; Cioffi, 1991; and Pennebaker and Hall, 1982 for excellent reviews), but the theory and findings suggest that response to somatic signals involves a multistage attributional process which is governed by cognitive and environmental factors.

First, as in the perception of any stimulus, whether or not an event is even noticed depends upon factors such as the degree of arousal of the individual and the salience of competing stimuli (which could mask the somatic stimulus). Second, once detected, explanations for the sensation are sought, which involves labeling the sensation and then deducing its cause. Social psychological research has shown that this inferential process is highly influenced by situational and experiential factors. In the classic studies in this area, subjects were injected with epinephrine to induce psychological and physiological arousal, but were uninformed about the effects. It was then demonstrated that self-labeling of the arousal state as euphoria or anger could be readily manipulated by exposure of the subjects to euphoric or angry confederates (Schachter and Singer, 1962). Importantly, this attributional process is understood to be a natural, probably hard-wired, and lawful process that has survival value for the organism (Chapter 3 of this volume; Pennebaker and Hall, 1982); i.e. it is normal to seek causal explanations for events in and around us, and to rely on contextual cues when the stimuli are ambiguous, which is often the case with somatic sensations.

In the current model of musculoskeletal disorders, it is suggested that somatic interpretation processes as discussed here (shaded area in Figure 1.2) mediate between biomechanical strain and musculoskeletal outcomes, and that these processes are influenced by various psychosocial factors (faint parallel inputs to the shaded processes in Figure 1.2). Within this framework, several effects of stress and psychosocial factors on musculoskeletal disorders seem plausible, although studies to confirm these effects have not been undertaken.

With regard to the detection of symptoms, it is possible that stress-related arousal may sharpen sensitivity to normally subthreshold musculoskeletal stimuli. Work organization might similarly influence the detection of musculoskeletal signals. For example, competition for attention to musculoskeletal stimuli may be considerably reduced in dull routine tasks in comparison to more varied, challenging tasks providing richer environmental stimulation. This may help to explain, for example, why clerical-level VDT jobs are associated with increased musculoskeletal symptoms in several studies (e.g. Canadian Labour Congress, 1982; Sauter *et al.*, 1983a, 1983b; Smith *et al.*, 1981), or why monotonous work was associated with neck symptoms in a Swedish working population (Linton, 1990). Ironically, as discussed by Pennebaker and Hall (1982), this mechanism might also increase the health risk for workers in more challenging, engrossing tasks by reducing their relative awareness to somatic danger signals. Could such a suppression phenomenon partially explain, for example, the reportedly high prevalence of musculoskeletal disorders among news editors (NIOSH, 1989, 1993)?

It is also possible to suggest ways in which psychosocial conditions might influence the labeling and attribution of musculoskeletal sensations. Assuming that people hold implicit hypotheses that stress promotes disease, it is predictable that musculoskeletal sensations arising in the context of stressful working conditions might be interpreted as signals of injury or disease. Further, attribution of these symptoms to the job might seem natural in the presence of adverse organizational conditions such as a negative safety climate. NIOSH (1993) found, for example, that perceived lack of management support for ergonomic programs nearly doubled the odds for neck symptoms among news editors.

Effects of personality or dispositional factors on musculoskeletal disorders in office work (Bergquist *et al.*, 1995a; Spillane and Deves, 1988) and in other occupations (Bigos *et al.*, 1991; Ursin *et al.*, 1988) might also be explained within the somatic interpretation framework. It is possible, for example, that negative affectivity, shown by Bergquist *et al.* (1995a) to predict neck and shoulder discomfort among VDT users, colors the labeling of sensations in negative (disease) terms. (Self-reports of working conditions might be similarly influenced adversely by negative affectivity, which would tend to inflate associations of organizational factors and musculoskeletal outcomes.)

Although the current model highlights somatic interpretations, it is important to emphasize that this process has not been investigated in the context of work-related musculoskeletal disorders, and thus the significance of this mechanism in comparison with other mechanisms suggested in the current model is unknown. It is very doubtful that this mechanism alone could fully explain the relationship between psychosocial factors and musculoskeletal disorders seen in the extant literature. Several studies have demonstrated significant associations between workplace psychosocial factors and more objective indices of musculoskeletal disorders involving clinical evaluation (Bergquist *et al.*, 1995a; Hales *et al.*, 1994; Leino, 1989; NIOSH, 1992; Ryan and Bampton, 1988; Toomingas, 1992). Use of more objective methods for assessment of musculoskeletal disorders obviates, to a considerable extent, the influence of cognitive processes which are integral to the somatic interpretation explanation.

Feedback Effects

Finally, the current model shows reciprocal effects of musculoskeletal disorders on psychological strain and work organization. This pathway is highly intuitive. For example, adjustments in job tasks such as assignment to 'light duty' or other forms of work redesign are commonly made for injured or symptomatic workers. With regard to effects on psychological strain, Ghiringhelli (1980) reported fear of health impairment to be an important source of stress among VDT users. However, evidence supporting such effects is quite limited. Sauter *et al.* (1983b) conducted a series of analyses showing reciprocal effects between illness symptoms and mood states in a sample of office workers, including VDT users. One other study, with a longitudinal design permitting stronger causal inference, reported this type of effect in a sample of office and production workers. Leino (1989) found that 1973–1978 stress symptom scores predicted rheumatic symptoms and clinically defined musculoskeletal disorders upon follow-up in 1983. However, among male workers, rheumatic symptoms and musculoskeletal disorders during 1973–1978 also predicted stress symptoms in 1983.

SUMMARY AND DIRECTION

A theoretical model suggesting multiple causal linkages between workplace psychosocial factors and musculoskeletal disorders in VDT work is discussed. This model and its linkages do not diminish the importance of physical environmental/ergonomic factors in the etiology of musculoskeletal disorders which is supported in prior research (Hunting *et al.*, 1981; Sauter *et al.*, 1991); rather, psychosocial effects are depicted as complementary to and interactive with effects of physical workplace demands. Further, the psychological mechanisms linking or mediating between psychosocial factors and musculoskeletal disorders are discussed as normal psychological processes, in contrast to clinical or abnormalistic characterizations by others (e.g. Luciere, 1986; Spillane and Deves, 1987).

Evidence presented in support of the psychosocial pathways suggested in these models is neither perfect nor complete. More powerful study methods employing longitudinal designs, improved exposure (to both psychosocial and ergonomic demands) and health assessment, and improved analytical schemes such as structural analysis would be useful in substantiating and isolating the effects of psychosocial factors. Further, research is needed to evaluate the strength of specific pathways postulated in the model. For example, to our knowledge, studies have not looked at the magnitude of static muscle loads during actual workplace exposure to known psychosocial stressors (e.g. deadline work, electronic monitoring, etc.). Thus, the need for further analytic study is evident.

But, from a prevention imperative, an additional course of investigation is worth consideration. Specifically, case studies of *organizational interventions* to prevent musculoskeletal disorders in VDT work suggest rather powerful effects of psychosocial factors. According to Westin (1990), for example the Federal Express Corporation has been able to maintain high levels of productivity with minimal experience of musculoskeletal disorders among VDT users by adopting a 'people-technology' philosophy that gives priority to improving job design to minimize monotony, by adoption of participative management practices, and by improved employee education, among other measures.

Intervention studies often do not permit the type of control or manipulation needed to define specific mechanisms or pathways of effect. Further, naturalistic interventions are not always pure enough to isolate specific causal factors. Indeed, the people-technology philosophy at Federal Express also included a commitment to improved ergonomics. Still, these types of studies have a high degree of ecological validity and can be much more powerful motivators of preventive actions than the more molecular investigations that have been examined in this paper.

NOTES

1 Although negative affectivity is commonly discussed as an individual or personality characteristic (e.g. see Watson and Pennebaker, 1989), it is plausible that, like job attitudes such as job dissatisfaction, negative affectivity could be shaped by chronic exposure to stressful working conditions. These two perspectives would have different implications (i.e. in terms of focusing on the person or the job) in attributing the cause of health outcomes associated with negative affectivity and in the design of interventions.

2 It should be noted, however, that the TNO authors were reluctant to represent this model as an 'explanatory' model. Rather they describe it as a vehicle for their extensive review of studies exploring associations between psychosocial factors and musculoskeletal disease.

3 However, this counterargument to the confounding hypothesis rests in part on the adequacy of the exposure assessment for physical demands, which has been a difficult issue and may be problematic in many studies.

REFERENCES

ARNDT, R. 1987 Work pace, stress, and cumulative trauma disorders, *The Journal of Hand Surgery*, **12A**, 866–9.

BAMMER, G. and MARTIN, B. 1988 The arguments about RSI: An examination, *Community Health Studies*, **12**, 348–58.

BELL, D. S. 1989 Repetition strain injury: An iatrogenic epidemic of simulated injury, *The Medical Journal of Australia*, **151**, 280–4.

BERGQUIST, U. 1984 Video display terminals and health, *Scandinavian Journal of Work, Environment and Health*, **10**(2), 68–77.

BERGQUIST, U., WOLGAAST, E., NILSSON, B. and VOSS, M. 1995a Musculoskeletal disorders among visual display terminal workers. Individual, ergonomic and work organizational factors, *Ergonomics*, **38**(4), 763–76.

BERGQUIST, U., WOLGAAST, E., NILSSON, B. and VOSS, M. 1995b The influence of VDT work on musculoskeletal disorders, *Ergonomics*, **38**(4), 754–62.

BIGOS, S. J., BATTIE, M. C., SPENGLER, D. M., FISHER, L. D., FORDYCE, W. E., HANSSON, T. H., NACHEMSON, A. L. and WORTLEY, M. D. 1991 A prospective study of work perceptions and psychosocial factors affecting the report of back injury, *Spine*, **16**(1), 1–6.

BONGERS, P. M. and DE WINTER, C. R. 1992 *Psychosocial Factor and Musculoskeletal Disease: A Report of the Literature* (Report 92.028), Netherlands: TNO Institute of Preventive Health Care.

BONGERS, P. M., DE WINTER, C. R., KOMPIER, M. J. and HILDEBRANDT, V. H. 1993 Psychosocial factors at work and musculoskeletal disease, *Scandinavian Journal of Work, Environment and Health*, **19**(5), 297–312.

BRIEF, A. P. and GEORGE, J. M. 1991 Psychological stress and the workplace: A brief comment on Lazarus' outlook, *Journal of Social Behavior and Personality*, **6**(7), 15–20.

CANADIAN LABOUR CONGRESS 1982 *Towards a More Humanized Technology: Exploring the Impact of Video Display Terminals on the Health and Working Conditions of Canadian Office Workers*, Ottawa: CLC Labour Education and Studies Centre.

CAPLAN, R. D., COBB, S., FRENCH, J. R., JR., VAN HARRISON, R. and PINNEAU, S. R., JR. 1975 *Job Demands and Worker Health: Main Effects and Occupational Differences*, Washington, DC: US Department of Health, Education, and Welfare.

CIOFFI, D. 1991 Beyond attentional strategies: A cognitive–perceptual model of somatic interpretation, *Psychological Bulletin*, **109**(1), 25–41.

CLELAND, L. G. 1987 'RSI': a model of social iatrogenesis, *The Medical Journal of Australia*, **147**, 236–9.

COHEN, S., GWALNEY, J. M., JR., DOYLE, W. J., SKONER, D. P., FIREMAN, P. and NEWSOM, J. T. 1994 'State and trait negative affect as predictors of objective and subjective symptoms of respiratory viral infections', presentation at the 102nd Annual convention of the American Psychological Association, Washington DC.

COOPER, C. L. and MARSHALL, J. 1976 Occupational sources of stress: A review of the literature relating to coronary heart disease and mental ill health, *Journal of Occupational Psychology*, **49**, 11–28.

EVANS, G. W., JOHANSSON, G. and CARRERE, S. 1994 Psychosocial factors and the physical environment: Inter-relations in the workplace, in COOPER, C. L. and ROBERTSON, I. T. (Eds), *International Review of Industrial and Organizational Psychology*, pp. 1–30, Chichester: John Wiley.

GHIRINGHELLI, L. 1980 Collection of subjective opinions on use of VDUs, in RANDJEAN, E. and VIGLIANI, E. (Eds), *Ergonomic Aspects of Visual Display Terminals*, pp. 227–31, London: Taylor and Francis.

GIULIANO, V. E. 1982 The mechanization of office work, *Scientific American*, **247**, 149–64.

GOMER, F., SILVERSTEIN, L. D., BERG, W. K. and LASSITER, D. L. 1987 Changes in electromyographic activity associated with occupational stress and poor performance in the workplace, *Human Factors*, **29**(2), 131–43.

GREEN, R. and BRIGGS, C. 1990 Prevalence of overuse injury among keyboard operators: Characteristics of the job, the operator and the work environment, *Journal of Occupational Health Safety*, **6**(6), 109–18.

HADLER, N. M. 1986 Industrial rheumatology: The Australian and New Zealand experiences with arm pain and backache in the workplace, *The Medical Journal of Australia*, **144**, 191–5.

HADLER, N. M. 1990 Cumulative trauma disorders, *Journal of Occupational Medicine*, **32**(1), 38–41.

HALES, T. R., SAUTER, S. L., PETERSEN, M. R., FINE, L. J., PUTZ-ANDERSON, V., SCHLEIFER, L. R., OCHS, T. T. and BERNARD, B. P. 1994 Musculoskeletal disorders among visual display terminal (VDT) users in a telecommunications company, *Ergonomics*, **37**(11), 1603–21.

HOCKING, B. 1987a Epidemiological aspects of 'repetition strain injury' in telecom Australia, *The Medical Journal of Australia*, **147**, 218–22.

HOCKING, B. 1987b Anthropologic aspects of occupational illness epidemics, *Journal of Occupational Medicine*, **29**(6), 526–30.

HOCKING, B. 1990 'The aftermath of RSI in Telecom Australia', unpublished report.

HOPKINS, A. 1990 Stress, the quality of work, and repetition strain injury in Australia, *Work and Stress*, **4**(2), 129–38.

HUNTING, W., LAUBLI, T. and GRANDJEAN, E. 1981 Postural and visual loads at VDT workplaces: I. Constrained postures, *Ergonomics*, **24**, 917–31.

HURRELL, JR., J. J. and MURPHY, L. R. 1992 Psychological job stress, in ROM, W. N. (Ed.), *Environmental and Occupational Medicine*, pp. 675–84, New York: Little, Brown.

INTERNATIONAL LABOUR OFFICE 1986 *Psychosocial Factors at Work: Recognition and Control*, Geneva: International Labour Office.

JOHANSSON, G., and ARONSSON, G. 1984 Stress reactions in computerized administrative work, *Journal of Occupational Behaviur*, **5**, 159–81.

JONSSON, B. 1978 Kinesiology – with special reference to electromyographic kinesiology, in COBB, W. A. and VAN DUIJN, H. (Eds), *Contemporary Clinical Neurophysiology*, EEG supplement no. 34, pp. 417–28, Amsterdam: Elsevier.

KAGAN, A. and LEVI, L. 1971 Adaptation of the psychosocial environment to man's abilities and needs, in LEVI, L. (Ed.), *Society, Stress and Disease*, pp. 399–404, New York: Oxford University Press.

KARASEK, R. and THEORELL, T. 1990 *Healthy Work: Stress, Productivity, and the Reconstruction of Working Life*, New York: Basic Books.

KASL, S. V. 1992 Surveillance of psychological disorders in the workplace panel, in KEITA, G. P. and SAUTER, S. L. (Eds), *Work and Well-being: An Agenda for the 1990s*, pp. 73–95, Washington, DC: American Psychological Association.

KOGI, K. 1982 Finding appropriate work-rest rhythm for occupational strain on the basis of electromyographic and behavioural changes, in BUSET, P. A., COBB, W. A. and OKUMA, T. (Eds), *Kyota Symposia: Electroenephalography and Clinical Neurophysiology*, **36**, pp. 738–49, Amsterdam: Elsevier Biomedical Press.

LAZARUS, R. S. 1966 *Psychological Stress and the Coping Process*, New York: McGraw-Hill.

LEINO, P. 1989 Symptoms of stress predict musculoskeletal disorders, *Journal of Epidemiology and Community Health*, **43**, 293–300.

LIM, S. Y. and CARAYON, P. 1993 An integrated approach to cumulative trauma disorders in computerized offices: The role of psychosocial work factors, psychological stress and ergonomic risk factors, in SMITH, M. J. and SALVENDY, G. (Eds), *Human Computer Interaction: Applications and Case Studies*, pp. 880–5, Amsterdam: Elsevier.

LINTON, S. J. 1990 Risk factors for neck and back pain in a working population in Sweden, *Work and Stress*, **4**(1), 41–9.

LINTON, S. J. and KAMWENDO, K. 1989 Risk factors in the psychosocial work environment for neck and shoulder pain in secretaries, *Journal of Occupational Medicine*, **31**(7), 609–13.

LUCIERE, Y. 1986 Neurosis in the workplace, *The Medical Journal of Australia*, **145**, 323–7.

LUNDERVOLD, A. 1951 Electromygraphic investigations during typewriting, *ACTA Physiologica Scandinavica*, **24**(84), 226–32.

MATTESON, M. T. and IVANCEVICH, J. M. 1989 *Controlling Work Stress: Effective Human Resource and Management Strategies*, San Fransisco, CA: Jossey-Bass.

MCGRATH, J. E. 1970 A conceptual formulation for research on stress, in MCGRATH, J. E. (Ed.), *Social and Psychological Factors in Stress*, pp. 10–21, New York: Holt, Rinehart and Winston.

MECHANIC, D. 1972 Social psychologic factors affecting the presentation of bodily complaints, *The New England Journal of Medicine*, **286**(21), 1132–9.

MULLALY, J. and GRIGG, L. 1988 RSI: Integrating the major theories, *Australian Journal of Psychology*, **40**(1), 19–33.

NATIONAL INSTITUTE FOR OCCUPATIONAL SAFETY AND HEALTH 1989 *HETA Report 89-250-2046*, Melville, NY: Newsday.

NATIONAL INSTITUTE FOR OCCUPATIONAL SAFETY AND HEALTH 1992 *HETA Report 90-013-2277*, Phoenix, AZ: US West Communications.

NATIONAL INSTITUTE FOR OCCUPATIONAL SAFETY AND HEALTH 1993 *HETA Report 90-013-2277*, Los Angeles, CA: Los Angeles Times.

NATIONAL OCCUPATIONAL HEALTH and SAFETY COMMISSION 1986 *Repetition Strain Injury: A Report and Model Code of Practice*, Canberra: Australian Government Publishing Service.

PAYNE, R. 1988 Individual differences in the study of occupational stress, in COOPER, C. L. and PAYNE, R. (Eds), *Causes, Coping and Consequences of Stress at Work*, pp. 209–32, Chichester: John Wiley.

PENNEBAKER, J. W. and HALL, G. 1982 The psychology of physical symptoms, New York: Springer-Verlag.

POT, F., PADMOS, P. and BROUWERS, A. 1986 Determinants of the VDU operator's well-being, in KNAVE, B. and WIDEBACK, P. G. (Eds), *Work with Display Units 1986*, pp. 16–25, Amsterdam: North-Holland.

RYAN, G. A. and BAMPTON, M. 1988 Comparison of data process operators with and without upper limb symptoms, *Community Health studies*, **XII**(1), 63–8.

SAUTER, S. L. 1991 'Ergonomics, stress, and the redesign of office work', presentation at The National Occupational Musculoskeletal Injury Conference, Ann Arbor, MI.

SAUTER, S. L., SCHLEIFER, L. M. and KNUTSON, S. J. 1991 Work posture, workstation design, and musculoskeletal discomfort in a VDT data entry task, *Human Factors*, **22**(2), 151–67.

SAUTER, S. L. and SWANSON, N. G. 1993 'An ecological model of musculoskeletal disorders in office work', presentation at The Duke University Conference Psychosocial Influence in Office Work CTDs, Raleigh-Durham, NC.

SAUTER, S. L., GOTTLIEB, M. S., JONES, K. C., DODSON, V. N. and ROHRER, K. M. 1983a Job and health implications of VDT use: Initial results of the Wisconsin–NIOSH study, *Communicaions of the Association for Computing Machinery*, **26**(4), 284–94.

SAUTER, S. L., GOTTLIEB, M. S., ROHRER, K. M. and DODSON, V. N. 1983b *The Well-Being of Video Display Terminal Users: An Exploratory Study*, Madison, WI: University of Wisconsin Department of Preventive Medicine.

SCHACHTER, S. and SINGER, J. E. 1962 Cognitive, social, and physiological determinants of emotional state, *Psychological Review*, **69**, 379–99.

SMITH, A. 1976 *An Inquiry into the Nature and Causes of the Wealth of Nations*, Chicago: University of Chicago Press.

SMITH, M. J. and CARAYON-SAINFORT, P. 1989 A balance theory of job design for stress reduction, *International Journal of Industrial Ergonomics*, **4**, 67–79.

SMITH, M. J., COHEN, B. G., STAMMERJOHN, L. W., JR. and HAPP, A. 1981 An investigation of health complaints and job stress in video display operations, *Human Factors*, **23**(4), 387–400.

Spillane, R. M. and Deves, L. A. 1987 RSI: Pain, pretence or patienthood?, *Journal of Industrial Relations*, **19**, 41–8.

Spillane, R. M. and Deves, L. A. 1988 Psychosocial correlates of RSI reporting, *Journal of Occupational Safety*, **4**(1), 21–7.

Stellman, J. M., Klitzman, S., Gordon, G. C. and Snow, B. R. 1987 Work environment and the well-being of clerical and VDT workers, *Journal of Occupational Behaviour*, **8**, 95–114.

Theorell, T., Harms-Ringdahl, K., Ahlberg-Hulten, G. and Westin, B. 1991 Psychosocial job factors and symptoms from the locomotor system: A multicausal analysis, *Scandinavian Journal of Rehabilitation Medicine*, **23**, 165–73.

Toomingas, A. 1992 Associations between perceived psychosocial job factors and prevalence of musculoskeletal disorders in the neck and shoulder regions, *Arbete och Hälsa*, **17**, 289–90.

Ursin, H., Endresen, I. M. and Ursin, G. 1988 Psychological factors and self-reports of muscle pain, *European Journal of Applied Physiology*, **57**, 282–90.

Ursin, H., Endresen, I. M., Svbak, S., Tellnes, G. and Mykletun, R. 1993 Muscle pain and coping with working life in Norway: A review, *Work and Stress*, **7**(3), 247–58.

Van Harrison, R. 1983 Job design and organizational variable, in National Research Council (Ed), *Video Displays, Work, and Vision*, pp. 173–93, Washington, DC: National Academy Press.

Waersted, M., Bjorklund, R. A. and Westgaard, R. H. 1987 Generation of muscle tension related to a demand of continuing attention, in Knave, B. and Wideback, P. G. (Eds), *Work with Display Units* 1986, pp. 288–93, Amsterdam: North-Holland.

Waersted, M., Bjorklund, R. A. and Westgaard, R. H. 1991 Shoulder muscle tension induced by two VDU-based tasks of different complexity, *Ergonomics*, **34**(2), 137–50.

Watson, D. and Pennebaker, J. W. 1989 Health complaints, stress, and distress: Exploring the central role of negative affectivity, *Psychological Review*, **96**(2), 234–54.

Westgaard, R. H. and Bjorklund, R. 1987 Generation of muscle tension additional to postural muscle load, *Ergonomics*, **30**(6), 911–23.

Westgaard, R. H., Jensen,L D. and Hansen, K. 1993 Individual and work-related risk factors associated with symptoms of musculoskeletal complaints, *International Archives of Environmental Health*, **64**, 405–13.

Westin, A. F. 1990 Organizational culture and VDT policies: A case study of the Federal Express Corporation, in Sauter, S. L., Dainoff, M. and Smith, M. (Eds), *Promoting Health and Productivity in the Computerized Office*, pp. 147–68, London: Taylor and Francis.

World Health Organization 1989 Work with visual display terminals: Psychosocial aspects and health, *Journal of Occupational Medicine*, **31**(12), 957–68.

CHAPTER TWO

Work organization, stress, and cumulative trauma disorders

MICHAEL J. SMITH and PASCALE CARAYON

INTRODUCTION

Since the turn of the century there have been many efforts to enhance the productivity of the workforce. The scientific management approach of Taylor (1947) and the introduction of the assembly line brought wholesale changes in the way that factory work was organized and supervised, and the way in which workers were paid. Research by the Gilbreths (Gilbreth, 1914) and Maynard (Maynard *et al.*, 1948) used scientific means to establish the most effective work methods. These could be considered early attempts at ergonomics. Other theorists and researchers added elements of psychological and social processes to define ways to make workers more motivated and productive (Roethlisberger and Dickson, 1964; McGregor, 1960; Herzberg, 1966; Hackman and Oldham, 1976; Lawler, 1986).

However, from the early days of factory automation there have been problems of employee dissatisfaction, psychological stress and ill health (Walker and Guest, 1952; OTA, 1985a). This led to theories concerned with the quality of working life (Kahn, 1981; French, 1963; Quinn and Staines, 1979). But these efforts have been overshadowed by additional attempts to improve worker contributions to productivity improvement (Deming, 1982; Drucker, 1980; Juran, 1951; Smith *et al.*, 1989).

Within the last few decades, office work has undergone a similar automation process to factories (OTA, 1985b). The stress and health problems encountered have been very similar to those found in manufacturing (Smith *et al.*, 1981; Sauter *et al.*, 1983; OTA, 1985b, 1987). The experiences with factory and office automation leave no question that the way in which work is organized can have substantial influences on workers' attitudes and motivation, and on their behavior at work. Research evidence has been accumulating about the relationship between the nature of work organization and stress-related diseases such as cardiovascular disorders and mental disturbances. (For reviews of this literature see House, 1981; Cooper and Marshall, 1976; Kasl, 1978; Smith, 1981, 1987). Recently, there has been an interest in the potential relationship between work organization, psychological stress and cumulative musculoskeletal disorders. This paper will discuss the various factors that have been associated with work organization and psychological distress, how these may be related to cumulative trauma disorders (CTDs), and potential psychological and physiological mechanisms through which psychological stress could influence CTDs.

CTDs represent a group of health problems that have the following three characteristics (Putz-Anderson, 1988). First, they are cumulative in that injuries develop over a long period of time as a result of repeated, continuous exposure of a particular body part to stressors. Second, this continuous exposure leads to trauma of tissues and joints. Third, CTDs are physical ailments or abnormal conditions. Putz-Anderson (1988) defined three types of upper-extremity CTDs: (1) tendon disorders (e.g. tendinitis), (2) nerve disorders (e.g. carpal tunnel syndrome), and (3) neurovascular disorders (e.g. thoracic outlet syndrome).

There is sufficient research and experiential evidence to be able to state that work organization can have profound effects on worker attitudes toward work, motivation to work, and behavior at work. (For detailed treatises on this see Dunnette and Hough, 1992 and Salvendy, 1992). Over the decade of the 1970s, the level of employee satisfaction with work decreased (Quinn and Staines, 1979), and there is no indication that this trend has stopped. During the 1980s the reported levels of job stress and CTDs have risen substantially (USDHHS, 1979; USBLS, 1992). Is there a possible link between these workplace problems?

We will first review theories of job stress and then propose a model of job stress and disease. This model is used to show the direct and indirect effects of work organization on CTDs. Work organization can affect CTDs indirectly via stress, which may have the potential to produce direct effects on the causation of CTDs. We will examine how physiological, psychological and behavioral stress reactions can be related to the causation of CTDs. Finally, a model of work organization will be described which can be used to identify and eliminate or reduce the ergonomic and psychosocial risk factors for CTDs.

THEORIES OF STRESS

It is essential to understand the underlying mechanisms of stress to understand how worker behavior and psychobiological processes may affect the risk of CTDs. According to Selye (1956), stress is a biological process by which the body attempts to adapt to some challenge by mobilizing its energy, disease-fighting and survival responses. This process of mobilization has the potential to increase the risk of CTDs through the physiological changes which may enhance the susceptibility of the organism as a whole to disease, or specific tissues to cumulative trauma.

In Selye's approach there are three stages that an organism undergoes in this syndrome. In the first, called the state of 'alarm', the body mobilizes biological defenses to resist the assault of an environmental demand. This stage is characterized by high levels of hormone production, energy release, muscle tension and increased heart rate. As discussed later, these physiological reactions can theoretically increase the susceptibility of nerves and muscles to damage. The stage of 'adaptation' is the second phase in which the body's biological processes appear to return to normal as it seems that the threat has been successfully dealt with. In this stage, the body is working very hard to maintain its 'homeostatic' balance, which often carries a high physiological cost. There is a third and final phase ('exhaustion') in which the biological integrity of the organism is in danger because most primary biological systems begin to fail from the overwork of trying to maintain homeostasis. This can result in serious disability or death.

The important concept from this theory is that physiological reactions to the stress of adaptation can affect the overall integrity of the organism and its 'heartiness'. In addition, it increases the sensitivity of the peripheral neuromuscular responses. Thus, 'stress–Selye' leads to increased muscle tension and pain, as well as feelings of muscular fatigue. These effects are similar to the early symptoms of CTDs.

There are also psychological and perceptual processes involved in stress. Lazarus (1974, 1977) has suggested that physiological changes arise from a need for action resulting from emotions. The quality and intensity of the emotional reaction and its resultant physiological and behavioral changes depend on cognitive appraisal of the present or anticipated significance of the interaction with the environment or its 'threat' to security and safety. Cognitive processes not only determine the quality and intensity of the emotional reaction, but also define coping activites which may affect the emotional reaction (Lazarus, 1974). Thus, the cognitive appraisal process defines the nature of physiological reactions and psychological perceptions of pain. Such appraisal processes are based on the individual's experience and personality, and the rewards of responding.

Stress can also influence worker behavior, specifically through coping strategies. There are different ways by which coping activities affect health (see Murphy, 1985). For instance, health outcomes may be affected by a coping style that influences the frequency, intensity and patterning of neuroendocrine stress responses. Particular coping styles in a certain context (e.g. problem-focused coping) are associated with increased physiological mobilization (Baum *et al.*, 1983), which can be maladaptive. Workers may engage in activities such as failing to take rest breaks to help keep output high, or using greater force than necessary to accomplish a task due to frustrations at work.

Levi (1972) has further developed the physiological approach to stress and also recognized the importance of psychological factors as primary determinants of the stress sources. He proposed a model that links 'psychosocial stimuli' with disease. In this model, any psychosocial stimulus (i.e. any event that takes place in the social environment at work as well as outside work) can act as a stressor. In accordance with the so-called 'psychobiological program', psychosocial stimuli may evoke physiological responses similar to those described by Selye. In turn, these physiological responses can lead to disease. Several intervening variables (individual characteristics, coping strategies, or social support) moderate the link between psychosocial stimuli and disease.

Levi (1972) emphasizes that the sequence of events described by the model is not a one-way process, but is a 'cybernetic system with continuous feedback'. Stress physiological responses and disease can feedback on the psychosocial stimuli, as well as the individual's psychobiological program. These feedback loops are important to understand why stress reactions and disease can act as stressors or mediate the effect of stressors on the individual. This may explain how stress can influence CTDs.

A MODEL OF JOB STRESS AND DISEASE

The job stress model in Figure 2.1 illustrates the relationship among work characteristics, individual stress responses and disease. (See Smith and Carayon-Sainfort, 1989 for a more detailed discussion of this model). In this model, job stressors, such as quantitative workload, lack of job control, and job future ambiguity, can produce short-term stress responses that increase the potential for ill health. These short-term responses can be classified as emotional (e.g. adverse mood states, job dissatisfaction), physiological (e.g. increased blood pressure, increased heart rate, increased catecholamine excretion, increased muscle tension), and behavioral (e.g. absenteeism, smoking, overeating, overuse of medication, using undue force).

Short-term stress responses can lead to illness or disease (e.g. hypertension, cardiovascular diseases, ulcers, neurosis, depression, alienation, withdrawal) if the individual is continuously exposed and is responsive to the job stressors. There are individual characteristics that influence the stress process; for instance, older individuals tend to be more satisfied with their job, but are more likely to suffer from hypertension. Personality characteristics may also moderate the effect of stressors on stress reactions, and the effect of short-term stress reaction on long-term health. For instance, when exposed to the same job stressors, Type A behavior individuals tend to have more negative short-term stress reactions and more ill health than Type B behavior individuals (Syme, 1987; Tyroler *et al.*, 1987).

The model also specifies 'feedback loops' between disease states, stress reactions, and stressors (Levi, 1972). For instance, individuals with chronic diseases may feel more dissatisfied at work or report more adverse mood states due to their inability to perform their job as well as desired. Conversely, adverse working conditions may exacerbate the symptoms of the disease and create poorer moods and increased pain. Stress reactions can also moderate or heighten the effect of stressors. For instance, individuals with adverse mood reactions may be more 'sensitive' to stress-

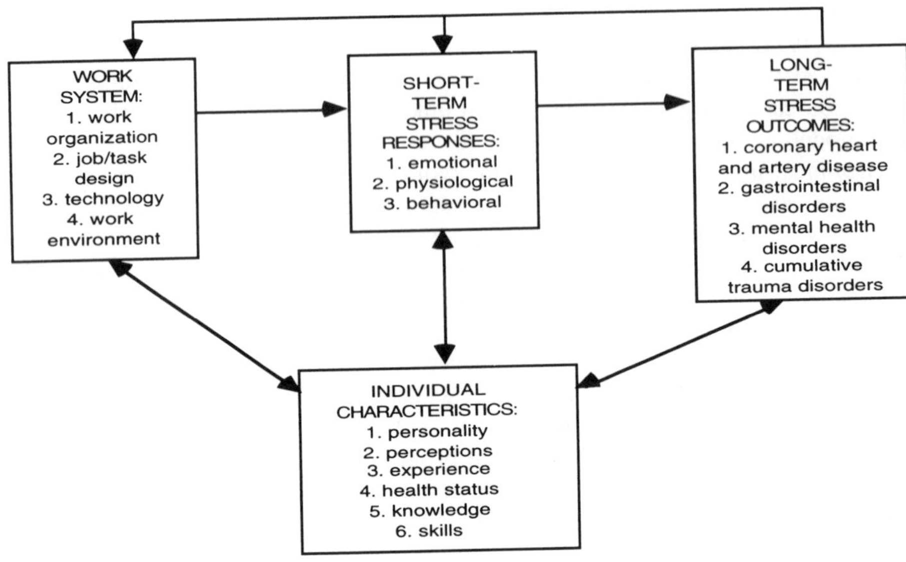

Figure 2.1 Model of job stress.

ors, that is they may have stronger physiological responses to stressors. Likewise, coping behaviors aimed at dealing with the stress reactions may be maladaptive and reinforce the individual's exposure or response to stressors.

WORK ORGANIZATION AND STRESS

Around the turn of the century the major innovation at the workplace concerned improvements in work methods and supervision. This changed during the Second World War, when substantial automation was introduced to counteract the shortage of workers in factories. The trend toward increasing factory automation has continued to the present (OTA, 1985a). Early automation efforts were seen as ways to enhance the physical capacity of the workforce and often added skill requirements to jobs.

Later, in the 1950s automation typically brought about psychological stress problems for workers due to job deskilling, job uncertainty, increased job demands, and organizational indifference to human resources (Walker and Guest, 1952; McGregor, 1960; Mann and Hoffman, 1960; Blauner, 1964; Hazelhurst *et al.*, 1971; Taylor, 1971). Today these same problems persist, but are seen in offices and service industries as well as factories (OTA, 1985a and 1985b; OTA, 1987; Smith, 1984, 1986; Cyert and Mowery, 1988; Smith and Carayon, 1995). Such problems have pertinence because they produce poorer worker health, decreased worker productivity, reduced product quality, increased worker absenteeism, and greater worker resistance to organizational change (Keita and Sauter, 1992; Smith, 1986, 1987).

Automation appears to be at the heart of many of the stress problems that employees have with work organization. Yet companies continue to rely on automation because it has the potential to improve their competitive status. New technology can provide many economic benefits such as lowered production costs, improved product or service quality and conformity, enhanced flexibility of the production system, and lowered insurance costs by reducing worker risks (Smith, 1986). Evidence from applications research indicates that many of the benefits of automation are realized (OTA, 1985a). However, there is also emerging evidence that technology can be detrimental to the production process and to the employees in an industry (OTA, 1984, 1985a and 1985b, 1987).

Automation often creates new production processes that cause stress due to tight scheduling demands, loss of task control, tasks with diminished content, fears of job loss, and new technological-based stressors such as electronic performance monitoring and equipment breakdowns. The way in which automation affects the nature of jobs, for instance the design of the tasks, supervisory style, and job loss, has been linked to psychological stress (Smith *et al.*, 1981, 1992; OTA, 1985a and 1985b; Cyert and Mowery, 1988; Majchrzak, 1988; Cooper and Smith, 1985).

Diminished worker control over task activities has been identified as a source of stress and ill health (Sainfort, 1991; Karasek, 1979; Smith, 1981, 1987). The design of jobs, and how jobs will be affected by advanced automation, is an important issue to workers. In general there is the concern that advanced automation will bring about a deskilling of jobs and little physical or intellectual challenge. The attitude that workers are merely an expendable resource to be allocated and used just as machines are allocated and used has produced many industrial relations problems (Cyert and Mowery, 1988).

Technological 'malfunctioning' is a trademark of complex systems, and computer breakdowns have their own unique stress aspects (Carayon-Sainfort, 1992). Technology can be unreliable or undependable which leads to downtime. Processes may be kept operational by having workers step in for the machines. However, if the system is designed primarily for the machinery needs, then workers may not fit into the process easily. Helander (1991) has discussed experiences in manufacturing processes where employees stepped in for broken technology and developed stress and cumulative trauma problems due to workplace design mismatches.

The following section will examine how work organization can affect CTDs.

MECHANISMS OF WORK ORGANIZATION, STRESS, AND CTDs

There are several ways in which work organization can influence the development of CTDs. First and foremost, work organization defines the physical levels of work activity that workers engage in. The organization determines the level of worker productivity that is acceptable, establishes output quotas and standards, and defines production incentives. Work organization can also affect the level of job stress experienced by workers through the various stressors that are defined by organization and job design. At the organizational level, the policies and procedures of a company can affect CTD risk through the design of jobs, the length of time of exposure to CTD risk factors, establishing work–rest cycles, defining the extent of work pressures, and establishing the psychological climate regarding socialization, career, and job security. In addition, the organization defines the nature of the task activities (specific work methods), employee training, availability of assistance and help, and supervisory relations with workers.

Work organization can contribute to CTD problems by defining job/task design and the physical requirements of work. These would include the nature of the work activities (variety or repetition), the extent of loads, the exposure to loads, the number and duration of actions, ergonomic considerations such as the workstation design, tool and equipment design, and environmental features of the work area. These factors interact as a system to produce an overall load on the person that can lead to both stress and CTDs.

Jobs that are lacking in challenge and meaningfulness, are boring, or have limited career opportunities and low compensation have been shown to produce worker apathy, alienation, and unproductive behavior (Kahn, 1981). When workers are apathetic it is likely that they will not be as careful of risks to their health, especially those that are more subtle, such as CTD risks. It is also possible that workers will engage in behaviors that will increase the risk of CTDs, such as using undue force or improper work methods in response to workplace frustrations. The psychosocial work environment affects an individual's motivation to work safely, the attitude toward personal health and safety, and willingness to seek health care.

A few studies have shown a link between work organization and CTD in service workers (Smith *et al.*, 1992; Sauter *et al.*, 1993). Smith *et al.* (1992) studied a group of 745 telecommunications workers from seven companies. The purpose of the study was to examine the link between job stress and electronic performance monitoring. Workers in monitored jobs reported higher levels of psychological stress, musculoskeletal symptoms and psychosomatic symptoms than workers in nonmonitored jobs. In particular, 49 per cent of the monitored workers complained of sore/stiff wrists as compared to 26 per cent for the nonmonitored workers. Other muscular health complaints showed similar differences, for instance for loss of feeling in fingers 41 per cent versus 29 per cent, shoulder soreness 79 per cent versus 54 per cent, and neck pressure 82 per cent versus 58 per cent.

Sauter *et al.* (1993) reported on two cross-sectional studies conducted by NIOSH that found a relationship between organizational factors and muscular health complaints. One examined telecommunications workers in five different jobs, and the other newspaper employees in four departments. Assessments of the upper-extremity musculoskeletal problems and of working conditions were done using questionnaires and medical examinations of a sample of employees. The results of the studies were consistent. Several measures of work organization were related to upper-extremity musculoskeletal symptoms. For the telecommunications workers, fear of being replaced by computers was related to increased neck and elbow symptoms, while high information-processing demands were related to increased neck and hand/wrist symptoms. In both studies, factors related to increased work pressure were 'salient' in predicting musculoskeletal health complaints of relevance to upper-extremity CTDs.

A review of studies on musculoskeletal disease (in particular back, neck, and shoulder symptoms) and psychosocial factors suggests that monotonous work, high workload, time pressure, lack of job control, and lack of social support are related to musculoskeletal symptoms (Bongers *et al.*, 1993). These same factors, as well as other job stressors, could also be related to upper-extremity CTDs.

We have identified two possible effects of work organization on CTDs. First, many work organization design factors have been linked to employees' short-term and long-term stress reactions, and therefore work organization could be related to CTD via employees' responses to stress. This potential linkage will be discussed later. Second, work organization can influence ergonomic risk factors, such as employee postures and duration of repetitive movements, which have been identified as risk factors of CTDs. Figure 2.2 displays these two mechanisms.

Work organization can define or influence recognized ergonomic risk factors of CTD, such as repetition, force, and posture (Armstrong *et al.*, 1993). Work organization can define the nature of, strength of, and exposure time to these ergonomic risk factors. Work organization, for instance, may define the degree of repetitiveness of the job. In a highly fractionalized job, the worker tends to do the same tasks over and over, making the actions of the upper extremities highly repetitive. Such repetitiveness has been defined as an ergonomic risk factor for CTDs (Silverstein *et al.*, 1987; Armstrong *et al.*, 1993).

Work organization can also define the duration of the exposures to the ergonomic risk factors. A work organization that does not encourage workers to take regular rest breaks and/or mini-breaks whenever needed, may create conditions where the employee is overworked. Alternatively, job designs that induce static postures may appear to underwork the person while overworking specific musculoskeletal structures.

Machine-paced work is a work organization design process where workers have no freedom in influencing the pace or duration of their work (Salvendy and Smith, 1981; Smith, 1985; Arndt, 1983). Such a system does not allow for any variation in work pace, and usually does not give time to workers to take mini-breaks when needed. This produces a rigid task structure that leads to repetitious movements

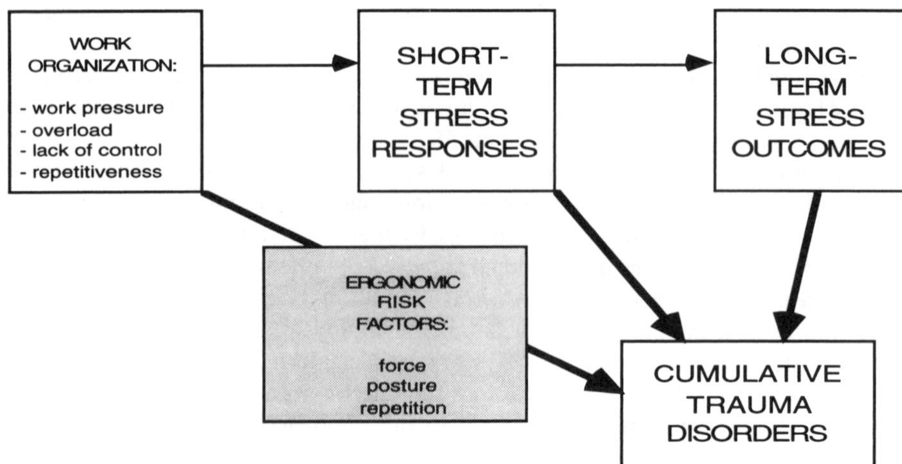

Figure 2.2 Work organization, ergonomic risk factors, and the stress/CTD relationship.

and boredom. Such work structures have been shown to produce job stress and related musculoskeletal and emotional discomfort (Smith, 1985; Salvendy and Smith, 1981; Arndt, 1983).

Work organization can also define the duration of exposure to the ergonomic risk factors by setting work and performance standards. If the worker is supposed to produce a specific number of products per time period, then this work standard will define the duration of exposure to, for instance, repetition, force, and posture. In addition, overtime work is a work organization factor that increases the duration of exposure to ergonomic risk factors, often when the employee is fatigued and likely to be more susceptible to strain.

We have shown that work organization design can affect ergonomic risk factors, which, in turn, are related to increased risk of CTDs. In the following two sections, we will describe how job stress and related psychological, physiological, and behavioral processes contribute to CTDs directly and indirectly. The role of job stress in the development and progression of CTDs is multifaceted. It can be due to:

biophysiological stress reactions;
behavioral stress effects;
general physical and psychological sensitization of the individual.

PSYCHOBIOLOGICAL MECHANISMS OF STRESS AND CTDs

When an individual is undergoing the psychological, physiological, and behavioral effects of job stress there are changes in body chemistry and neurophysiology that may increase the risk of CTDs. These changes include: increased blood pressure, increases in corticosteroids, increases in peripheral neurotransmitters, increases in muscle tension, and increased immune system response. Figure 2.3 shows how these short-term biological reactions to stress may contribute to increased CTD risk.

The organism's basic reaction to external threat and internal psychological stress is to mobilize energy resources for defensive actions and to 'shut down' response

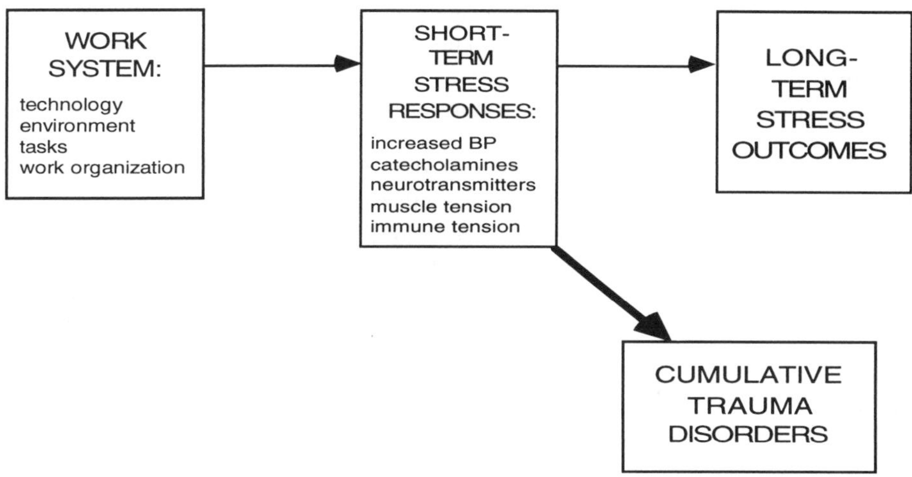

Figure 2.3 Psychobiological mechanisms of the stress/CTD relationship.

mechanisms that could compromise the organism's survival if injured (Selye, 1956). When this reaction occurs, there is less blood flow to the extremities. This is to protect the organism by reducing blood loss if an extremity is cut and bleeds, and to provide more blood for vital organs. This also means that when a worker is under stress there is the potential for less blood flow to the muscles and tendons of the extremities when they most need it during repetitive work.

Several studies have shown a link between increased blood pressure and job stress. In particular, workload, work pressure, and lack of job control have been related to increased blood pressure (Rose *et al.*, 1978; Matthews *et al.*, 1987). Recent studies performed by researches at the Cornell University Medical College have further demonstrated the link between hypertension and job stress (Schnall *et al.*, 1990), and between emotions (e.g. anger and anxiety) and increased blood pressure (James *et al.*, 1986). Individuals with high blood pressure may be more likely to experience CTDs because high blood pressure produces a higher pressure in the internal carpal tunnel canal (Armstrong *et al.*, 1993; Szabo and Gelberman, 1987).

A second physiological reaction to stress that occurs is an increase in corticosteroids (Frankenhaeuser, 1986; Finestone, 1986; Daleva, 1987). These, in particular cortisol, can lead to an increase in fluid retention in peripheral body tissues. This could be an important CTD risk factor since several upper-extremity CTDs are due to nerve compression that is compounded by fluid retention. An analogy would be the increased fluid production and tissue swelling due to repeated friction of the tendon body within the tendon sheath. This can create pressure on and pinching of the nerve(s) that can cause the paresthesia and pain associated with peripheral neuropathy (Armstrong *et al.*, 1993).

Another biochemical reaction that occurs when an organism is under stress is the increase in peripheral neurotransmitters (in particular norepinepherine) (Levi, 1972; Frankenhaeuser, 1986). This creates an increased sensitivity of the neuromuscular synapses due to greater availability of norepinephrine. Those persons under acute psychological stress have the potential to perform faster than when not under stress due to this increased sensitivity. This effect is observed in athletic competition where stress motivates high performance. However, if this increased performance is sustained over a long period of time, it could lead to a substantially higher level of repetitive loading of the muscles, tendons, ligaments, and joints which could be detrimental. This increased sensitivity may also make workers more prone to feel pain.

Frankenhaeuser and her colleagues have developed a psychobiological model of stress that specifies the psychosocial factors more likely to induce increases in cortisol and catecholamines (Frankenhaeuser, 1986; Lundberg and Frankenhaeuser, 1980; Frankenhaeuser and Johansson, 1986). There are two different neuroendocrine responses to the psychosocial environment: (1) secretion of catecholamines via the sympathetic–adrenal medullary system, and (2) secretion of corticosteroids via the pituitary–adrenal–cortical system. They observed that different patterns of neuroendocrine stress responses occur depending on the psychosocial characteristics of the environment. These psychosocial factors are effort and distress. The effort factor 'involves elements of interest, engagements, and determination,' while the distress factor 'involves elements of dissatisfaction, boredom, uncertainty and anxiety' (Frankenhaeuser, 1986).

Effort with distress is accompanied by increases in both catecholamine and cortisol secretion. Effort without distress is characterized by increased catecholamine secretion, but no change in cortisol secretion. Distress without effort in generally accompanied by increased cortisol secretion, with a slight elevation of catecholamines. This model emphasizes two important issues. The first is the interaction between personal effort (behavior) and distress in creating a combined physiological reaction (catecholamine and cortisol production). The second is the role of personal control in mediating the biological responses to stress. A lack of control is almost always related to distress, whereas personal control tends to stimulate effort. Studies performed by Frankenhaeuser and Johansson (1986) found that overload can lead to increased catecholamine secretion, but not to increased cortisol when control is high.

Another consideration related to physiological stress is the amount of tension in the muscles. As Westgaard (Chapter 5 of this volume) has shown, there are direct nerve pathways between the emotional center of the brain and peripheral muscles. When persons are under emotional stress, the level of muscle tension increases. This is independent of the biomechanical loading of the muscle. In addition, with increased levels of norepinepherine, the tension in muscles has the potential to be greater, and the amount of force generated by the muscles in performing an activity may be greater. This heightened muscle tension is increased by adverse psychological moods such as anxiety or anger (Jacobson, 1932; Chapter 5 of this volume). Thus, when the person is angry or frightened the muscles are more tense. This same heightened muscle tension and excessive muscular force may be present during stressful working conditions that create negative emotions.

A few studies have suggested that increased muscle tension may be a mediating variable between job stressors and psychological stress on the one hand, and musculoskeletal symptoms on the other hand (Ursin *et al.*, 1988; Theorell *et al.*, 1991). Theorell *et al.* (1991) studied the effects of work stressors on emotions, psychosomatic reactions, muscle tension, and musculoskeletal symptoms (back, neck, shoulders, and other joints) in a group of 207 workers in six occupations. Work stressors were related to negative emotions (e.g. worry), psychosomatic reactions (e.g. tiredness and sleep disturbance), and self-reported muscle tension. Muscle tension was strongly related to back, neck, and shoulders symptoms and to emotions. The authors argued that muscle tension may be an important pathway from psychosocially adverse job conditions to musculoskeletal symptoms.

At some point in the stress syndrome the organism is unable to continue to respond normally and exhaustion occurs (Selye, 1956). During this stress-induced exhaustion, the immune system is not able to function normally and thus cannot provide the typical resources for repairing damaged tissues. Studies by Vaernes *et al.* (1991) and Endresen *et al.* (1991) have shown that job stress, anxiety and depression were correlated with changes in the immune system. Chronic exposure to cumulative trauma stressors while the organism is undergoing psychological stress may create micro damage that cannot be fully repaired due to the impaired immune response, and over time this may lead to permanent tissue damage. Stress may influence this process by limiting the ability of the immune system to respond positively for repairing tissue damaged by micro trauma caused by physical work demands.

PSYCHOLOGICAL AND BEHAVIORAL REACTIONS TO STRESS

A second major way in which stress can influence the occurrence of CTDs is through its effects on a person's psychological and behavioral reactions. Stress can affect psychological moods, work behavior, coping style and actions, motivation to report injury, and motivation to seek treatment for a CTD injury or symptoms of impending injury.

Upper-extremity CTDs are disorders that involve significant pain. Many times, diagnosis of a disorder is based on the nature and extent of pain subjectively reported by the person. Stress may serve to increase the frequency of reporting of upper-extremity pain because of a general increase in personal sensitivity to pain brought on by negative psychological moods. Thus, pain that is really nonclinical and a normal part of the general adaptation process to work activity may be perceived by the employee as much more significant due to heightened psychological stress. If this same person were not under psychological stress the pain may not be perceived as significant and go unreported and untreated. Many cases of reported pain end up being treated as CTDs, and continued psychological stress may cause continued pain in spite of treatment(s). This may lead to more substantial treatment(s) such as surgical interventions. Figure 2.4 displays this psychological mechanism that may explain the relationship between stress and CTD.

A related issue is a social psychological aspect of illness behavior. It is possible that a person under psychological stress could develop specific physical symptoms (such as sore wrists) that would 'legitimate' their general psychological discomfort and pain (see Figure 2.5). Having pains in the wrists and fingers is a socially acceptable disorder, while feeling depressed is not. Thus, the effects of psychological disturbances may be reflected in physical disorders of the musculoskeletal system. This is much like mass psychogenic illness or psychosomatic disorders where psychologically induced disturbances lead to physical impairment. There has been some conjecture that upper-extremity CTD outbreaks have similarities to mass psychogenic illness (Kiesler and Finholt, 1988). However, we feel that this characterization is incorrect since CTD outbreaks have not been shown to have 'triggering' events or immediate social contagion reactions. Rather, the CTD outbreaks seem to have

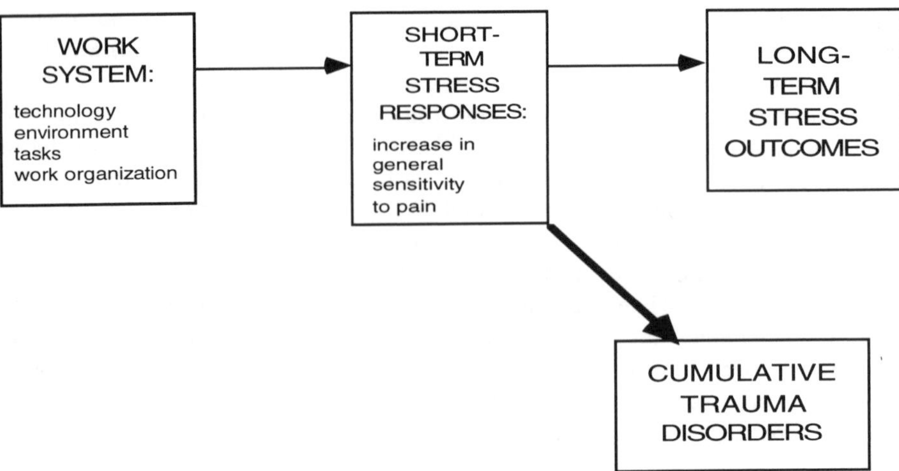

Figure 2.4 Psychological mechanism of the stress/CTD relationship.

occurred over a substantial period of time (often months) with a different social contagion dynamic than mass psychogenic illness (Schmitt *et al.*, 1980).

Mass psychogenic illness has been defined as 'the collective occurrence of a set of physical symptoms and related beliefs among two or more individuals in the absence of an identifiable pathogen' (Colligan and Murphy, 1979). The presence of a physical or chemical agent (e.g. odor) often serves as a trigger for the outbreak of physical symptoms. The illness is perceived as being caused by a physical or chemical agent and the affected individual can then escape the hazardous environment (Colligan and Murphy, 1979). A review of eight NIOSH investigations of unexplained physical symptoms show that these symptoms are related to job and organizational characteristics that are well-known stressors (Schmitt *et al.*, 1980).

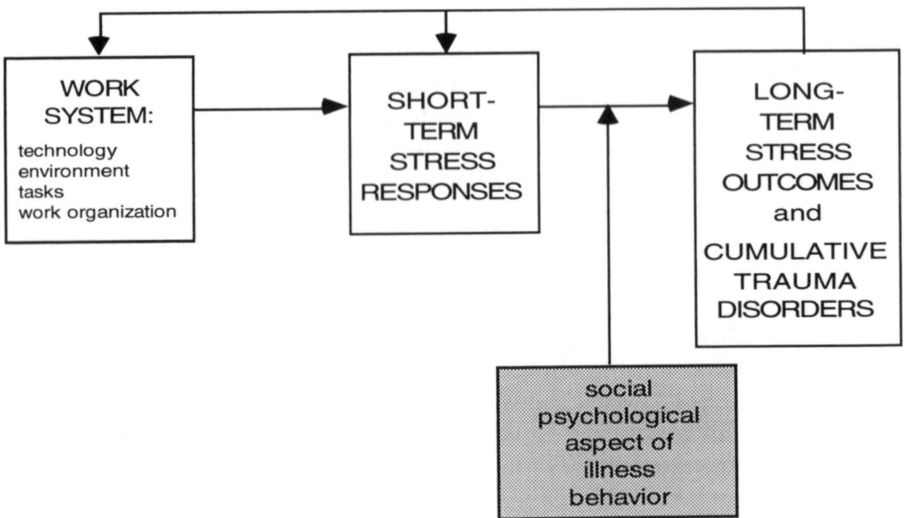

Figure 2.5 Social psychological aspect of illness behavior in the stress/CTD relationship.

Individuals with low-paid, high-pressure, repetitive jobs are more likely to report these physical symptoms.

The emergence of group outbreaks of CTDs in Australia (Kiesler and Finholt, 1988) and the United States (NIOSH, 1992) may have some similarities to cases of mass psychogenic illness observed in the 1960s and 1970s, and stuffy office syndrome of the 1980s. For instance, reporting a CTD which is a physical disorder with a known ergonomic cause may be more socially acceptable than reporting emotional stress reactions. Like mass psychogenic illness, CTDs have often been observed in low-paid, high-pressure, repetitive jobs (Putz-Anderson, 1988; Silverstein *et al.*, 1987; NIOSH, 1990, 1992). There most likely were social contagion aspects of the upper-extremity CTD outbreaks in Australia and the United States (NIOSH, 1992; Kiesler and Finholt, 1988), but the timing of the responses of the affected employees was quite different than the more acute reactions that occur with mass psychogenic illness.

As shown is Figure 2.5, the occurrence of a CTD may itself act as a source of emotional stress that leads to heightened physical and pain symptoms (i.e. feedback loop). Experiencing a CTD or observing a co-worker with a CTD may trigger emotional stress reactions that lead to CTD symptoms in the observer. The observer logically speculates that he or she may be exposed to the same working conditions that produced the symptoms in the co-worker which also leads to emotional stress.

We know that job stress can affect the behaviour of a person in dealing with the work environment (Smith, 1987). For instance, a person who is stressed may become angry and this could lead to using improper work methods, or using excessive force in performing a work activity, or gripping a tool too tightly. Persons under stress often develop poor attitudes and motivation about the job and about personal health and well-being (Kahn, 1981; Caplan *et al.*, 1975; Landy, 1989). They become apathetic, and it is difficult to get them to take positive action even when it affects their health. These same people are not likely to seek medical assistance until a serious health condition interferes with their ability to do their job duties. They are

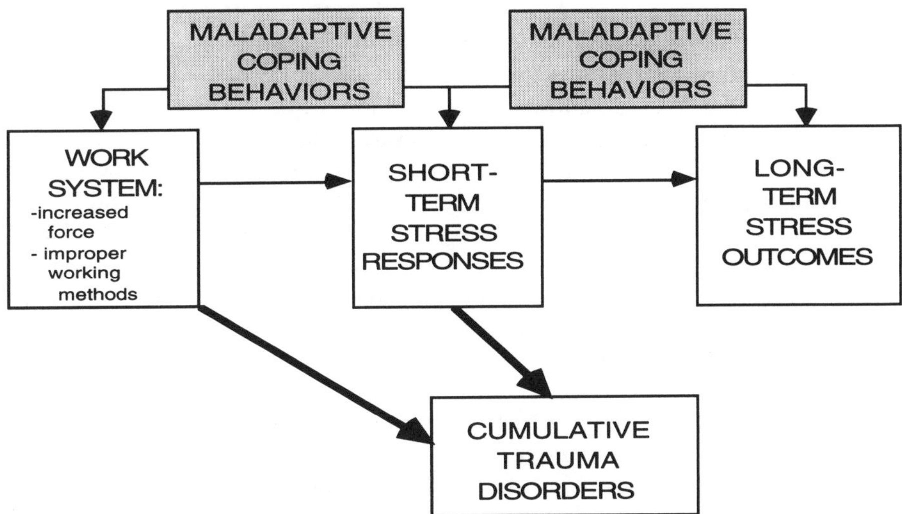

Figure 2.6 Maladaptive coping behaviors and the stress/CTD relationship.

more likely to be absent from work because of sickness (USDHHS, 1979). Generally, maladaptive coping behaviors have been related to poorer overall health, less energy, and greater general fatigue. This could make people more susceptible to injury or disease and lead to a diminished capacity to work, both conditions that increase the potential for CTDs. The relationships between these maladaptive coping behaviors, stress, and CTDs are displayed in Figure 2.6.

In summary, there are potentially many ways that job stress can affect the risk of CTDs. At the individual's level, the first influence is the biophysiological stress reactions that can exacerbate the effects of physical strain and/or limit the ability of the body's defense and repair systems to deal with micro trauma. The second influence is the effect of stress on the behavior of the individual that may increase exposures to CTD risk factors or which decreases the motivation to seek help. The third is the general sensitization of the individual psychologically and physically to pain by exposure to emotional stress. These processes may lead to greater perceived pain and poorer overall health and lower vital capacity to deal with work demands. These can lead to the development of CTDs.

CONCEPTUAL FRAMEWORK FOR EXAMINING JOB STRESS AND CTDs

A conceptual framework for examining job stress and CTDs should have the following characteristics. First, the conceptual framework should give a central place to emotional stress. Second, it should include both physical ergonomic stressors and work organization stressors as potential causes of CTDs. There currently is no scientific evidence or valid hypothetical biological mechanisms that can logically define physical stressors as superordinate to work organization stressors in causing CTDs, or inversely, as subordinate to work organization stressors in causing CTDs. It is very likely that CTDs develop because of the joint influence of both types of stressor, but it is possible that CTDs may develop from exposure to either source of stressors. We have shown how work organization factors can directly and indirectly influence CTDs by affecting physical ergonomic stressors and emotional stressors. The model of CTD causation that we are proposing allows for interactions between the various job factors that produce physical and emotional stressors.

Third, the conceptual framework should not be limited to select work organization factors. Many of the jobs linked to high incidence of CTDs are jobs with characteristics that are well-known sources of job stress, such as work overload, work pressure, and lack of control. However, other jobs, such as journalism (NIOSH, 1990), that do not have these same characteristics have also been related to a high incidence of CTDs. Therefore, the conceptual framework should be holistic enough to include a large variety of job factors. We believe that the balance theory of job design and stress as defined by Smith and Carayon-Sainfort (1989) can provide a useful framework for examining the relationships and interactions between work organization, ergonomics, job stress, and CTDs. It is a systems approach that includes both work organization and ergonomic factors as potential sources of job stress.

The balance theory developed by Smith and Carayon-Sainfort (1989) provides a useful framework to examine relationships and interactions between work organization and ergonomic factors, and their effect on worker stress. According to this theory, stress is a result of an imbalance between elements of the work system. This imbalance produces a 'load' on the human response mechanisms that can produce adverse reactions, both psychological and physiological. The human response mechanisms, which include behavior, physiological reactions, and cognition, act to bring control over the environmental factors that are creating an imbalance. These efforts, coupled with an inability to achieve balance, produce overloading of the response mechanisms that lead to mental and physical fatigue. Prolonged exposure and fatigue leads to strain and disease.

This model emphasizes the definition of sources of occupational stress (stressors) that can produce an imbalance in the work system. These stressors can be categorized into one of the following elements of the work system: (1) job/task design, (2) the organizational context, (3) technology, (4) work environment, and (5) the individual. Figure 2.7 displays the model of the work system. The imbalance in the work system leads to stress and strain responses which are caused by physical, ergonomic loads and psychological loads. The persistence of these loads defines the extent of the psychobiological and behavioral adaptive responses in attempting to restore balance in the system.

Balance can also be disturbed or enhanced through actions taken by the work organization in controlling stressors. When the work organization imposes excessive demands, especially those related to ergonomic misfit, then the results can be increased exposure to CTD risk factors and increased psychological distress. In combination, it is postulated that the risk for CTDs is greatly increased through

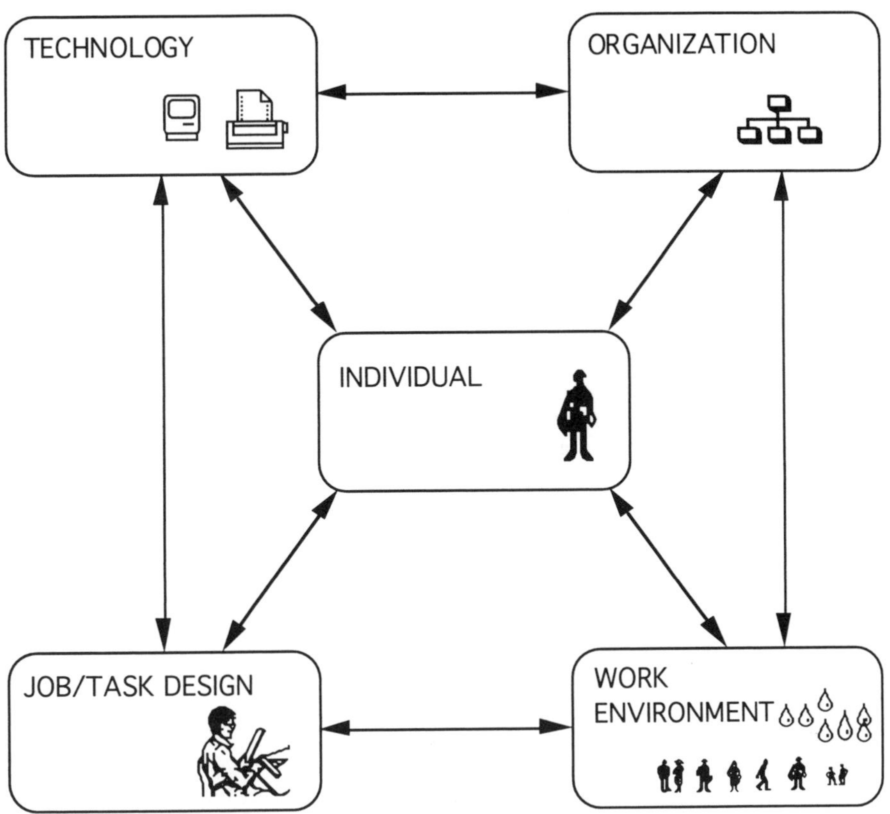

Figure 2.7 Model of the work system.

adverse psychobiological reactions and maladaptive coping behavior. Smith and Carayon-Sainfort (1989) have proposed ways to achieve better balance in the work system to decrease the level of stress and to enhance health. Many of these strategies would also be effective for reducing ergonomic risk factors for CTDs.

CONCLUSION

Much of this discussion has been speculative and has been presented to illustrate that there is some potential for work organization factors to contribute directly and indirectly to the risk of CTDs. There is inadequate research to know precisely what this role is, and whether it is significant. Yet, there are very plausible physiological mechanisms through which work organization considerations that create job stress can have a major influence on the development and severity of upper-extremity CTDs. These mechanisms have as much 'face validity' as biomechanical theories.

Traditional ergonomic risk factors such as repetition, force, and posture have been postulated as the major contributors to CTDs (Putz-Anderson, 1988; Silverstein *et al.*, 1987; Armstrong *et al.*, 1993). This paper has demonstrated that work organization factors can also have direct effects on CTDs through psychobiological mechanisms of stress, and can also have direct effects by defining the levels of exposures to the biomechanical CTD risk factors. However, we feel that to fully understand the etiology of CTDs and to prevent or control CTDs, it is necessary to examine simultaneously physical ergonomic, work organization factors and stress (Smith and Carayon-Sainfort, 1989; Carayon-Sainfort, 1992; Carayon, 1993). We feel that the Smith and Carayon-Sainfort (1989) balance model that describes how the work system influences job stress and health provides a useful framework to conceptualize the totality of work-related factors that contribute to CTDs, and the relationship between job stress, biomechanics and CTDs.

REFERENCES

ARMSTRONG, T. J., BUCKLE, P., FINE, L. J., HAGBERG, M., JONSSON, B., KILBORN, A., KUONINKA, I., SILVERSTEIN, B. A., SJOGAARD, G. and VIIKARI-JUNTURA, E. 1993 A conceptual model for work-related neck and upper limb musculoskeletal disorders, *Scandinavian Journal of Work, Environment and Health*, **79**, 73–84.

ARNDT, R. 1983 Working posture and musculoskeletal problems of video display terminal operators: Review and appraisal, *American Industrial Hygiene Association Journal*, **44**, 437–46.

BAUM, A., FLEMING, R. and SINGER, J. E. 1983 Coping with victimization by technological disaster, *Journal of Social Issues*, **39**(2), 117–38.

BLAUNER, R. 1964 *Alienation and Freedom*, Chicago: University of Chicago Press.

BONGERS, P. M., DE WINTER, C. R., KOMPIER, M. A. and HILDEBRANDT, V. H. 1993 Psychosocial factors at work and musculoskeletal disease, *Scandinavian Journal of Work, Environment and Health*, **19**, 297–312.

CAPLAN, R. D., COBB, S., FRENCH, J. R. JR., VAN HARRISON, R. and PINNEAU, S. R. 1975 *Job Demands and Worker Health*, Washington, DC: US Government Printing Office.

CARAYON, P. 1993 Job design and job stress in office workers, *Ergonomics*, **36**(5), 463–77.

CARAYON-SAINFORT, P. 1992 The use of computers in offices: Impact on task characteristics and worker stress, *The International Journal of Human–Computer Interaction*, **4**(3), 245–61.

COLLIGAN, M. J. and MURPHY, L. R. 1979 Mass psychogenic illness in organizations: An overview, *Journal of Occupational Psychology*, **52**, 77–90.

COOPER, C. L. and MARSHALL, J. 1976 Occupational sources of stress: A review of the literature relating to coronary heart disease and mental ill health, *Journal of Occupational Psychology*, **49**, 11–28.

COOPER, C. L. and SMITH, M. J. 1985 *Job Stress in Blue Collar Work*, London: John Wiley.

CYERT, R. M. and MOWERY, D. C. 1988 *The Impact of Technological Change on Employment and Economic Growth*, Cambridge, MA: Ballinger.

DALEVA, M. 1987 Metabolic and neurohormonal reactions to occupational stress, in KALIMO, R., EL-BATAWI M. A. and COOPER C. L., (Eds), Psychosocial factors at work and their relation to health, pp. 48–63, Geneva: World Health Organization.

DEMING, W. E. 1982 *Quality, Productivity, and Competitive Position*, Cambridge, MA: MIT Press.

DRUCKER, P. F. 1980 *Managing in Turbulent Times*, New York: Harper & Row.

DUNNETTE, M. and HOUGH, L. M. (Eds) 1992 *Handbook of Industrial and Organizational Psychology*, 2nd Edn, Palo Alto, CA: Consulting Psychologist Press.

ENDRESEN, I. M., ELLERTSEN, B., ENDRESEN, C., HJELMEN, A. M., MATRE, R. and URSIN, H. 1991 Stress at work and psychological and immunological parameters in a group of Norwegian female bank employees, *Work and Stress*, **5**(3), 217–27.

FINESTONE, A. J. 1986 Neurohumoral mediators of emotional stress, in WOLF, S. and FINESTONE, A. J. (Eds), *Occupational Stress Health and Performance*, pp. 34–42, Littleton, MA: PSG.

FRANKENHAEUSER, M. 1986 A psychobiological framework for research on human stress and coping, in APPLEY, M. H. and TRUMBULL, R. (Eds), *Dynamics of Stress: Physiological Psychological and Social Perspectives*, pp. 101–16, New York: Plenum Press.

FRANKENHAEUSER, M. and JOHANSSON, G. 1986 Stress at work: Psychobiological and psychosocial aspects, *International Review of Applied Psychology*, **35**, 287–99.

FRENCH, J. R. P., Jr. 1963 The social environment and mental health, *Journal of Social Issues*, **19**, 39–56.

GILBRETH, F. B. 1914 *Primer of Scientific Management*, New York: Van Nostrand.

HACKMAN, J. R. and OLDHAM, G. R. 1976 Motivation through the design of work: Test of a theory, *Organizational Behavior and Human Performance*, **16**, 250–79.

HAZLEHURST, R. J., BRADBURY, R. J. and CORLETT, E. N. 1971 A comparison of the skills of machinists on numerically controlled and conventional machines, *Occupational Psychology*, **43**, 169–82.

HELANDER, M. 1991 Human factors in manufacturing, presentation at The Symposium on the Effects on New Technology, Uppsala, Sweden.

HERZBERG, F. 1966 *Work and the Nature of Man*, New York: Thomas Y. Crowell.

HOUSE, J. 1981 *Work, Stress, and Social Support*, Reading, MA: Addison-Wesley.

JACOBSON, E. 1932 Electrophysiology of mental activities, *American Journal of Psychology*, **44**, 677–94.

JAMES, G. D., YEE, L. S., HARSHFIELD, G. A., BLANK, S. G. and PICKERING, T. G. 1986 The influence of happiness, anger, and anxiety on the blood pressure of borderline hypertensives, *Psychosomatic Medicine*, **48**(7), 502–8.

JURAN, J. M. 1951 *Quality Control Handbook*, New York: McGraw-Hill.

KAHN, R. 1981 *Work and Health*, New York: John Wiley.

KARASEK, R. 1979 Job demands, job decision latitude, and mental strain: implications for job redesign, *Administrative Science Quarterly*, **24**, 295–308.

KASL, S. V. 1978 Epidemiological contributions to the study of work stress, in COOPER, C. L. and PAYNE, R. (Eds), *Stress at Work*, pp. 3–48, Chichester: John Wiley.

KEITA, G. P. and SAUTER, S. L. 1992 *Work and Well Being*, Washington DC: American Psychological Association.

KIESLER, S. and FINHOLT, T. 1988 The mystery of RSI, *American Psychologist*, **43**(12), 1004–15.

LANDY, F. J. 1989 *The Psychology of Work Behavior*, 4th Edn, Monterey, CA: Brooks/Cole.

LAWLER, E. E. 1986 *High Involvement Management*, San Francisco, CA: Jossey-Bass.

LAZARUS, R. S. 1974 Psychological stress and coping in adaptation and illness, *International Journal of Psychiatry in Medicine*, **5**, 321–33.

LAZARUS, R. S. 1977 Cognitive and coping processes in emotion, in MONAT, A. and LAZARUS, R. S. (Eds), *Stress and Coping: An Anthology*, pp. 145–58, New York: Columbia University Press.

LEVI, L. 1972 Stress and distress in response to psychosocial stimuli, *Acta Medica Scandinavia*, **191**, suppl. 528.

LUNDBERG, U. and FRANKENHAEUSER, M. 1980 Pituitary-adrenal and sympathetic-adrenal correlates of distress and effort, *Journal of Psychosomatic Research*, **24**, 125–30.

MAJCHRZAK, A. 1988 *The Human Side of Factory Automation*, San Francisco, CA: Jossey-Bass.

MANN, F. C. and HOFFMAN, L. R. 1960 *Automation and the Worker*, New York: Henry Holt.

MATTHEWS, K. A., COTTINGTON, E. M., TALBOTT, E., KULLER, L. H. and SIEGEL, J. M. 1987 Stressful work conditions and diastolic blood pressure among blue collar factory workers, *American Journal of Epidemiology*, **126**(2), 280–91.

MAYNARD, H. B., STEGEMERTEN, G. J. and SCHWAB, J. L. 1948 *Methods-Time Measurement*, New York: McGraw-Hill.

MCGREGOR, D. 1960 *The Human Side of Enterprise*, New York: McGraw-Hill.

MURPHY, L. R. 1985 Individual coping strategies, in COOPER, C. L. and SMITH, M. J. (Eds), *Job Stress and Blue-Collar Work*, pp. 225–39, Chichester: John Wiley.

NIOSH 1990 *Health Hazard Evaluation Report: HETA 89-250-2046*, Washington, DC: Newsday.

NIOSH 1992 *Health Hazard Evaluation Report: HETA 89-299-2230*, Washington, DC: US West Communications.

OTA 1984 *Computerized Manufacturing Automation: Employment, Education and the Workplace*, Washington, DC: Office of Technology Assessment, US Congress.

OTA 1985a *Preventing Illness and Injury in the Workplace*, Washington, DC: Office of Technology Assessment, US.

OTA 1985b *Automation of America's Offices*, Washington, DC: Office of Technology Assessment, US Congress.

OTA 1987 *The Electronic Supervisor*, Washington, DC: Office of Technology Assessment, US Congress.

PUTZ-ANDERSON, V. (Ed.) 1988 *Cumulative Trauma Disorders: A Manual for Musculoskeletal Diseases of the Upper Limbs*, London: Taylor & Francis.

QUINN, R. P. and STAINES, G. L. 1979 *The 1977 Quality of Employment Survey: Descriptive Statistics, With Comparison Data from the 1969–70 and the 1972–73 Survey*, Ann Arbor, MI: University of Michigan Survey Research Center.

ROETHLISBERGER, F. J. and DICKSON, W. J. 1964 *Management and the Worker*, 13th Edn, Cambridge, MA: Harvard University Press.

ROSE, R. M., JENKINS, C. D. and HURST, M. W. 1978 *Air Traffic Controller Health Change Study*, Washington, DC: US Department of Transportation, Federal Aviation Administration, Office of Aviation Medicine.

SAINFORT, P. CARAYON 1991 Stress, job control and other job elements: A study of office workers, *International Journal of Industrial Ergonomics*, **7**, 11–23.

SALVENDY, G. (Ed.) 1992 *Handbook of Industrial Engineering*, New York: John Wiley.

SALVENDY, G. and SMITH, M. J. 1981 *Machine Pacing and Occupational Stress*, London: Taylor & Francis.

SAUTER, S. L., GOTTLIEB, M. S., ROHRER, K. M. and DODSON, V. N. 1983 *The Well-Being of Video Display Terminal Users*, Madison, WI: Department of Preventive Medicine, University of Wisconsin.

SAUTER, S., HALES, T., BERNARD, B., FINE, L., PETERSEN, M., PUTZ-ANDERSON, V., SCHLEIFER, L. and OCHS, T. 1993 Summary of two NIOSH field studies of musculoskeletal disorders and VDT work among telecommunications and newspaper workers, in LUCZAK, H. CAKIR, A. and CAKIR, G. (Eds.) *Work With Display Units 92*, pp. 229–34, Amsterdam: North-Holland.

SCHMITT, N., COLLIGAN, M. J. and FITZGERALD, M. 1980 Unexplained physical symptoms in eight organizations: Individual and organizational analyses, *Journal of Occupational Psychology*, **53**, 305–17.

SCHNALL, P. L., PIEPER, C., SCHWARTZ, J. E., KARASEK, R. A., SCHLUSSEL, Y., DEVEREUX, R. B., GANAU, A., ALDERMAN, M., WARREN, K. and PICKERING, T. G. 1990 The relationship between 'Job Strain', workplace diastolic blood pressure, and left ventricular mass index, *Journal of the American Medical Association*, **263**, 1929–35.

SELYE, H. 1956 *The Stress of Life*, New York: McGraw-Hill.

SILVERSTEIN, B., FINE, L. and ARMSTRONG, T. 1987 Occupational factors and the carpal tunnel syndrome, *American Journal of Industrial Medicine*, **11**, 343–58.

SMITH, M. J. 1981 Occupational stress, in SALVENDY, G. and SMITH, M. J. (Eds), *Machine Pacing and Occupational Stress*, pp. 13–19, London: Taylor & Francis.

SMITH, M. J. 1984 Health issues in VDT work, in BENNETT, J., CASE, D., SANDELIN, J. and SMITH, M. J. (Eds), *Visual Display Terminals*, pp. 193–228, Englewood Cliffs, NJ: Prentice-Hall.

SMITH, M. J. 1985 Machine paced work and stress, in COOPER, C. and SMITH, M. J. (Eds) *Job Stress in Blue Collar Work*, pp. 51–64, London: John Wiley.

SMITH, M. J. 1986 Sociotechnical considerations in robotics and automation, *Proceedings of the IEEE International Conference on Robotics and Automation*, **2**, 1112–20.

SMITH, M. J. 1987 Occupational stress, in SALVENDY, G. (Ed.), *Handbook of Ergonomics/Human Factors*, pp. 844–60, New York: John Wiley.

SMITH, M. J. and CARAYON, P. 1995 New technology, automation and work organization: Stress problems and improved technology implementation strategies, *International Journal of Human Factors in Manufacturing*, **5**, 99–116.

SMITH, M. J., CARAYON, P., SANDERS, K. J., LIM, S-Y. and LEGRANDE, D. 1992 Employee stress and health complaints in jobs with and without electronic performance monitoring, *Applied Ergonomics*, **23**, 17–27.

SMITH, M. J. and CARAYON-SAINFORT, P. 1989 A balance theory of job design for stress reduction, *International Journal of Industrial Ergonomics*, **4**, 67–79.

SMITH, M. J., COHEN, B. G. F., STAMMERJOHN, L. and HAPP, A. 1981 An investigation of health complaints and job stress in video display operations, *Human Factors*, **23**, 387–400.

SMITH, M. J., SAINFORT, F., CARAYON-SAINFORT, P. and FUNG, C. 1989 Efforts to solve quality problems, in *Investing in People: A Strategy to Address America's Workforce Crisis*, pp. 1949–2002, Washington, DC: Commission on Workforce Quality and Labor Market Efficiency, US Department of Labor.

SYME, S. L. 1987 Coronary artery disease: A sociocultural perspective, *Circulation* (supplement), **76**(1), 112–6.

SZABO, R. M. and GELBERMAN, R. H. 1987 The pathophysiology of nerve entrapment syndromes, *Journal of Hand Surgery*, **12A**(5), 880–4.

TAYLOR, F. W. 1947 *Scientific Management*, London: Harper & Row (originally published in 1911).

TAYLOR, J. C. 1971 Some effects of technology in organizational change, *Human Relations*, **24**, 105–23.

Theorell, T., Ringdahl-Harms, K., Ahlberg-Hulten, G. and Westin, B. 1991 Psychosocial job factors and symptoms from the locomotor system: A multicausal analysis, *Scandinavian Journal of Rehabilitation Medicine*, **23**, 165–73.

Tyroler, H. A., Haynes, S. G., Irvin, C. W., James, S. A., Kuller, L. H., Miller, R. E., Shumaker, S. A., Syme, S. L. and Wolf, W. 1987 Task force 1: Environmental risk factors in coronary artery disease, *Circulation* (supplement), **76**(1), 139–44.

Ursin, H., Endresen, I. M. and Ursin, G. 1988 Psychological factors and self-reports of muscles pain, *European Journal of Applied Physiology*, **57**, 282–90.

USBLS (US Bureau of Labor Statistics) 1992 *BLS News–USDL-92-731*, Washington, DC: Bureau of Labor Statistics News, US Department of Labor.

USDHHS (US Department of Health and Human Services) 1979 *Healthy People: The Surgeon General's Report on Health Promotion and Disease Prevention*, Washington, DC: Publication no. 79-55071, US Government Printing Office.

Vaernes, R. J., Myhre, G., Aas, H., Homnes, T., Hansen, I. and Tonder, O. 1991 Relationships between stress, psychological factors, health and immune levels among military aviators, *Work and Stress*, **5**(1), 5–16.

Walker, C. R. and Guest, R. H. 1952 *The Man on The Assembly Line*, Cambridge, MA: Harvard University Press.

CHAPTER THREE

Somatic interpretation in cumulative trauma disorders

A Social Cognitive Analysis

DELIA CIOFFI

INTRODUCTION

Cumulative trauma disorders (CTDs) pose significant problems for US business and industry (Roughton, 1993). The workshop upon which this volume is based attests to the multifaceted nature of the problem; most researchers now believe that CTDs implicate ergometric, psychosocial, and organizational factors (e.g. Pransky, see Chapter 15 of this volume). This implies that CTD disabilities arise in part from the process by which people make sense of their physical sensations, and by the social environment in which that process takes place. In other words, some portion of CTD phenomena is governed by social cognitions.

In this chapter, I summarize social–cognitive research on somatic interpretation, and advance three major theses along the way. First, somatic interpretation is guided by people's implicit theories about their physical symptoms, and in particular by assumed cause-and-effect relationships between these symptoms and the events that could potentially explain them. Second, because the content of these implicit theories and the process of forming them are greatly affected by the social milieu, somatic interpretation itself will be heavily influenced by the features of one's social situation. Third, these principles imply that the most powerful level of analysis of psychological factors in CTDs will be at that of the individual's social dynamic – that is, where personal, biomechanical, social, and organizational factors converge and interact; constructs such as work environment, organizational climate, social norms for work, and illness reporting are likely to be the most powerful types of descriptive and explanatory constructs in CTD research, prevention, and intervention.

A sidebar about my background may be an appropriate reference point for this discussion. I am an experimental social psychologist whose work has concerned somatic interpretation but who has just recently begun to consider the interesting and important topic of CTDs in the workplace. Thus, my discussion is based on only a recent exposure to and virtually no direct experience with the issues faced by many readers who have long grappled with this problem in their research or practical lives. Moreover, I approach the CTD issue with all the biases and assumptions that the label of 'experimental social psychologist' implies. These biases show themselves in the sorts of hypotheses I generate for CTD phenomena and the methods and approaches I recommend for studying them. I expect both biasing factors will become clear in the course of this discussion. Still, I hope these will not be limiting factors to the reader, but will instead present some additional perspectives with which to approach repetitive use disorders in the workplace.

WHAT IS SOCIAL COGNITION?

Social cognition has been the predominant paradigm of experimental social psychology for the past 25 years (Fiske and Taylor, 1984; Higgins and Bargh, 1987; Schneider, 1991; Sherman *et al.*, 1989). However, those outside the discipline may know little of its assumptions and findings. To facilitate an understanding of how social cognition applies to somatic interpretation in general and to CTD phenomena in particular, a brief exposition is presented here.

In the following two sections I outline two important components to the social cognitive approach. The first subsumes the premises of social psychology in general; that situational features are usually more powerful explanations of behavior and beliefs than are individual labels of traits or dispositions. The second component is the additional, specific premise of social cognition; that information about the social world and about the self is processed in stages, each of which can be influenced or directed by a host of environmental or contextual factors.

The Assumptions of Social Psychology

Social cognition is a subdiscipline of social psychology, and social psychology is primarily a situationist doctrine. That is, the history, tradition, and findings of social psychology predominantly address how even small or subtle situational manipulations can overwhelm the most entrenched traits or proclivities of the individual. Indeed, most of social psychology's best-known studies are classic parables of this point – as when Milgram's 'normal' subjects were induced to administer severe shocks to another study participant (Milgram, 1963, 1965), Zimbardo's college students adopted the passive or the vicious behaviors of their assigned roles of prisoners or guards (Zimbardo, 1972), and Darley and Batson's experimental 'bystanders' failed to come to the aid of others in an emergency situation (Darley and Batson, 1973).

The point of these classic studies is not to deny that people are different from one another in sometimes stunning and important ways. Rather, we find that the true explanatory power for many important social behaviors comes not from a label for any *particular* individual's behavior but from understanding what *most* individuals would see, believe, and do in certain social situations (Fiske and Taylor, 1984). The social psychologists believes, for example, that the question 'why did that person come to another's aid?' is not really answered with 'because she's courageous;' such an 'explanation' merely redescribes the observed behavior of labeling it. We will come to a deeper explanation of that behavior if it is understood in terms of how the actor read the pressures, sanctions, signals, and features of the situation (Cantor *et al.*, 1982; Cantor, 1990). In this sense, social psychologists speak not to how people are different from one another – i.e. how people vary on some stable trait such as 'courage' – but to how most people are similar to one another – i.e. how the 'average' person can be induced to act courageously *or* timidly given particular contextual features and social dynamics.

Social psychologists are wary of trait 'explanations' for another reason as well; our research has discovered that people are overwhelmingly prone to rely on such explanations in their everyday lives, even when they are patently less informative than are those that take situational or contextual features into account. A very large body of research shows that people consistently make the 'fundamental attribution error' of evoking dispositional explanations for others' behavior while ignoring or underweighting situational or transient forces on that behavior, and this tendency is extremely robust and resistant to change (Ross, 1977; Ross *et al.*, 1977). Thus, social psychologists shy away from personology accounts of social phenomena both because they are most widely and inappropriately used by social perceivers and because they have been repeatedly found to account for less variance in behavior than have situational analyses of behavior (Mischel, 1984).

It should come as no surprise then that a social psychological approach to somatic interpretation and CTDs will not rely on an individual-level analysis. Rather, we will be interested in trait labels mainly to the extent that they describe features of the situation that allow, induce, or encourage the observed behavior in the 'average' person or in a large proportion of individuals across a sample of many.

The Information-processing Model of Social Inference

Social cognition brings additional features to the study of social behavior, and these concern the particular processes by which people come to make inferences about themselves and their social world (Fiske and Taylor, 1984). People's social inferences are based on information that has been processed in stages, and people possess habitual processing rules or algorithms for each stage. Although these heuristics usually result in correct and efficient judgements, they can also be biased by contextual or situational features, resulting in systematic errors (Kahneman *et al.*, 1982; Nisbett and Ross, 1980).

Imagine for example that Joe is estimating the likelihood that he will get mugged if he ventures into a particular neighborhood. This inference will be based on how the actor has gathered 'data' pertaining to this hypothesis, how that information was interpreted and stored in memory, how it was retrieved, and how it was weighted and used in his inference (Kahneman *et al.*, 1982). Joe's estimate of the frequency of crime in that neighborhood will depend in part on the ease with which crime events in that neighborhood can be easily recalled from his memory (Tversky and Kahneman, 1973, 1981). Thus, recent media reports of crime in that part of town will cause crime instances to be more available in his memory, and will therefore cause him to inflate his subjective sense of risk – even if the frequency of media reports is uncorrelated to any actual increase in crime. He will also be much more likely to notice, retain, and use confirmatory data for his inferences – that is, occasions when someone did go to that neighborhood and was mugged – than he is to notice, retain, and use nonevents which should also bear on his decision – that is, occasions when someone passed through the neighborhood unscathed (Kahneman *et al.*, 1982).

It is important to emphasize that the same processing algorithms that can result in a faulty judgment are responsible for our usually correct and efficient ones. Take for example Joe's use of memory retrievability as an estimate of frequency. It is often and naturally true that the more frequently one 'sees' an event, the more frequently it has actually occurred. It is only when the frequency of reporting is elevated for other reasons – as it is with media attention – that the heuristic will run afoul of objective reality and result in an incorrectly inflated estimate of risk. Research in social cognition has time and again demonstrated that human 'irrationality' is often cut from the same cloth as efficient, adaptive functioning (Kahneman *et al.*, 1982; Nisbett and Ross, 1980). Note also that this approach concerns the ways in which people are similar to each other rather than how they differ, because it concerns the cognitive processes that are common to all people, or those that have the greatest average effect across many types of people. If and when stable individual differences in inference are found to exist, they will likely be analyzed for how various inferential processes have been 'loaded' by information or influence in the person's social environment (Anderson and Weiner, in press; Cantor *et al.*, 1982).

A SOCIAL COGNITIVE ANALYSIS OF SOMATIC INTERPRETATION

The Tools of Somatic Inference

To the social cognitive psychologist, the processing of somatic information is posited to proceed along the same basic routes as is the processing of other types of social information; physical sensations will be noticed, labeled, explained, stored in memory, recalled, and used as the basis for subsequent inference, and all of these processing stages can be influenced by the situation, by the behavior and beliefs of others, and by the assumptions and attributions of the perceiver. Thus, somatic interpretation is viewed not as a direct and predetermined response to some physical event, but as a highly plastic process; the same objective physical stimulus can produce highly variant interpretations, not only across different individuals given the same circumstances, but also *within* the same individual *across* different circumstances (Cioffi, 1991b, 1991c).

What are the tools of this interpretive process? Twenty-five years of social cognitive research in health psychology has identified two mechanisms as particularly influential in guiding and shaping somatic inference. They are the rules by which people go about making attributions for somatic events in their lives (attribution theory), and the common-sense way that people represent and think about their physical status (mental representations of illness and symptoms).

Attribution theory

Humans are meaning-making organisms; we do not go about buffeted at random by events and by our moment-to-moment evaluation of them. Rather, we seek to find meaningful relationships between occurrences, form coherent pictures of their nature, and develop cause-and-effect theories about them (Bohner *et al.*, 1988; Jones *et al.*, 1971; Jones and Harris, 1967; Kelley and Michela, 1980). Did Susan lose her temper because she is a nasty person, or because she is currently under stress? Did Joseph fail his bar exam because of innate inability, or because he didn't study? Do my fingers tingle because I have a circulatory disorder, or because it is cold in my office? Posing and answering such attributional questions is a highly adaptive enterprise; causal analyses are initiated by people's need to predict and control future events, and causal analyses also contribute to the sense that desirable future outcomes are achievable and undesirable outcomes can be avoided or minimized (Jones *et al.*, 1971; Kelley and Michela, 1980). And as with all attributions, those made for somatic sensations provide the basis for action, and become a powerful template for the interpretation of new somatic information.

Consider for example cardiac rehabilitation Patients X and Y. Both have had a myocardial infarction from which medical recovery is complete – that is, there is no remaining organic impediment to full functioning – and both have been prescribed a jogging program to improve cardiovascular fitness and to minimize risk for future problems. If we discover that Patient X adheres to this jogging program and Patient Y does not, how might we explain this difference? It is illogical by medical standards as both patients have the same aerobic and physical capacities. But the behavioral difference between them would make more sense if we discovered the different attributions that each makes for the physical sensations of exercise; Patient X views rapid heart rate and heavy breathing as the functional response of a robust, healthy heart to the demands of exertion: Patient Y attributes the same sensations to a heart that is overtaxed, weak, and impaired. In this example, the same 'objective' stimuli (i.e. breathlessness, increased heart rate) can have entirely divergent motivational, affective, and behavioral consequences (i.e. compliance or noncompliance) depending on how the actor explains them.

We may of course be tempted to recategorize these different attributional systems as differences in the patient's personalities or traits, and indeed the robustness of the 'fundamental attribution error' predicts that we will overwhelmingly do just that (Ross, 1977). This, however, would cause us to miss a deeper understanding of what such labels might *mean*. In this example, which is taken from an actual research program (Ewart *et al.*, 1983; Taylor *et al.*, 1985), the patients who feared the sensations of exercise had spouses who were themselves fearful of the same thing, and who communicated trepidation about the patient's exertion in several life domains. In contrast, patients who exercised regularly had spouses who held adaptive construals of the patient's exercise and who saw the patient's exertion as evidence of recovery and increased capacity. Moreover, training the noncompliant patients to make more adaptive attributions for their exercise sensations positively affected future attitudes and behavior regarding exercise, but only if their spouses were part of the same training. The attributions that people make for their physical symptoms are profoundly influenced by the social and situational milieu.

Mental representations of illness and symptoms

Does this mean that people go from moment to moment adopting the somatic interpretations suggested by their immediate environment, with attributions arising *de novo* from situation to situation? No: attributions take place within and are guided by larger *models* or *schemata* for how the world (including the somatobiological world) is put together. Illness schemata are cognitive structures that organize and represent knowledge about complex biological concepts in an abstracted or prototypical way (Fiske and Linville, 1980). Thus, Patient X's belief that a rapid heart rate is due to impaired cardiac functioning makes sense only because she believes that there is a covariation between elevated heart rate and cardiac stress – because, in other words, she holds a *mental representation* of cardiac functioning that implicates heart rate through some meaningful, substantive relationship. It is unlikely that she would view an earache or dry skin as diagnostic of her cardiac condition, no matter how forcefully her spouse suggests that she should. Thus, situational forces on somatic attributions are constrained by the larger mental models that people hold of the disease or biological process under consideration. Social forces influence somatic attributions either because they help form, shape, or change a representation, or because they highlight, support, or make salient some aspect of a preexisting one. In either case, attributions are significant because they are the pivot point of an illness schemata.

The schema notion is at the center of much recent work in health psychology. Several researchers have explored the properties of people's implicit 'common-sense' models of health and illness, discovering how we collect somatic and medical information, how we organize it through elaborated associations, and the processes by which this organized knowledge is used to make inferences about a symptom or a diagnosis (Skelton and Croyle, 1991). We hold health-related schemata about social roles and types of people (i.e. doctors, patients), situations (i.e. clinics, hospitals), and events (i.e. particular injuries and diseases), and these schemata include both information about the concept's attributes and information about the relationships among them (Leventhal *et al.*, 1980). Thus, for example, a schema for a particular medical illness will include attribute knowledge about its symptoms and the physical processes that produce them, as well as cause-and-effect relationship knowledge regarding how they work together, unfold over time, and respond to treatment (Bishop, 1991; Leventhal *et al.*, 1986). It has been demonstrated that these mental models are the primary shapers of illness-related behavior, and they also function as a set of expectations which guide the encoding of new information (Leventhal and Diefenbach, 1991; Leventhal *et al.*, 1980; Leventhal *et al.*, 1986; Leventhal *et al.*, 1982).

Although people's common-sense mental representations of illness do not always conform to objective medical or physiological knowledge, they are not random or irrational at bottom. Instead, they follow certain systematic laws or principles that are themselves generally adaptive and reasonable. For example, one particularly powerful law is that of symmetry between physical symptoms and an illness label. When people are provided with a medical diagnosis or label – either by a medical professional or through their own inferential processes – they seek out and pay attention to the symptoms that are the natural consequences of this state – according to their representation of it. Likewise, if they experience symptoms with any degree of regularity or severity, they will seek out a label that explains them (Croyle and Jemmott, 1991; Easterling and Leventhal, 1989; Leventhal *et al.*, 1982; Pennebaker, 1982; Zimmerman *et al.*, 1984).

Again, it is worth pointing out that this 'symmetry law' is not an irrational belief; it is an offshoot of the stable and very robust tendency to perceive, find, or create cause-and-effect relationships – a construction that is both highly adaptive and usually accurate (Kahneman *et al.*, 1982; Nisbett and Ross, 1980). But as with other general processing heuristics described above, it can result in maladaptive judgment on the occasions when facts run afoul of it. This is illustrated by research on people with hypertension, a condition that produces no systematic physical symptoms (Baumann and Leventhal, 1985; Meyer *et al.*, 1985). Many hypertension patients take their prescribed medicine only some portion of the time, and medical professionals used to categorize this self-medication as 'erratic', that is, possessing no rhyme or reason. It was found, however, that these people medicate themselves mainly when their 'symptoms' (such as flushed face and headaches) were particularly severe. In fact, these symptoms covaried more reliably with emotions and moods than with actual blood pressure, but the patients themselves labeled them as hypertension indices. Interestingly, most of the patients believed the medically accurate representation of the disorder; 80 per cent of them accepted that hypertension was in fact an asymptomatic condition – a fact that they had been told over and over by their physician. However, the need for illness-label symmetry is so robust that 88 per cent of these patients believed that *they* were the *exception* to this rule, and that *their* symptoms were indeed valid indicators of their blood pressure levels. This example highlights that people who are 'noncompliant' with medical prescription may be responding to their own internal representation of their condition which, although medically inaccurate, is neither unpredictable nor inexplicable.

There are many such stable and robust 'laws' that guide somatic construals. Research on these in care-seeking patterns, risk behaviors, and responses to diagnostic tests have demonstrated that therapeutic goals are best served by learning more about the patient's illness representations than by aggressively defending the physician's (Cioffi, 1991a, 1991b, 1994; Leventhal and Gutmann, 1984; Sanders, 1982; Skelton and Croyle, 1991).

A Process Model of Somatic Interpretation

Process features

In this section I derive a model of somatic interpretation based on social cognitive principles and on what is known about people's representations of somatic events. It is a model of the process by which individuals find, label, interpret, and act upon their somatic sensations, and about the mediators and moderators that are at work at each process stage.

I begin by illustrating certain key process features of this model with an analogy from medicine. If one wanted to understand the process by which the organism produces any given blood pressure value, one would invoke the model of the cardiovascular system. This system contains certain variables (e.g. blood volume, the elasticity of capillaries, heart stroke or cardiac output, kidney function) which combine to produce any particular outcome or endpoint (e.g. blood pressure). That is, any outcome is a function of the configuration of the system as a whole (Guyton, 1982). Note that we will use this *same system* to explain hypertension, to explain hypotension, or to explain normotension. That is, the cardiovascular system is a description of the *machine*, not of the disease; any particular outcome is described by specifying certain values of the system variables. Note also that any particular state (such as high sodium intake) might predict multiple possible outcomes (it might result in high, low, or normal blood pressure) depending on values of other variables in the system (such as kidney function, peripheral resistance, the efficacy of compensatory or regulatory responses, and so on). Finally, given any particular observed outcome (such as hypertension), we understand there are *multiple processes by which* the outcome could have obtained (i.e. as a function of blood volume, secondary to cardiac impairment, malfunctioning of central sympathetic regulators). In a complex regulatory system, there is any number of routes to a particular outcome.

These same features define a process model of somatic interpretation. First, it too identifies key variables in an interactive, regulatory system, a system that can describe the person who vehemently complains of discomfort and the person who does not. Second, it shows that any particular physical state (i.e. inflammation in the joints) might result in one of any number of outcomes – no complaint, temporary discomfort, a self-diagnosis of CTD – depending on the values of other variables in the system. Third, it illustrates that any particular measured outcome (i.e. symptom complaint) can implicate multiple *processes by which* the outcome occurred. In other words, like all process models, it is a picture of *how* rather than of *what*.

Model components

A hypothetical CTD-related scenario will be used to illustrate the model components (see Figure 3.1), which appear in italics in the following text. The model itself is adapted from Cioffi (1991b), to which the reader is referred for a more detailed explication of the model and the research evidence upon which it is based.

Consider an individual who is working at a computer display terminal, and in whom a *somatic event* occurs; some mild nerve constriction in the wrist area. Will this somatic event result in a *somatic label*? That is, will she even notice or encode any somatic signals at all from this event? It depends. If she is deeply engrossed in her work or in some other compelling stimuli (either environmental or internal), the somatic signals from her wrist may not even emerge above other events that are competing for her attention. In this case, a particular somatic event will not even progress through the interpretive system far enough to be labeled as such (McCaul and Malott, 1984; Pennebaker and Lightner, 1980; Pennebaker and Skelton, 1981; Skelton and Pennebaker, 1982; Suls and Fletcher, 1985).

But let us assume that it does. At this point some preliminary linguistic encoding of this signal will occur. She may label the signal as an 'ache' or a 'tingling' or a 'pain,' for example. Which label she applies in particular will be influenced both 'bottom-up' (i.e. by the physical properties of the sensation) and 'top-down' (i.e. by higher-order cognitive processes), a point that is expanded upon shortly. In any event, we simply note for now that many somatic events can be labeled in a variety of ways.

Note also that this labeling process can occur even in the absence of somatic *change per se*. All people at all times possess a host of somatic sensations that are candidates for labeling; we experience a baseline cacophony of itches, tingles, aches, and fatigues which can become the starting-point for an elaborated somatic inference (Pennebaker and Skelton, 1981). This is why self-monitoring can be pernicious; self-awareness makes one aware of somatic states which, given the right higher-order interpretive influence, can set the meaning-making machine in motion (Cioffi, 1991b, 1991c).

Once a basic label has been attached to a somatic sensation, it is almost immediately (if not instantaneously) *attributed* to something. For example, the person may believe that this ache is due to the position of her hands – a relatively acute and situational representation that does not imply anything like a disorder or a

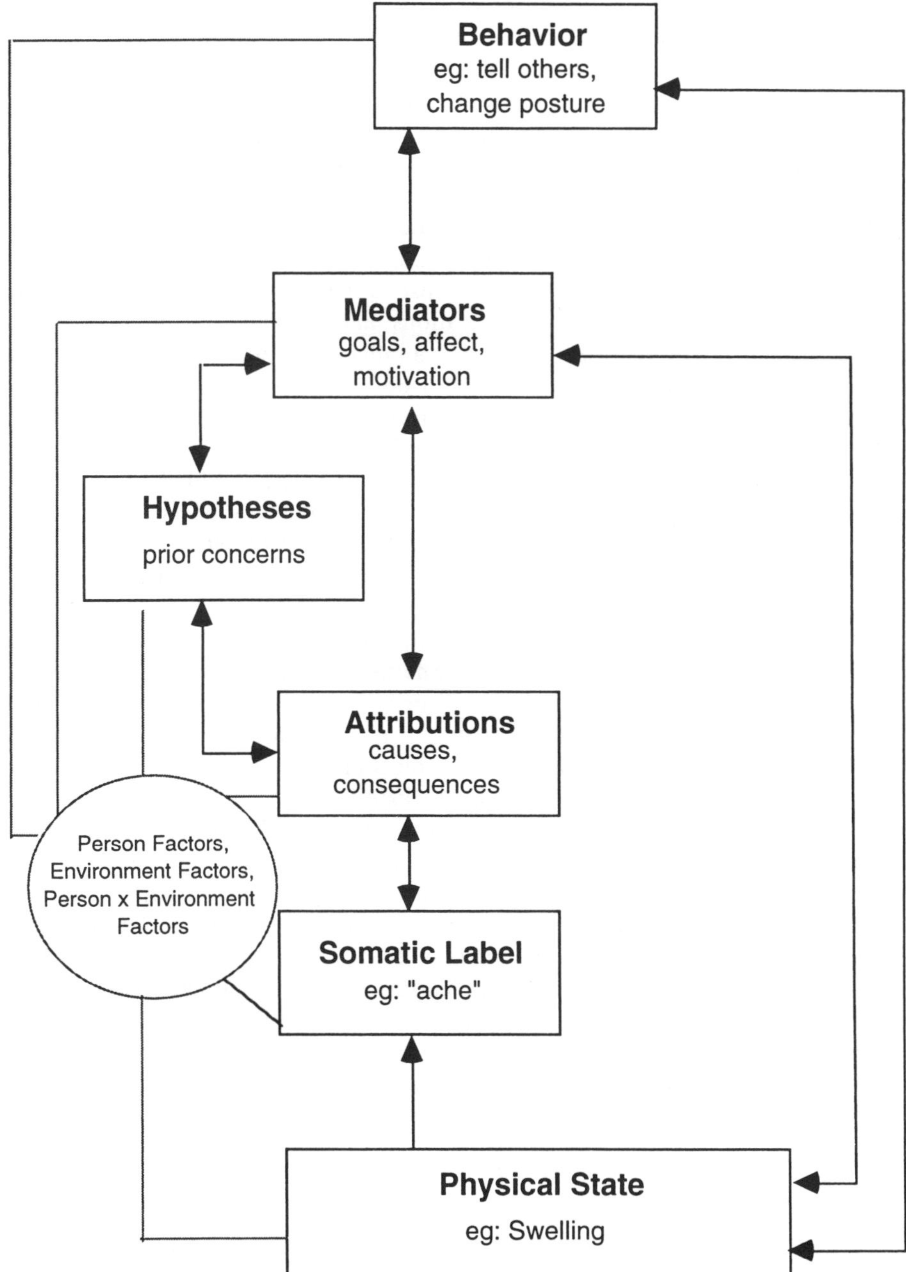

Figure 3.1 A process model of somatic interpretation (adapted from Cioffi, 1991b).

disease. Alternately, she could attribute the now-labeled sensation to something outside of the workplace, such as to some activity of the day before. Another alternative is that she suspects that it may indicate something 'serious' – that is, a relatively stable or chronic disorder of some physiological or biological process. It is at this point that mental representations of illness and symptoms can be particularly influential. If, for example, her label for the sensation (e.g. 'tingling fingers') provides a good fit to a symptom of some well-developed or momentarily salient mental representation (e.g. 'carpal tunnel causes tingling fingers'), then the tentative *hypothesis* she holds for the sensation means that she is no longer experiencing a mere basic somatic state ('tingle') or a benign and transient condition (i.e. 'cold fingers') but a *symptom* of a particular condition ('carpal tunnel syndrome'; Leventhal *et al.*, 1982; Chapter 8 of this volume; Nerenz and Leventhal, 1983).

At this level of the system, it is easy to appreciate the 'two-way' influence that occurs between sensations and cognitions. Just as the stimulus properties of somatic events can drive higher-order interpretations and attributions in a bottom-up fashion, there is also a great deal of top-down influence as well. Attributions for and prior hypotheses about a sensation will not only affect further 'upward' cognitive elaboration, but it can also launch a 'downward' search for somatic information relevant to those attributions and hypotheses. That is, if this individual suspects that her tingling fingers are due to carpal tunnel syndrome, she will likely develop extra vigilance to any and all somatic information that could be labeled as this or another symptom of the same disorder. In this way, a hypothesis-driven selective attention to somatic events can both heighten detection *for* those events and bias the interpretation *of* them (Cioffi, 1991b; Ingram, 1990).

Let us assume that our hypothetical employee has formed a provisional hypothesis that she may have a chronic disorder. She may be actively scanning her sensations for symptoms pertaining to this disorder, especially vigilant to any such sensations, and prone to interpret them as possible further evidence that her hypothesis is correct. There are still several points of variance between this construal and any particular *behavior*. Whether she seeks out social comparison information from co-workers, approaches a supervisor, reads up on CTDs, or does nothing at all will depend on a host of behavioral *mediators*, such as her social and personal goals, mood, motivations, efficacies, and so on. For example, stress or a negative mood will probably elevate her estimation of the seriousness of her 'disorder', thus providing impetus for seeking care or relief (Cioffi, 1991c; Salovey and Birnbaum, 1989; Salovey *et al.*, 1991). Likewise, if she is fearful of the medical profession she will likely turn to 'lay conferral' with friends and family (Sanders, 1982). Similarly, her motivations for this or that course of action will be affected by various social and interpersonal sanctions or incentives for particular overt actions (Sanders and Suls, 1982).

Some derivations of the model

The process model of somatic interpretation accommodates many different outcomes; it is a model of the machine that generates interpretations, not a model of any single interpretation itself. This means that *adaptive* as well as maladaptive response take place with the same system; the same attentional, attributional, and interpretive mechanisms that can produce a belief that one has carpal tunnel syndrome are those that, under different circumstances, produce the postural adjustments by which chronic problems are avoided (Kirschenbaum, 1984; Morgan and Pollock, 1977; Morgan, 1981).

The model also illustrates the regulatory nature of the entire system; people *will* make sense of their physical sensations, and attempts to block this sense-making process will not stop the process, but will simply become a part of it. Thus, effective interventions will seek to alter the content and process components of the interpretive system rather than to shut it down. This logic provides the basis for many clinical interventions for somatic discomfort; the most effective of these do not merely 'forbid' or disallow particular conclusions of a maladaptive or medically inaccurate interpretive system, but are instead designed to 'rebuild' entire new ones from the bottom up (Feuerstein, 1991; Fordyce, 1976; Kabat-Zinn *et al.*, 1985; Keefe, 1982; Keefe and Williams, 1990; Keller *et al.*, 1989; Turk *et al.*, 1983).

Finally, even though there is great potential for variation in somatic interpretation, the system can be 'loaded', that is, driven top-down through so many inputs that a particular somatic interpretation is overdetermined (Cioffi, 1991b, 1991d). Athletes, for instance, commonly experience somatic sensations that nonathletes would interpret with great distress. But because the athlete's interpretive system is positively 'loaded' at every point – through attributions, motivations, mood, goals, and monitoring strategies – his or her overall construal and experience of the sensations are instrumentally adaptive and subjectively benign. Similarly, even the most ambiguous of somatic sensations will be viewed with distress and worry if negative hypotheses for it are available, the person's mood is chronically negative or stress levels high, and goals and motivations are primarily directed toward obtaining relief (Baumeister, 1984; Cioffi, 1991b, 1991c; Cioffi and Holloway, 1993; Nideffer, 1976).

This implies that whatever affects the greatest number of system components will have the greatest influence over its operation and outcome. Somatic interpretation is the result of the cumulative and interactive system of the 'two-way' influence of multifaceted psychosocial and physical events. Its outcome is most affected by factors that load this system the most consistently and at many points of influence.

IMPLICATIONS FOR CTD PHENOMENA

The Interactive Level of Analysis

So where *are* these points of greatest interpretive influence, and how might we measure them for CTD research, and affect them for intervention and prevention? I would like to address this question by comparing the view of somatic interpretation derived in this paper with current strategies in CTD research, and I will suggest that these strategies may obscure rather than reveal the psychosocial mediators and moderators of work-related somatic disorders.

Current research on psychosocial factors in CTD accept that traditional biomedical assumptions provide an insufficient account of CTDs in the workplace, and investigations now commonly employ a 'psychosocial model' in its stead. Such studies assume that CTD symptoms and signs are a function of both 'physical' factors (e.g. ergonomics) and 'psychosocial' factors (e.g. psychological stress), and seek to establish the relative contributions of each factor type to CTD pathology and complaint. Yet the model advanced in this paper slices the somatointerpretive process into different conceptual segments altogether; it is virtually impossible to locate person or situation variables in Figure 3.1, or to identify influences on these variables as predominantly 'psychological' or 'environmental'. This is because *each* of these process stages can be and will be affected by person variables, by situation variables, by a combination of these, and by an interaction of these. And if any *component* of the interpretive process can be multiply determined in this way, then certainly any *outcome* of the process – such as behavior, complaint, or disability – will be even more so.

Consider for example the powerful influence that prior hypotheses have on the interpretive system. Where do these prior hypotheses come from? They may certainly be influenced by individual history or idiosyncratic traits, but they will also be shaped by a host of other factors such as social norms, mood, motivation, and the availability of information in the immediate situational context. These 'person' and 'environment' influences, in turn, are themselves shaped by a combination of and interaction between psychological, social, and physical states. Mood, for example – which can exert a powerful influence on somatic attention, interpretation, and action – may be a function of the person (i.e. personal depression), the social milieu (i.e. stress), and the physical environment (suboptimal ergonomics). Much more likely, it will be a function of their interaction and combination; bad ergonomics will have relatively less mood-altering power in an otherwise efficient and comfortable organizational environment than it will in a stressful and chaotic one, and even the most depressed individual is less likely to generate a somatic complaint over time if there is literally no objective baseline of somatic discomfort to base it on and few environmental factors that encourage or support the elaboration of distress (Anderson and Weiner, forthcoming; Cantor, 1990; Higgins and Wells, 1986). In sum, over large numbers of people and across time, single environmental and personal variables are important mainly to the extent that they are co-occuring with other facilitating or inhibiting forces to create the multidimensional constructs that are the truly influential inputs into the somatic interpretation system.

This places the traditional dependent variables of CTD research in a slightly new light. It suggests that many of these measures are important to the extent that they are tapping into larger multidimensional constructs made up of personal, social, and physical variables. Consider for example the measure of 'job dissatisfaction'. There is no discrete place in the model of Figure 3.1 where we can locate this construct, and researchers should probably be interested in the measured construct of job dissatisfaction to the extent that it *either influences or taps into* some component of the interpretive process – through, for example, its relationship to biases in top-down somatic interpretation, its co-occurrence with mood states, or its interaction with and exacerbation of physical tension or fatigue. There are many ways in which job dissatisfaction could relate to the somatic interpretation system, but its conceptual identification as a 'psychological' variable mutes the lion's share of its likely significance; it is probably valuable not because of any unique property of job dissatisfaction *per se*, but because it influences or reflects some portion of the multidimensional constructs that are the true muscle in the somatic interpretation process.

Implications for research theory and method

It is ironic that the most common methods used to explore CTD phenomena may prohibit this multidimensional conceptualization, as they force a segregation rather than an integration of psychosocial and biomechanical variables. They do so in large part because they are based on techniques that assume a dichotomization between variables rather than on a principled theory for how they interact. In other words, several common methodological approaches are limited to exploring the unique, nonrelated aspects of measured variables rather than the relationships between them.

Figure 3.2 illustrates a hypothetical example of such a 'multiple predictors' approach, in which observed variables are subjected to exploratory factor analysis, the results of which are used to statistically account for variance in one or more outcome measures. The observed variables are represented by the small boxes at the bottom of the figure (the small circles attached to each observed variable represent residual or unique variance associated with each measure). Observed variables may include measures of ergonomic factors, workplace variables, individual stress levels or perceptions of job characteristics, and are chosen for use on face-valid assumptions; the investigator imagines that they might or should affect some outcome of interest, although their precise relationship is not specified a priori. The large circles in the center of Figure 3.2 represent the *common factors* that are extracted from exploratory factor analysis, which are named by the experimenter on face-valid criteria. Each individual in the sample can then be given scores (usually factor loadings) representing each common factor, which are then used via regression analyses to statistically predict *outcome variables* of interest (the overlapping ovals at the top of Figure 3.2).

Because these analyses are called 'exploratory,' it is easy to overlook that they are not really exploratory at all; they are in fact based on several explicit assumptions about now the variables relate to one another. Moreover, the particular assumptions made by these analyses actually prohibit the sorts of interaction between variables that are most likely to occur in CTD phenomena. In other words, they are 'exploratory' only in the sense that the *researcher* has not defined a set of statistical constraints and assumptions based on a priori theory, but has opted instead for the constraints and assumptions of the 'exploratory' techniques. A statistical treatise on these assumptions is beyond the scope of this article (readers interested in same are

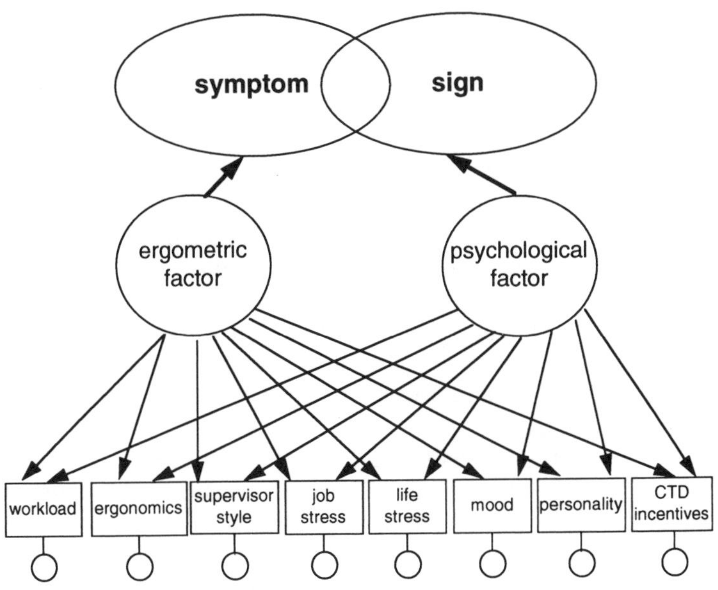

Figure 3.2 A hypothetical 'multiple predictors' model of CTD symptoms and signs.

referred to Hull *et al.*, 1991, and Long, 1983a, 1983b), but their nature can be illustrated with a few examples. Exploratory factor analyses and multiple regressions assume that:

1. All observed variables are directly affected by all common factors, and a measured item is identified as due to one and only one of the common factors based on its relative goodness of fit; those items that fit poorly with all common factors are dropped from use, and they are not allowed to exert independent influence on outcome measures. Thus, for example, the relationship between an observed variable and a common factor must be direct, without any mediating influence of any other observed or unobserved construct.
2. All unique factors (residual variance) are uncorrelated with each other. Thus, there can be no direct relationship between observed measures except through the common factors.
3. No unique factor is correlated directly with any common factor or with an outcome variable. Thus, it cannot be the case that the residual variance associated with any particular measure could act directly on an outcome variable.

These few examples illustrate that the multidimensional and interactive theories that CTD researchers may be most interested in exploring are based on the very sorts of relationship that are prohibited by exploratory techniques.

Many analytic techniques are more conducive to CTD theories that posit interactive constructs and multiple points of influence. In all cases, however, they first require that the researcher specify this theory through an a priori hypothesis that becomes the guide for analytic assumptions and constraints. At the most rudimentary level, this might simply mean employing certain types of cross-level analyses – specifying, for example, that the norms for CTD reporting (the aggregate reporting measures of a particular worksite or workgroup) can predict any individual's reporting probability to some degree above and beyond that made by the individual's unique scores on reporting predictors alone (Baratta and McManus, 1992). Even more powerful analytic options can be found in structural modeling and confirmatory factor analyses techniques, which are designed to study complex systems involving multiple latent constructs (Anderson and Gerbing, 1988; Baron and Kenny, 1986; Bollen, 1989; Dillon and Goldstein, 1984; Long, 1983a, 1983b). The approach begins with a hypothesized structural relationship for CTD outcomes, and statistics on this theory-driven model reveal the extent to which observed subcomponents cohere as indicators of an unobserved latent variable, and how the latent variables relate to each other and to the outcome variables. In other words, structural models are based on the question: to what extent do the observed subcomponents (such as workload, supervisor style, and worker stress levels) correlate with one another *because they share* a common source; latent, underlying (unobserved), and multifaceted constructs that are themselves the likely 'drivers' of symptom complaint and pathology?

Figure 3.3 is an entirely hypothetical structural model of CTD, constructed purely for the sake of illustration. The observed measures are represented by the labeled rectangles, and the unique variance associated with each by the small circles attached. In this model I have specified a 'work environment' latent construct (larger circle near the center of the figure), which contributes to observed variables such as workload, job stress, and supervisory style. I have also posited a latent construct

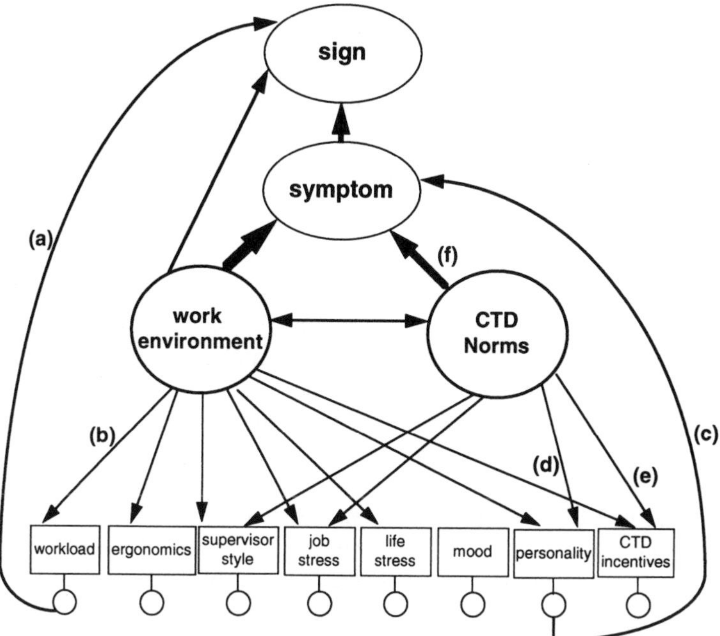

Figure 3.3 A hypothetical structural model of CTD symptoms and signs.

that specifically relates to norms regarding CTD in that particular environment (second center circle). This may be reflected in aggregate measures of CTD reporting in that workplace, indices of economic incentive, and measures of stress, supervisor style, and individual differences of various sorts (Chapter 14 of this volume).

If this model were to be tested and supported, what sort of information would it convey? For example, would lowering workers' keystrokes per hour diminish joint disorders? This model would suggest that there *is* some influence of workload on CTD signs that is not sufficiently accounted for by its relationship with other submeasures (line 'a'), and this represents the 'specific' effect of the observed variable on an outcome measure (again, an effect that is forbidden by exploratory factor analysis). However, we would also note that this specific effect of workload is trivial compared to workload's effect on pathology *through the mediating construct* of work environment (line 'b'). In other words, workload exerts its greatest influence in combination with other factors, and is important mainly to the extent that it 'echoes' a small piece of this real multidimensional muscle behind the outcome. Similarly, we might ask if individual neuroticism contributes to CTD outcomes. This model suggests that certain personality factors do have a specific effect on symptom complaint (line 'c'), but again it is shown to be relatively trivial; if individual neuroticism is important at all, it is mainly through the mediating construct of CTD norms (line 'd'). Finally, economic incentives for CTD disability to constitute part of the CTD norms of the workplace (line 'e'), but they affect symptom reports (line 'f') only *through* that mediating construct – that is, to the extent that they coexist with other facilitating and inhibiting forces such as job stress and supervisory style. Finally, note that two latent constructs can relate to one another, some variables may relate to one, two, or no latent factors, multiple outcome measures (and the relationship between them) can be built into the model, and both latent and observed variables may relate either directly or indirectly to one, both, or none of the outcomes – all possibilities that are prohibited by the model represented in Figure 3.2.

In sum, it is likely that CTD phenomena are a function of physical, social, and personal factors interacting with one another in some complex but knowable ways. Techniques that facilitate rather than prohibit such a conceptualization are likely to be the most fruitful when studying them.

Implications for intervention and prevention

The crux of this discussion suggests that it is at the highest levels of organizational structures that CTD phenomena are best conceptualized, because it is at this level that personal, social, and physical factors in the workplace interact. What might this conceptualization imply for CTD intervention and prevention? I suggest that it primarily implies that the most effective interventions will be those that address several workplace factors (i.e. ergometrics, communications, group structures, organizational practices) at once.

One rationale for multifaceted interventions is that they are statistically prudent, as even confirmed structural models cannot establish the causal relationship between variables. Thus, for example, Figure 3.2 might indicate that worker mood affects the work environment, that work environment affects worker mood, or that both affect each other. In the absence of controlled experimentation on causal mechanisms, the action that is most likely to be effective is that which accounts for all possible causal relationships, including reciprocal ones (Davis, 1985).[1]

The second rationale for systemic interventions for CTD stems from the interactive nature of the phenomena itself. That is, the principles behind the models of Figure 3.3 and Figure 3.1 suggest that the drivers of CTD complaint and pathology will be multiply determined – dependent on the co-occurrence of many facultative, inhibitive, and interactive factors – changing mood, for example. At best, then, piecemeal interventions may simply be ineffective.

At worst, however, individual or isolated interventions may do more harm than good. This is because *all* events in the individual's milieu – physical, social, and organizational – are coordinated within the meaning-making process of interpreting somatic sensations. Consider for instance a workplace in which ergonomic factors are found to be part of the CTD problem, but so too are larger factors such as supervisory style or organizational climate. Suppose that money is allocated to replace the old workstations with ergonomically efficient ones, but for one reason or another the organizational issues are left unaddressed. Isn't attacking at least one piece of the problem better than doing nothing at all? Perhaps not, *if* the workforce construes this selective action as indicating management's disregard for social psychological issues or as an example of a 'mechanical' organizational climate; such a construal could easily exacerbate other (nonergometric) negative influences on somatic interpretation. In other words, single actions are likely to be interpreted not in isolation but in coordination with other actions (or nonactions), and it is for this reason that 'minimum guidelines' for CTD prevention be carefully examined before implementation for their possible systemic consequences.

To people who are struggling to deal with severe resource limitations in business and industry, there certainly could be something disquieting about the notion that the most effective interventions for CTD may be at the most complex organizational levels. By similar lights, it may also be appealing to view multipronged and multilevel interventions as 'kitchen-sink' strategies, likely to work thorough 'placebo effects' alone. I have tried to advance a principled argument for considering an organizational and multipronged analysis, and perhaps that same argument suggests a slightly enlarged interpretation of what a 'placebo effect' is. The classic illustration of the placebo effect comes from the Hawthorne studies of the 1930s (Roethlisberger and Dickson, 1939). Workers were found to increase their productivity every time the light bulbs were changed in their workspace, even when the 'change' was to replace a bulb with one of the identical wattage. From this it was concluded that increased productivity was due, not to any actual change on illumination, but to the mere illusion on the part of the employees that such a change had occurred. In other words, people had responded 'irrationally' because 'nothing' had really been done. However, although the claim that 'nothing' had been done may make sense to the visual physiologist, it is resoundly rejected by the social psychologist! The individual who witnesses something being done on his or her behalf has not witnessed a 'placebic' or empty action by any means; the action would substantively alter the social dynamics of the workplace in ways that would reasonably and rationally improve workers' productivity according to dozens of psychosocial principles – principles that are no more illusory (and which are often far more powerful) than those of visual acuity (Ross and Nisbett, 1991).

CONCLUSION

In this chapter, I have suggested that effective interventions and preventions regarding CTD disorders are likely to be at least as complex as the psychosocial processes that govern their development. The good news is that this converges on directions that many businesses have embraced for a host of other reasons, and perhaps the whole of this discussion has been a long-winded way of saying what successful industries already know; a humane, efficient, comfortable, and coordinated workplace is going to be the most effective workplace, in both human and functional terms. Of course, further research on CTDs will be the ultimate judge of this claim. But odds are good that the results will support the preexisting goal of all effective industries; to build a healthy workplace, not just one designed to minimize ills.

NOTE

1 Indeed, there are other reasons that particular caution should attend the use of any measurement at the individual level to predict future somatic complaint, no matter how 'perfect' the relationship is found to be. Let us assume for example that the trait of 'X-ness' is found to correlate 0.80 with future CTD complaint, and that a causal relationship (X-ness causes complaint) has also been established through experimentation. This is about as close to an iron-clad support of a theory as science ever receives, yet it would still be inappropriate to use any one individual's score of X-ness to predict that individual's future complaint. This is because the 'iron-clad' support was obtained across a sample of many individuals, and any single individual may or may not conform to the group average. Even if the correlation was found to be a perfect 1.0 (virtually impossible in practice), random variance and measurement error would still forbid using this statistic to predict any individual outcome. *Post-hoc* explanations for why someone has registered a

somatic complaint (i.e. he or she is high in X-ness) is similarly inappropriate. These are the same statistical and probalistic principles that severely limit the use of expert psychological testimony and 'profiles' in legal trials, parole hearings, and insurance claims (Wrightsman, 1991); even theories with strong empirical support are based on average outcomes across many people, using variables with some measurement error, and in a world where random variance is assured. Thus, they cannot be used with confidence to predict or explain the single, individual act (Kahneman *et al.*, 1982; Nisbett and Ross, 1980; Schwartz and Griffin, 1986).

REFERENCES

ANDERSON, C. A. and WEINER, B. 1992 Attribution and attributional processes in personality, in CAPRARA, G. and HECK, G. (Eds), *Modern Personality Psychology: Critical Reviews and New Directions*, pp. 295–324, New York: Harvester Wheatsheaf.

ANDERSON, J. and GERBING, D. 1988 Structural equation modeling in practice: A review and recommended two-step approach, *Psychological Bulletin*, **103**, 411–23.

BARATTA, J. and McMANUS, M. 1992 The effect of contextual factors on individuals' job performance, *Journal of Applied Social Psychology*, **22**, 1702–10.

BARON, R. and KENNY, D. 1986 The moderator-mediator variable distinction in social psychological research: Conceptual, strategic, and statistical considerations, *Journal of Personality and Social Psychology*, **51**, 1173–82.

BAUMANN, L. and LEVENTHAL, H. 1985 'I can tell when my blood pressure is up: Can't I?' *Health Psychology*, **4**, 203–18.

BAUMEISTER, R. 1984 Choking under pressure: Self-consciousness and paradoxical effects of incentives on skillful performance, *Journal of Personality and Social Psychology*, **46**, 610–20.

BISHOP, G. 1991 Understanding the understanding of illness: Lay disease representations, in SKELTON, J. A. and CROYLE, R. T. (Eds), *Mental Representations in Health and Illness*, New York: Springer Verlag.

BOHNER, G., BLESS, H., SCHWARZ, N. and STRACK, F. 1988 What triggers causal attributions? The impact of valence and subjective probability, *European Journal of Social Psychology*, **18**, 335–45.

BOLLEN, K. 1989 *Structural Equations with Latent Variables*, New York: John Wiley.

CANTOR, N. 1990 From thought to behavior: 'Having' and 'doing' in the study of personality and cognition, *American Psychologist*, **45**, 735–50.

CANTOR, N., MISCHEL, W. and SCHWARTZ, J. 1982 A prototype analysis of psychological situations, *Cognitive Psychology*, **14**, 45–77.

CIOFFI, D. 1991a Asymmetry of doubt in medical self-diagnosis: The ambiguity of 'uncertain wellness,' *Journal of Personality and Social Psychology*, **61**, 969–80.

CIOFFI, D. 1991b Beyond attentional strategies: A cognitive-perceptual model of somatic interpretation, *Psychological Bulletin*, **109**, 25–41.

CIOFFI, D. 1991c Sensory awareness versus sensory impression: Affect and attention interact to produce somatic meaning, *Cognition and Emotion*, **5**, 275–94.

CIOFFI, D. 1994 When good news is bad news: Medical wellness as a non-event, *Health Psychology*, **13**, 63–72.

CIOFFI, D. and HOLLOWAY, J. 1993 The delayed costs of suppressed pain, *Journal of Personality and Social Psychology*, **64**, 274–8.

CROYLE, R. and JEMMOTT, J. 1991 Psychological reactions to risk factor testing, in SKELTON, J. A. and CROYLE, R. T. (Eds), *The Mental Representation of Health and Illness*, ch. 5, New York: Springer Verlag.

DARLEY, J. and BATSON, C. 1973 'From Jerusalem to Jericho:' A study of situational and dispositional variables in helping behavior, *Journal of Personality and Social Psychology*, **27**, 100–19.

DAVIS, J. 1985 *The Logic of Causal Order*, Beverly Hills, CA: Sage.

DILLON, W. and GOLDSTEIN, M. 1984 *Multivariate Analysis: Methods and Applications*, ch. 12, New York: John Wiley.

EASTERLING, D. and LEVENTHAL, H. 1989 Contribution of concrete cognition to emotion: Neutral symptoms as elicitors of worry about cancer, *Journal of Applied Psychology*, **74**, 787–96.

EWART, C., TAYLOR, C., REESE, L. and DE BUSK, R. 1983 Effects of early postmyocardial infarction exercise testing on self-perception and subsequent physical activity, *The American Journal of Cardiology*, **51**, 1076–80.

FEUERSTEIN, M. 1991 A multidisciplinary approach to the prevention, evaluation, and management of work disability, *Journal of Occupational Rehabilitation*, **1**, 5–12.

FISKE, S. and LINVILLE, P. 1980 What does the schema concept buy us?, *Personality and Social Psychology Bulletin*, **6**, 543–57.

FISKE, S. and TAYLOR, S. 1984 *Social Cognition*, New York: Random House.

FORDYCE, W. 1976 *Behavioral Methods for Chronic Pain and Illness*, St Louis, MO: Mosby.

GUYTON, A. 1982 *Human Physiology and Mechanisms of Disease*, Philadelphia, PA: W. B. Saunders.

HIGGINS, E. and BARGH, J. 1987 Social cognition and social perception, *Annual Review of Psychology*, **38**, 369–425.

HIGGINS, E. and WELLS, R. 1986 Social construct availability and accessibility as a function of social life phase: Emphasizing the 'how' versus the 'can' of social cognition, special issue: Developmental perspectives on social-cognitive theories, *Social Cognition*, **4**, 201–26.

HULL, J., LEHN, D. and TEDLIE, J. 1991 A general approach to testing multifaceted personality constructs, *Journal of Personality and Social Psychology*, **61**, 932–45.

INGRAM, R. 1990 Self-focused attention in clinical disorders: Review and conceptual model, *Psychological Bulletin*, **107**, 156–76.

JONES, E. and HARRIS, V. 1967 The attribution of attitudes, *Journal of Experimental Social Psychology*, **3**, 1–24.

JONES, E., KANOUSE, D., KELLY, H., NISBETT, R., VALINS, S. and WEINER, B. 1971 *Attribution: Perceiving the Causes of Behavior*, Morristown, NJ: General Learning Press.

KABAT-ZINN, J., LIPWORTH, L. and BURNEY, R. 1985 The clinical use of mindfulness meditation for the self-regulation of chronic pain, *Journal of Behavioral Medicine*, **8**, 163–90.

KAHNEMAN, D., SLOVIC, P. and TVERSKY, A. 1982 *Judgment under Uncertainty: Heuristics and Biases*, New York: Cambridge University Press.

KEEFE, F. 1982 Behavioral assessment and treatment of chronic pain: Current status and future direction, *Journal of Consulting and Clinical Psychology*, **50**, 896–911.

KEEFE, F. and WILLIAMS, D. 1990 A comparison of coping strategies in chronic pain patients in different age groups, *Journals of Gerontology*, **45**, 161–5.

KELLER, M., WARD, S. and BAUMANN, L. 1989 Processes of self-care: Monitoring sensations and symptoms, *Advances in Nursing Science*, **12**, 54–66.

KELLEY, H. and MICHELA, J. 1980 Attribution theory and research, *Annual Review of Psychology*, **31**, 457–501.

KIRSCHENBAUM, D. 1984 Self-regulation and sport psychology: Nurturing an emerging symbiosis, *Journal of Sport Psychology*, **6**, 159–83.

LEVENTHAL, H. and DIEFENBACH, M. 1991 The active side of illness cognition, in SKELTON, J. A. and CROYLE, R. T. (Eds), *Mental Representations in Health and Illness*, New York: Springer Verlag.

LEVENTHAL, H. and GUTMANN, M. 1984 Compliance: A self-regulatory approach, in

GENTRY, W. D. (Ed.), *Handbook of Behavioral Medicine*, pp. 369–436, New York: Guilford.

LEVENTHAL, H., MEYER, D. and NERENZ, D. 1980 The common sense representation of illness danger, in RACHMAN, S. (Ed.), *Contributions to Medical Psychology*, Vol. 2, pp. 7–30, New York: Pergamon.

LEVENTHAL, H., NERENZ, D. and STEELE, D. 1986 Illness representations and coping with health threats, in BAUM, A. and SINGER J. (Eds), *A Handbook of Psychology and Health*, Vol. 4, pp. 219–52, Hillsdale, NJ: Erlbaum.

LEVENTHAL, H., NERENZ, D. and STRAUSS, A. 1982 Self-regulation and the mechanisms for symptom appraisal, in MECHANIC, D. (Ed.), *Psychosocial Epidemiology*, pp. 58–86, New York: Neal Watson Academic Publications.

LONG, J. 1983a *Confirmatory Factor Analysis: A Preface to LISREL*, Beverly Hills, CA: Sage.

LONG, J. 1983b *Covariance Structure Models: An Introduction to LISREL*, Beverly Hills, CA: Sage.

MCCAUL, K. and MALOTT, J. 1984 Distraction and coping with pain, *Psychological Bulletin*, **95**, 516–33.

MEYER, D., LEVENTHAL, H. and GUTMANN, M. 1985 Commonsense models of illness: The example of hypertension, *Health Psychology*, **4**, 115–35.

MILGRAM, S. 1963 Behavioral study of obedience, *Journal of Abnormal and Social Psychology*, **67**, 371–8.

MILGRAM, S. 1965 Some conditions of obedience and disobedience to authority, *Human Relations*, **18**, 57–76.

MISCHEL, W. 1984 Convergences and challenges in the search for consistency, *American Psychologist*, **39**, 351–64.

MORGAN, W. 1981 Psychophysiology of self-awareness during vigorous physical activity, *Research Quarterly for Exercise and Sport*, **52**, 385–427.

MORGAN, W. and POLLOCK, M. 1977 Psychologic characterization of the elite distance runner, *Annals of the New York Academy of Sciences*, **301**, 382–403.

NERENZ, D. and LEVENTHAL, H. 1983 Self-regulation theory in chronic illness, in BURISH, T. and BRADLEY, L. (Eds), *Coping with Chronic Disease: Research and Applications*, pp. 13–38, New York: Academic Press.

NIDEFFER, R. 1976 The relationship of attention and anxiety to performance, in STRAUB, W. (Ed.), *Sport Psychology: An Analysis of Athlete Behavior*, pp. 231–5, Ithaca, NY: Mouvement.

NISBETT, R. and ROSS, L. 1980 *Human Inference: Strategies and Shortcomings of Social Judgment*, Englewood Cliffs, NJ: Prentice–Hall.

PENNEBAKER, J. 1982 *The Psychology of Physical Symptoms*, New York: Springer Verlag.

PENNEBAKER, J. and LIGHTNER, J. 1980 Competition of internal and external information in an exercise setting, *Journal of Personality and Social Psychology*, **39**, 165–74.

PENNEBAKER, J. and SKELTON, J. 1981 Selective monitoring of physical sensations, *Journal of Personality and Social Psychology*, **41**, 213–23.

ROETHLISBERGER, F. and DICKSON, W. 1939 *Management and the Worker*, Cambridge, MA: Harvard University Press.

ROSS, L. 1977 The intuitive psychologist and his shortcomings: Distortions in the attribution process, in BERKOWITZ, L. (Ed.), *Advances in Experimental Social Psychology*, Vol. 10, pp. 173–220, New York: Academic Press.

ROSS, L., AMABILE, T. and STEINMETZ, J. 1977 Social roles, social control, and biases in social-perception processes, *Journal of Personality and Social Psychology*, **35**, 485–94.

ROSS, L. and NISBETT, R. 1991 *The Person and the Situation: Perspectives of Social Psychology*, New York: McGraw-Hill.

ROUGHTON, J. 1993 Cumulative trauma disorders: The newest business liability, *Professional Safety*, **38**, 29–35.

Salovey, P. and Birnbaum, D. 1989 Influence of mood on health-related cognition, *Journal of Personality and Social Psychology*, **57**, 539–51.

Salovey, P., O'Leary, A., Stretton, M. S., Fishkin, S. A. and Drake, C. A. 1991 Influence of mood on judgments about health and illness, in Forgas, J. P. (Ed.), *Emotion and Social Judgment*, pp. 241–62, New York: Pergamon.

Sanders, G. 1982 Social comparison and perceptions of health and illness, in Sanders, G. S. and Suls, J. (Eds), *Social Psychology of Health and Illness*, pp. 129–57, Hillsdale, NJ: Erlbaum.

Sanders, G. and Suls, J. 1982 *Social Psychology of Health and Illness*, Hillsdale, NJ: Erlbaum.

Schneider, D. 1991 Social cognition, *Annual Review of Psychology*, **42**, 527–61.

Schwartz, S. and Griffin, T. 1986 *Medical Thinking: The Psychology of Medical Judgment and Decision Making*, New York: Springer Verlag.

Sherman, S., Judd, C. and Park, B. 1989 Social cognition, *Annual Review of Psychology*, **40**, 281–326.

Skelton, J. and Croyle, R. 1991 *The Mental Representation of Health and Illness*, New York: Springer Verlag.

Skelton, J. and Pennebaker, J. 1982 The psychology of physical symptoms and sensations, in Sanders, G. S. and Suls, J. (Eds), *Social Psychology of Health and Illness*, pp. 99–128, Hillsdale, NJ: Erlbaum.

Suls, J. and Fletcher, B. 1985 The relative efficacy of avoidant and non-avoidant coping strategies: A meta-analysis, *Health Psychology*, **4**, 249–88.

Taylor, C., Bandura, A., Ewart, C., Miller, N. and De Busk, R. 1985 Raising spouse's and patient's perception of his cardiac capabilities after clinically uncomplicated myocardial infarction, *American Journal of Cardiology*, **55**, 635–8.

Turk, D., Meichenbaum, D. and Genest, M. 1983 *Pain and Behavioral Medicine*, New York: Guilford.

Tversky, A. and Kahneman, D. 1973 Availability: A heuristic for judging frequency and probability, *Cognitive psychology*, **5**, 207–32.

Tversky, A. and Kahneman, D. 1981 The framing of decisions and the psychology of choice, *Science*, **211**, 453–8.

Wrightsman, L. 1991 *Psychology and the Legal System*, Pacific Grove, CA: Brooks-Cole.

Zimbardo, P. 1972 Pathology of imprisonment, *Transaction Society*, April, 4–8.

Zimmerman, R., Linz, D., Leventhal, H. and Penrod, S. 1984 Illness schemata and the symmetry of labels and symptoms, unpublished manuscript, University of Wisconsin-Madison.

CHAPTER FOUR

Possible mechanisms behind the relationship between the demand–control–support model and disorders of the locomotor system

TÖRES THEORELL

As reported elsewhere in this book, many studies have been published in which psychosocial working conditions have been related to locomotor disorders. In the present review, possible mechanisms underlying observed relationships are examined. The decision to use the demand–control–support model as theoretical basis in the present review is arbitrary. Other models could have been used as well, and the concepts that will be discussed could be translated into similar ones in other theoretical models.

DEMAND–CONTROL–SUPPORT

The demand–control–support model was originally introduced by Karasek (1979) and further developed by Karasek and Theorell (1990) as well as by Johnson and Hall (1988). According to this model, psychological demands (both quantitative and qualitative) have more adverse consequences if they occur jointly with lack of possibility to influence decisions regarding the job (low decision latitude). This dimension in turn has two components, namely *authority over decisions* – which is the immediate possibility that the individual has to influence decisions regarding what to do and how to do it at work – and *intellectual discretion* – which is the opportunity that the organization gives the individual to use and develop skills at work so that he or she can develop the possibility of control in the work situation. Social support, finally, refers to the social climate in the worksite. Both decision latitude and social support are factors that can be influenced by changes in work organization. Possibilities for employees to improve skill development (for instance by increasing job variability and development of competence) and decreased hierarchy as well as improved democracy in the worksite are examples of changes that increase decision latitude of employees. Social support is also heavily influenced by work organization factors, for instance payment systems. A payment system that increases competition may have adverse consequences for social support in the worksite, for instance.

EPIDEMIOLOGICAL STUDIES

Bongers and de Winter (1992) have recently published an extensive review of epidemiological studies in this field. Some articles have been published after this review. The global concepts of demands, decision latitude, and social support at work have been used in many studies. The design of these studies has varied considerably. Most of them have been cross-sectional – which limits the possibilities to draw final conclusions since recall bias may be a problem. Only a few of them have simultaneously included physical load and ergonomy factors on the one hand and psychosocial factors on the other hand. Physiological factors that explore possible mechanisms have not been studied to any great extent.

In some studies psychological demands, in others decision latitude and in a third group social support at work are of significance to symptoms from the locomotor system although there is also overlap between these groups of studies. The differences seem to be determined by the variance of these factors in the different groups. Differences between the psychosocial risk patterns associated with low back pain versus neck–shoulder pain have not been found so far, although such differences may be discovered in more systematic studies in the future.

The relative risks associated with adverse psychosocial job factors seem to be comparable to those associated with adverse physical ergonomy (Holmstrom *et al.*, 1992; Johansson and Rubenowitz, 1992; Kamwendo *et al.*, 1991; Linton, 1991; Rundcrantz, 1991; Tola *et al.*, 1988). In most of the studies that have data on demands, decision latitude, and support at work, at least one of the three dimensions shows an odds ratio of at least 2.0 in relation to either low back pain or neck–shoulder pain. The exceptions to this seem to be in studies of mixed populations in which the relative risks are often lower (Karasek *et al.*, 1987; see Bongers and de Winter, 1992). The precision of the outcome variable, as expected, is of importance to the reported magnitudes of association. Toomingas *et al.* (1992), on the basis of the Stockholm MUSIC study, showed that there was a prevalence rate ratio of 2.0 (95 per cent confidence limits ranging from 1.1 to 3.7) of having tender points either in the trapezius region or in the neck if there was a high level (worst third compared with the most favoured third of the subjects studied) of self-reported job strain. Physicians doing the medical examinations had no information regarding working conditions; calculations were adjusted for gender, age and ergonomic conditions at work.

Combinations for instance between high psychological demands and low decision latitude do not seem to have the importance that has been observed in relation to cardiovascular illness. It has been suspected that different psychosocial factors are of importance to different kinds of locomotor disorders, but so far no strong consistent findings of this kind have been made across different study groups either.

MECHANISMS

Psychosocial factors may comprise anything from personality to job organization. The situation is further complicated by the fact that there are three different end-points, one social (disability), one psychological (illness), and one medical/physiological (disorder). Although these are interrelated it creates confusion in the literature that they are often mixed. Similarly there are three different kinds of mechanism that may tie psychosocial factors to symptoms in the locomotor system (see below). To complicate matters even more, the mechanisms generating acute conditions in the locomotor system are to a great extent other than those perpetuating pain and creating chronic conditions. Often these two groups of mechanisms are mixed.

1. Physiological mechanisms which lead to *organic changes*. An old theory that has been formulated in psychophysiology states that long-lasting adverse life conditions enforce energy mobilization, *catabolism*, at the expense of restoring and rebuilding activities in the body, *anabolism*. The importance of anabolism for protecting the body against adverse effects of energy mobilization could be understood when I mention that the white blood cells that are responsible for our protection against infections have a half life of ten days. This means that a person who does not produce any new white blood cells today will only have half the number of his white blood cells left in ten days. There are similar effects on the locomotor system. Thus, the skeleton and the muscles are constantly being rebuilt to be adapted to the pattern of movements that the individual has. Muscles cells are being worn out and have to be replaced. Interestingly, several of the hormones that stimulate anabolism have their peak activity during the deep phases of sleeping. When sleep becomes more shallow, the activity of these hormones diminish. This may show the importance of deep sleep to our possibility to protect our body from the adverse effects of long-lasting energy mobilization.

   Apart from the effects of the combined action of high demands and low decision latitude, there may also be an independent effect of a low decision latitude on catabolism, reflected in increased catecholamine output (Härenstam and Theorell, 1988). But it has been shown that job strain increases sleep disturbance (Theorell *et al.*, 1988) – and sleep disturbance inhibits anabolism. Decreasing anabolism could be reflected for instance in decreasing plasma concentrations of testosterone and growth hormone.

   Lack of social support has been shown to have sympatho–adreno–medullary correlates. This system consists of the adrenal medulla and the sympathic nervous system. These two stimulate the release of adrenaline and noradrenaline which help the body to mobilize energy. This is reflected in increasing concentrations of carbohydrate and lipid in the blood and also results in increased heart rate and blood pressure. Persons who report low social support at work have a high heart rate throughout day and night (Undén *et al.*, 1991) and a decreasing social support at work has been shown to be associated with rising systolic blood pressure levels in a longitudinal study (Theorell, 1990).

   Long-lasting inhibition of anabolism may adversely effect the vulnerability of several organ systems such as skeletal muscles, immune cells, and gastrointestinal functions. This may certainly have significance for the development of acute organic conditions in the musculoskeletal system. If it is correct, a relatively small mechanical load that does not cause injury under normal conditions may do so during such a period. For instance, a worker who has had adverse psychosocial conditions at work during several months may develop an injury at home when he or she rises from bed in the morning. Unfortunately this mechanism has been explored to a very limited extent in the literature, and the findings are not clear. Theorell *et al.* (1991), for instance, showed that high psychological demands were associated with high plasma cortisol levels (an indication of high energy mobilization) which were correlated with high subjective indices of muscle tension. Although high psychological demands were associated with pain in back, neck or shoulders, no significant relationship was found between high plasma cortisol concentration and pain. Furthermore, a high concentration of plasma testosterone in the male participants in this study was significantly associated with a high frequency of worries and self-reported muscle tension as well as conflicts, low authority over decisions, and low social support at work. These latter findings are even against the hypothesis – which states that adverse conditions should be correlated with low testosterone concentration. More sophisticated studies will be needed in this field. In a longitudinal study of *variations* in plasma total testosterone concentrations in relation to changes in job strain (Theorell *et al.*, 1990) it was shown that increasing levels of job strain were associated in the expected way with decreasing testosterone concentration, but changes in symptoms in the locomotor system were not analysed. Thus, the crucial object to analyze is the regulation of endocrine functions in future studies.

Muscle tension that is reflected in electrical activity in muscles (electromyography, EMG) is another important possible mechanism that may tie the psychosocial situation to risk of developing disorders in the locomotor system. Recent psychophysiological studies of monotonous work have indicated that the ergonomic loads typical of this kind of work elicit increased electrical muscle activity (EMG). However, when psychological loads are added, the electrical muscle activity increases considerably (Lundberg *et al.*, 1994). This illustrates that psychological and physical demands may interact in complex ways in generating locomotor disorder.

Several indirect pathways may also be of importance of the relationship between psychosocial job factors and the development of acute locomotor disorders, such as sleep disturbance with resulting lack of concentration which may increase the risk of injury.

Organic changes are also discussed in relation to chronic conditions in the locomotor system. There is evidence that even the idiopathic or chronic pain syndromes with atypical localization of pain that constitute a major part of patients in rehabilitation may arise in well-defined physiological processes, for instance spread of muscle tension which causes metabolic changes which may facilitate further spread of muscle tension, etc. (see Johansson and Sjölander, 1993). Unfortunately this has been insufficiently studied in relation to the locomotor system.

2. Physiological mechanisms that influence *pain perception*. According to a rapidly growing literature, there is in chronic pain syndromes a strong element of psychological depression which influences the adrenocortical axis as well as hormonal systems such as the dopamin-sensitive prolactin levels. The turnover of endorphins may also be influenced. There is evidence from psychological liter-

ature that feelings of lack of control in the general life situation may increase pain sensitivity (see Maier *et al.*, 1982; Feuerstein *et al.*, 1987; Reesor and Craig, 1987).

A recent study by our group has shown that pain threshold may be related to the demand–control–support model in a very complex way. Randomly selected men and women were asked to fill out questionnaires about these dimensions in the description of their work. Their pain thresholds were measured on six different points in the neck and shoulders: first at rest before anything else happened in the laboratory, second in conjunction with an experimental stress test (the Stroop test), and finally after a new resting period. Our analyses indicated that, as expected, the pain threshold increased during acute stress, that those who reported a habitually high level of psychological demands at work had higher pain thresholds than others (i.e. were less pain-sensitive than others), and finally that those who reported a low level of decision latitude in their habitual working situation had a lower pain threshold during experimental stress than others (Theorell *et al.*, 1993). The interpretation of these findings is very difficult. It seems plausible that subjects with high psychological demand levels who mobilize energy to be able to meet demands may also repress feelings of pain. This may increase risks of long-term development of pathological changes in locomotor tissues. On the other hand it is also plausible to assume that long-term exposure to low decision latitude may increase the risk of depression (Turk *et al.*, 1993) and that this could explain why some subjects who describe their jobs in these terms are unable to raise their pain thresholds during acute stress situations.

3. Sociopsychological conditions that are of significance to the individual's *possibility to cope with the illness.* Such conditions are of central importance in the rehabilitation of subjects who suffer from pain in the locomotor system. Of particular interest for subject in working ages is illness behavior in relation to sick leave. In the study by Theorell *et al.* (1991), psychosocial working conditions were studied in relation to outcome variables on three different levels, namely

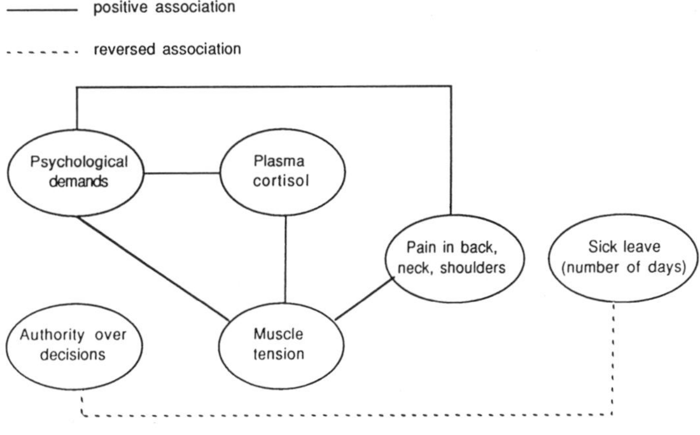

Figure 4.1 Significant associations (after adjustment for age, gender, body mass index, and physical stressors) between psychosocial environment, physiological state, locomotor pain, and sick leave in working men and women, (Source: Theorell *et al.*, 1991.)

psychophysiological correlates (muscle tension, plasma cortisol, sleep disturbance), pain in the locomotor system, and finally sick leave. Several interrelationships were found (after adjustment for gender, age, weight in relation to height, and physical demands at work) both between factors in the three levels of outcome and between psychosocial factors and factors in the three outcome levels. A statistically significant relationship was found between lack of opportunity to influence decisions at work (authority over decisions) and sick leave – the lower the opportunity to influence decisions, the more sick leave, and this relationship was not medicated by psychophysiological reactions or pain. Thus, some of the illness behavior variables may actually be in the web of factors although they are independent of physiology and pain perception (see Figure 4.1).

PSYCHOSOCIAL FACTORS OUTSIDE WORK

A small percentage of patients with pain in the locomotor system develop long-lasting chronic pain syndromes. In these cases person characteristics are important. There is agreement in the literature that psychological individual characteristics are less important to the development of acute conditions in the locomotor system. Interactions between individuals and environment may be decisive.

Psychosocial factors are defined as social organization factors that influence the psychological states at the worksite. Psychosocial factors outside work, for instance when a spouse becomes ill (Theorell *et al.*, 1975) may be of importance to organic changes. Worries about the spouse lead to increased energy mobilization and catabolism and decreased anabolism as well as increased muscular tension. Movements in awkward positions (which become more common in this situation since the healthy spouse may have to do work at home that he or she has not been doing to any great extent before!) may create iterated trauma to and vulnerability in the musculoskeletal system. This may increase the likelihood that injury may arise at work. It may also affect pain perception (depression may lower pain thresholds) and illness behavior (there is increased need to stay home to help the spouse).

PHYSICAL LOAD AND PSYCHOSOCIAL FACTORS

One of the reasons for the inconsistent findings in different studies may be that groups with markedly different amounts and kinds of ergonomic and psychosocial stressors have been studied. Efforts have sometimes been made to adjust statistically for ergonomic load in this study of locomotor symptoms in relation to psychosocial stressors (see, for instance, Theorell *et al.*, 1991). If strong interactions take place between ergonomic and psychosocial stressors, adjustment is of no help in the analysis. An example from an ongoing study is the following.

A study of the determinants of frequency of pain in shoulders and lower back, respectively, in a sample of female health-care personnel was based primarily upon a questionnaire (Ahlberg-Hultén *et al.*, 1993). Information regarding demands, decision latitude, and support as well as social relationships between workmates and with superiors was included as well as estimations of ergonomic load in the various wards (outpatient care of pediatric children, infectious ward, and emergency ward), marital state, and number of children. Multivariate analyses (multiple logistic regression) showed that low authority over decisions was a statistically significant determinant of lower back pain, regardless of other determinants – the less authority the employee felt that she had, the higher the likelihood that she would report lower back pain. Similarly, a measure of social support at work was the only statistically significant determinant of pain in the shoulders – the poorer the support at work, the greater the likelihood that an employee would report pain in her shoulders. In univariate analyses the group (after trichotomy of the study group) of women with the least authority over decisions had a likelihood 3.0 times higher of reporting lower back pain and the group of women with the worst social support (also trichotomy) had a likelihood 4.4 times higher of reporting shoulder pain than other women. There was only marginal overlap between the groups, the relationship between reporting lower pack pain and shoulder pain was not statistically significant, and the contingency coefficient (roughly corresponding to correlation) was trivial (= 0.15). Accordingly we are dealing for the most part with two different groups of subjects. Further analysis would require detailed information that we do not have regarding the situations in which lower back pain and shoulder pain arose. A resonable speculation, however, is that emotionally loaded situations often arise when ill patients are moved from supine to sitting positions or from one bed to another. These situations require skillful cooperation between patient and personnel but also between staff members. If the social atmosphere in the ward is poor, these situations may become more unpredictable and the likelihood of sudden unexpected physical load during lifting increases. This may be more likely to occur in the neck–shoulder region when forward bending positions and use of arms and shoulders are common. Lower back pain may arise on other kinds of situations with heavy lifting of objects in which the social atmosphere may be less important but in which feelings of frustration created by poor possibilities to influence decisions may play a role.

CONCLUSIONS

The following general conclusions were made:

1. Different theoretical models have to be used in the study of etiology of locomotor disorders versus long-term outcome of these disorders.
2. The global concepts of psychological demands, decision latitude, and social support at work seem to be useful, and there is empirical support for the assumption that these dimensions are of relevance to the development of locomotor disorders and symptoms. Relatively simple theoretical models are preferable in preventive practical work.
3. Despite the fact that psychosocial measures have been relatively vague in many studies, the relative risks associated with psychosocially adverse job conditions are not clearly lower than those associated with physically adverse conditions. There is a complex interaction between physical and psychosocial job conditions.
4. Different parts of the demand–control–support model are of importance in different populations and possibly also to different diagnostic categories within the locomotor system.
5. More physiological studies are needed in the exploration of possible pathways.

6. Both cross-sectional and longitudinal studies will be needed – recall bias is a problem in cross-sectional studies and lack of relevant information for the most recent period preceding the onset of locomotor disorders or symptoms is a problem in longitudinal studies.
7. Precision in the psychosocial exposure measurements need to be developed, preferably by means of direct comparisons between observations, interviews, and questionnaires. The subjective component is always important in psychosocial descriptions, however, and accordingly it is meaningless to express the relationship between observation and questionnaire, for instance, as correlations.

REFERENCES

Ahlberg-Hultén, G., Sigala, F. and Theorell, T. 1993 Social support, job strain and pain in the locomotor system among female health care personnel, *Scand. J. Work Environ. Health.*

Bongers, P. M. and de Winter, C. R. 1992 Psychosocial factors and musculoskeletal disease, mimeograph, Nederlands Instituute voor Praeventieve Gezondheidszorg TNO.

Feuerstein, M., Papciak, A. S. and Hoon, P. E. 1987 Biobehavioral mechanisms of chronic low back pain, *Clinical Psychological Review*, **7**, 243–73.

Härenstam, A. and Theorell, T. 1988 Work conditions and urinary excretion of catecholamines: a study of prison staff in Sweden, *Scandinavian Journal of Work and Environmental Health*, **14**, 257–64.

Holmström, E. B., Lindell, J. and Moritz, U. 1992 Low back and neck/shoulder pain in construction workers: Occupational workload and psychosocial risk factors, *Spine*, **17**, 672–7.

Johansson, H. and Sjölander, P. 1993 Neurophysiology of joints, in Wright, V. and Radin, E. L. (Eds), *Mechanics of Human Joints*, New York: Dekker.

Johansson, J. Å. and Rubenowitz, S. 1992 *Arbete och besvär i nacke, skuldra och rygg, mineograph*, Institute of Psychology, University of Göteborg.

Johnson, J. V. and Hall, E. M. 1988 Job strain, workplace social support and cardiovascular disease: A cross-sectional, study of a random sample of the Swedish working population, *American Journal of Public Health*, **78**, 1336–42.

Karasek, R. A. 1979 Job demands, job decision latitude, and mental strain: Implications for job redesign, *Administrative Science Quarterly*, **24**, 285–307.

Karasek, R. A. and Theorell, T. 1990 *Healthy Work*, New York: Basic Books.

Karasek, R. A., Gardell, B. and Lindell, J. 1987 Work and non-work correlates of illness and behaviour in male and female Swedish white-collar workers, *Journal of Occupation and Behaviour*, **8**, 187–207.

Kamwendo, K., Linton, S. and Moritz, U. 1991 Neck and shoulder disorder in medical secretaries, *Scandinavian Journal of Rehabilitation Medicine*, **23**, 127–33.

Linton, S. J. 1990 Risk factors for neck and back pain in a working population in Sweden, *Work and Stress*, **4**, 41–9.

Lundberg, U., Kadefors, R., Melin, B., Palmerud, G., Hassmén, P., Engström, M. and Elfsberg Dohns, I. 1994 Stress, muscular tension and musculoskeletal disorders, Third International Congress on Behavioral Medicine, Amsterdam, 1994, Book of abstracts, p. 55, and 1994, *International Journal of Behavioural Medicine*, **1**, 354–70.

Maier, S. F., Dragan, R. C. and Oran, J. W. 1982 Controllability, coping behaviour and stress-induced analgesia in the rat, *Pain*, **12**, 47–56.

Reesor, K. and Craig, K. P. 1987 Medically incongruent chronic back pain: Physical limitation, suffering and ineffective coping, *Pain*, **32**, 35–45.

RUNDCRANTZ, B-L. 1991 Pain and discomfort in the musculoskeletal system among dentists, Doctoral dissertation, Department of Physical Therapy, University of Lund, Sweden.

THEORELL, T. 1990 Socialt stöd i arbetet (Social support at work), *Scialmed Tidskr*, **67**(1–2), 27–31.

THEORELL, T., FLODÉRUS, B. and LIND, E. 1975 The relationship of disturbing life-changes and emotions to the early development of myocardial infarction and other serious illnesses, *International Journal of Epidemiology*, **4**, 281–96.

THEORELL, T., KARASEK, R. A. and ENEROTH, P. 1990 Job strain variations in relation to plasma testosterone fluctuations in working men: A longitudinal study, *Journal of International Medicine*, **227**, 31–6.

THEORELL, T., NORDEMAR, R., MICHÉLSEN, H. and STOCKHOLM MUSIC STUDY GROUP 1993 Pain thresholds during standardized psychological stress in relation to perceived psychosocial work situation, *Journal of Psychosomatic Research*, **37**, 299–305.

THEORELL, T., PERSKI, A., ÅKERSTEDT, T., SIGALA, F., AHLBERG-HULTÉN, G., SVENSSON, J. and ENEROTH, P. 1988 Changes in job strain in relation to changes in physiological states: a longitudinal study, *Scandinavian Journal of Work and Environmental Health*, **14**, 189–96.

THEORELL, T., HARMS-RINGDAHL, K., AHLBERG-HULTÉN, G. and WESTIN, B. 1991 Psychosocial job factors and symptoms from the locomotor system: A multicausal analysis, *Scandinavian Journal of Rehabilitation Medicine*, **23**, 165–73.

TOLA, S., RIIHIMÄKI, H., VIDEMAN, T., VILKARI-JUNTURA, E. and HÄNNINEN, K. 1988 Neck and shoulder symptoms among men in machine-operating, dynamic physical work and sedentary work, *Scandinavian Journal of Work, Environment and Health*, **14**, 299–305.

TOOMINGAS, A., THEORELL, T. and the STOCKHOLM MUSIC STUDY GROUP 1992 On the relationship between psychosocial working conditions and symptoms/signs of locomotor disorders in the neck/shoulder region, lecture at the PREMUS, Stockholm, May 1992.

TURK, D. C., MEICHENBAUM, D. and GENEST, M. 1983 *Pain and Behavioral Medicine*, New York: Guilford Press.

UNDÉN, A.-L., ORTH-GOMÉR, K. and ELOFSSON, S. 1991 Cardiovascular effects of social support in the work place: twenty-four hour ECG monitoring of men and women, *Psychomatic Medicine*, **53**, 50–60.

CHAPTER FIVE

Effects of psychological demand and stress on neuromuscular function

R. H. WESTGAARD

INTRODUCTION

The term 'cumulative trauma disorder' (CTD) implies damage to the musculoskeletal system associated with extensive usage or 'strain' of this system. Additional to the more generally accepted relationship between CTD and biomechanical stressors, e.g. damage to the wrist in repetitive work tasks, the phenomenon of many office workers developing musculoskeletal pain syndromes without any striking evidence of physical exertions at work is becoming increasingly noticeable. These pain syndromes are often located in the upper trunk, neck, shoulders, and facial muscles. They have long been recognized in the clinical literature and are classified in a group of suboccipital pain syndromes and as tension headache by the International Association for the Study of Pain (Mersky, 1986).

There is a vast literature on pain syndromes of presumed musculoskeletal origin in journals of pain syndromes (e.g. headache), psychophysiology, psychology, psychosomatic and behavioral medicine, and stress research, besides those dealing with the work environment. In this literature conditions at work are mentioned as a possible etiological factor, however, psychological factors and a negative emotional state of the patient feature prominently. Many patients with these syndromes describe themselves as tense, and muscle activity is assumed to initiate the pathophysiological process.

Much of the research has been directed toward showing an increase in muscle activity associated with these pain syndromes. This has proved difficult, to the extent that the International Headache Association in its classification system has renamed tension headache as tension-type headache to emphasize this uncertainty. In a critical review of psychophysiological literature Flor and Turk (1989) concluded that, on balance, there was evidence that muscle tension is elevated among tension headache sufferers compared to healthy controls during stressful conditions, but not at rest. However, this evidence is not clear cut. Thus, in the more limited context of CTD and psychosocial factors in office work we need to know whether 'cumulative trauma' is a valid concept in terms of psychosocial factors causing muscle pain, and if so, how this strain comes about. We also want to identify the specific pathophysiological mechanisms involved.

MUSCLE ACTIVITY AS A PATHOPHYSIOLOGICAL FACTOR IN THE DEVELOPMENT OF MUSCLE PAIN SYNDROMES

This paper holds that there must be a physiological correlate to the association between psychosocial factors and the development of muscle pain syndromes in trunk, neck, and shoulders, pointed out in epidemiological studies. I feel that the evidence of an association between psychosocial factors and pain syndromes in the extremities is less compelling and the arguments presented here are conceptually limited to the former muscle group, using trapezius myalgia as a specific model.

A critical question is whether muscle pain associated with psychosocial factors is mediated through increased muscle activity (Figure 5.1A), by modifying the effect of muscle activity occurring due to work demands (Figure 5.1B), or by influencing the health status independently of muscle activity (Figure 5.1C). Furthermore, we need to know the physical exposure dose–effect relationship, and whether selective muscle activation patterns (e.g. low-threshold motor units) must be considered. If so, the muscle activity of interest may not be readily observable in recordings with conventional surface electromyography (EMG).

In a review of studies aiming to observe long-term health effects in the shoulder-neck region of physical exposure at the workplace, Winkel and Westgaard (1992) suggested that the physical exposure dose at the workplace should be quantified by a combination of the variables level, repetitiveness, and duration. It was concluded in the review that physical exposure at a high or medium level should be reduced to a low level for reduced risk of muscle pain syndromes. However, the

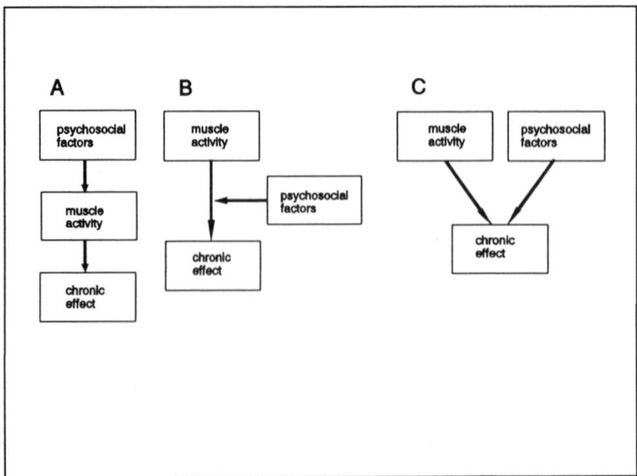

Figure 5.1 Possible relationship between muscle activity, psychosocial risk factors and cumulative trauma disorders. Psychosocial risk factors may act through a general increase in the muscle activity (A), through an interaction with muscle activity due to work demands (B), or through some mechanism independent of muscle activity (C). Both overall activity and selected activity patterns (e.g. in low-threshold motor units) must be considered.

A

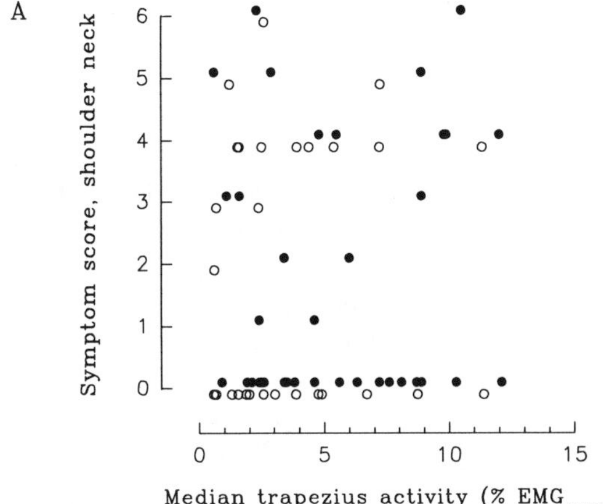

B

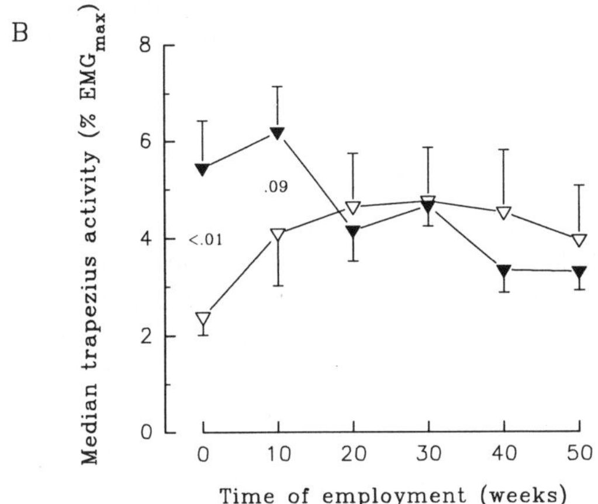

Figure 5.2 A. Scatter plot of median activity in the trapezius from vocational recordings versus complaint level in the shoulder in the last 12 months before the interview. Complaint level is determined on the basis of intensity and frequency of symptoms, scoring from 0 to 6 (Westgaard and Jansen, 1992a). Individual data from two groups of female workers performing light, repetitive manual work (●) and general office work (○) are shown. One data point corresponding to 19.7 per cent EMG and a symptom score of 5 is not shown for the office group. Redrawn from Jensen *et al.*, 1993. B. Median trapezius activity level of workers developing acute trapezius myalgia (▼) and workers remaining healthy (▽) as a function of employment time. P-values for Mann–Whitney tests are shown between the means of considerable difference. The workers performed light, repetitive work tasks and were without such symptoms at employment (time 0). From Veiersted *et al.*, 1993.

repetitiveness or lack of variation in the muscle usage contributed significantly to a high risk also at low activity levels.

We have looked at this in more detail by comparing muscle activity in the trapezius, measured by surface EMG, and muscle pain symptoms in the shoulder region for groups of workers performing the same work tasks and by that exposed to similar external demands. One group performed office work including administrative and clerical duties. Their work duties involved the use of video display terminals (VDTs) in a dialog mode, telephones, etc., but the work tasks could not be considered repetitive as in high-speed typing or data keying. The other group performed the highly repetitive tasks of chocolate manufacturing or packing. The work tasks of both groups were light with respect to load on the shoulder, with group mean values for the median load on the trapezius being 4.1 per cent and 5.3 per cent of the EMG signal at maximal voluntary contraction (EMG_{max}). These values correspond approximately to the same relative muscle force levels. Individual values of median trapezius activity varied widely, from 0.6 per cent to 12.1 per cent EMG_{max} for the production workers and 0.6 per cent to 19.7 per cent EMG_{max} for the office workers. There was no correlation between median muscle activity and pain symptoms for the last 12 months within either group (Jensen *et al.*, 1993; see Figure 5.2A).

In a separate study with a longitudinal design, healthy young females recruited to another chocolate manufacturing plant were followed for at least half a year until some workers developed acute trapezius myalgia. The future patients did not show higher muscle activity levels than those remaining healthy. This was true both before and after the change in patient status, but not for the first recording when the future patients recorded a significantly higher activity level (Veiersted *et al.*, 1993; Figure 5.2B).

Those reporting psychosocial stresses at work in the cross-sectional study recorded a higher pain symptom score, but there were no differences in the EMG variables between those reporting and not reporting such stress (Jensen *et al.*, 1993). In a recent case-control study with matching for physical exposure, cases of office workers with musculoskeletal complaints and performing office work were differentiated from their controls on the basis of psychosocial variables, but recorded the same physical load (Vasseljen and Westgaard, 1995; Vasseljen *et al.*, 1995). Subjectively reported stress at work also proved a risk factor for trapezius myalgia in the longitudinal study (Veiersted and Westgaard, 1994).

In summary, there appears to be a correlation between muscle activity level and pain when considering the wider variation in activity level between different occupational groups (e.g. comparing median muscle activity in the range zero to 30 per cent EMG_{max}; Westgaard *et al.*, 1993a). This correlation is more difficult to show within the span of median load levels represented in the same occupational group with light work. In particular, some workers with very low EMG levels develop muscle pain symptoms and subjectively relate these to conditions at work.

MUSCLE ACTIVITY RELATED TO MENTAL DEMANDS AND PSYCHOSOCIAL FACTORS

The findings of musculoskeletal symptoms being associated with negative psychosocial factors, negative psychological factors, and the subjectively reported tendency of developing muscle tension (Kamwendo *et al.*, 1991; Westgaard and Jensen, 1992b; Westgaard *et al.*, 1993a) has aroused our interest in non-voluntary or psychogenic muscle tension. This is a well-established phenomenon first measured electromyographically by Jacobson (1927, 1930) who showed that muscle activity may result in situations where a conscious movement was not supposed to take place. Subsequent studies showed such muscle activity to be associated with effort (Eason and White, 1961), motivation (Malmo, 1965, 1975), and personality (Rimehaug and Sveback, 1987) among many other variables (Goldstein, 1972).

These associations, implicating muscle activation mechanisms and pointing to muscular reactions as a response of the individual to adverse psychosocial conditions at work, have prompted us to perform further experiments to show that factors in the work environment can initiate non-voluntary muscle activation (Westgaard and Bjørklund, 1987; Wærsted *et al.*, 1991; 1994).

The muscle activity patterns observed in our experimental setting, a two-choice reaction time test presented on a VDT screen and requiring only minimal finger movement to respond, is typically very stable, with a variation pattern of only a few tenths of 1 per cent EMG_{max} (see Figure 5.3). The mean EMG level, when the response is present, may vary from less than five to 100 μV, corresponding to less than 0.5 to about 10 per cent EMG_{max}. These levels are similar to the muscle activ-

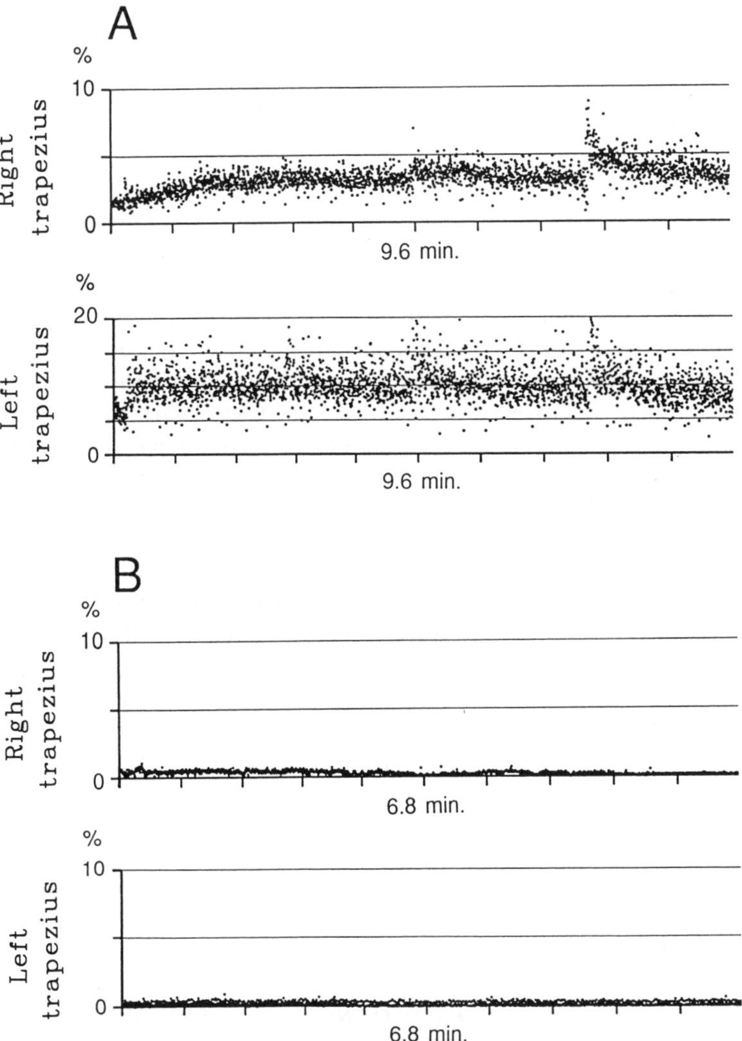

Figure 5.3 Muscle activity patterns from right and left trapezius of two subjects responding and not responding while performing an attention-demanding reaction–time test. From Westgaard *et al.*, 1993b.

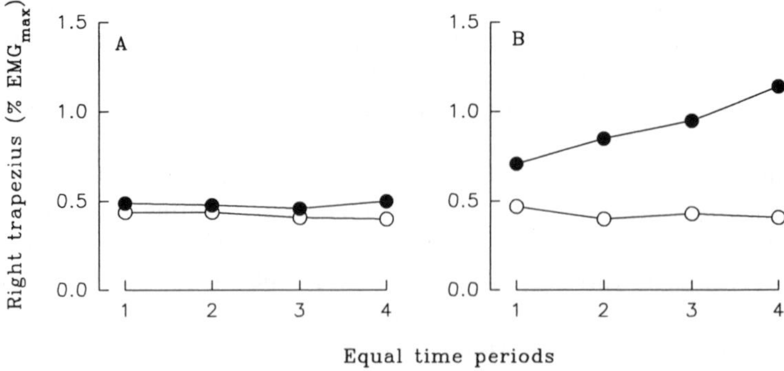

Figure 5.4 A. EMG responses in the right trapezius during the reaction–time test in a control condition (○) and a condition with feedback on results (●). Error rate 8.9 per cent and 12.7 per cent, reaction time 1.6s and 1.3s in control and feedback condition, respectively. B. Same as part A, except a financial reward for good performance (~US$30) was introduced. Error rate 12.7 per cent and 12.2 per cent, reaction time 1.5s and 1.2s in control and feedback condition, respectively. Redrawn from Wærsted *et al.*, 1994.

ity levels observed in the vocational recordings from office work, but have a more static appearance. The mean value may remain stable, show a gradual increase or decrease, or a sudden shift in mean level. Such features can be simultaneously present in recordings from several muscles.

In a series of experiments we have looked at the effect of feedback of results with and without an added incentive (money reward) for good performance. Feedback without the added incentive resulted in faster response time, more errors and no change in the level of muscle tension (see Figure 5.4A). When performing the task with the added incentive of a money reward, the result was a faster response time and no increase in the number of errors, but with a significant increase in muscle tension (see Figure 5.4B).

We have also shown that prolonged activation of single motor units is a prominent feature in this form of nonvoluntary muscle activity (Wærsted *et al.*, 1993). This is shown by direct observation of single motor units, probably recruited at low threshold in voluntary activation, remaining active throughout the experimental period. An observed modulation of the firing frequency of the motor units coincided with a similar modulation of the surface EMG response, suggesting simultaneous activation of a small number of motor units.

These and other results of laboratory studies show that motivational factors common in working life affect performance and have distinct psychophysiological effects. Other psychosocial factors can be postulated to result in a similar reaction, on the basis of studies showing that anger, hostility, or fear can cause an increase in muscle tension (Holmes and Wolff, 1952; Sainsbury and Gibson, 1954).

THE NEUROPHYSIOLOGICAL BASIS OF NONVOLUNTARY MUSCLE ACTIVITY

The neurophysiological basis for nonvoluntary muscle activation is not known with certainty. Postural activity to stabilize head and arms cannot be excluded. However, recent advances in the understanding of the functional anatomy of the motor system point to another neural system as a possible contributor. A system of predominantly monoaminergic descending pathways from the brain stem, including serotonergic neurons from the raphe nuclei and noradrenergic neurons from the locus coeruleus and subcoeruleus, appears to initiate or control motor responses to emotive stimuli. Many neurons in the same pathways contain other neuropeptides that are candidate neurotransmitters or modulators of motoneuron excitability, in part coexisting with serotonin in the same cells.

This system of small-diameter nerve fibres has only recently been demonstrated by immunohistochemical techniques, and is termed the third motor system by Holstege (1991). (The first system consists of interneurons and propriospinal neurons and provides integration of motor activity at the spinal cord and medullary level. The second somatic system controls voluntary movement including posture and the integration of body and limb movement.) The understanding of the neurophysiology of these neurons is continuously updated in this very active research field.

The pre-motor neurons of the third motor system have a diffuse projection, with single cells projecting to the motor nuclei in the caudal brain stem as well as to many levels of the spinal cord. They can be monosynaptic to motoneurons (Alstermark *et al.*, 1987), but serotonergic nerve fibers may also terminate near motoneurons without synaptic specializations (Ulfhake *et al.*, 1987). There is evidence to suggest that the third motor system is involved in level-setting of the motoneurons in the caudal brain stem and the spinal cord (Barbeau and Bédard, 1981; Hansen *et al.*, 1983), possibly mediated through long-lasting 'plateau-potentials' in the spinal cord motoneurons (Hounsgaard *et al.*, 1984; Hounsgaard and Kiehn, 1985). These potentials may be implicated in the switching between states of low and high motoneuron activity (Eken *et al.*, 1989).

The same brain stem structures, i.e. the raphe nuclei and the loceus coeruleus/subcoeruleus, also project to the autonomic preganglionic cell groups (raphe nuclei) and to cells in the dorsal horn. They inhibit ascending sensory systems, in particular nociception (Dostrovsky *et al.*, 1983; Mokha *et al.*, 1986). Thus, activation of these brain stem structures facilitates the motor responses and depresses sensory input, as typified by the classic 'fight or flight' response. Neurons in locus coeruleus have been shown to respond to stressful conditions in experiments with awake animals (Jacobs, 1986).

These brain stem nuclei receive strong input from the limbic system, especially from the medial hypothalamic area and the paraventricular hypothalamic nucleus, providing the emotional brain with direct pathways and a controlling influence over the motor system (Holstege, 1991). The paraventricular hypothalamic nucleus also controls parasympathetic and sympathetic innervation of the body and initiates a variety of hormonal responses through its projection to the hypophysis.

THE MODIFICATION OF SENSORY-MOTOR REFLEXES ASSOCIATED WITH MUSCLE PAIN SYNDROMES

This new insight in the functioning of the motor system and its control by the emotional brain has the potential of providing a neural substrate for the association between psychosocial factors and muscle pain syndromes. Is there any evidence for muscle pain syndromes somehow associated with the activation of motor systems by limbic influences? One line of evidence relates to the finding that the second temporalis exteroceptive suppression period (ES2), a polysynaptic facial reflex, is reduced in patients with chronic and episodic tension headache (Schoenen *et al.*, 1987; Wallasch *et al.*, 1991). The reflex is elicited by painful peri- or intraoral stimulation which in humans produces two successive suppressions of voluntary masseter and temporalis activity, termed exteroceptive suppressions. It is part of the jaw opening reflex (JOR), used in animal models to study pain mechanisms (Mason *et al.*, 1985).

Stimulation of the raphe magnus and periaqueductal grey matter is shown in animal experiments to inhibit the JOR (Sessle and Hu, 1981; Dostrovsky *et al.*, 1982). In humans the ES2 reflex is increased by 5-HT antagonists and reduced by a 5-HT reuptake blocker, indicating that serotonin-dependent pathways take part in the modulation of this reflex (Schoenen *et al.*, 1991). The effect on the ES2 reflex in tension headache can, in view of these findings, be considered indirect evidence of abnormal functioning of serotonergic pathways in this muscle pain syndrome (Schoenen, 1993). Preliminary data from one of our experimental series show marked depression of pain level in patients with tension headache during a one-hour experiment where they performed the choice–reaction time task. The experimental condition with nonvoluntary motor activity thus suppresses nociceptive sensory input, an effect presumably due to gating effects of ascending sensory pathways, occurring simultaneously with motoneuron activation. This is consistent with a general activation of serotonergic pathways.

The effect on the ES2 in other pain states is variable, the ES2 is reported reduced in patients with thoracic neuralgia and lower back pain, but not in patients with migraine (Schoenen *et al.*, 1987; Wallasch and Göbel, 1993). There are also reports that the ES2 reflex is influenced by the state of well-being (Wallasch *et al.*, 1993). However, no definite conclusions can yet be drawn regarding neurophysiological substrate and pathophysiological mechanisms to explain the modulation of this reflex.

The excitability of motoneurons as studied by segmental reflexes is enhanced in subjects performing cognitive tasks (Brunia and Boelhouwer, 1988). This effect is present in motoneurons many spinal cord segments away from those participating in response execution, and appears to be in part related to general activation mechanisms underlying information processing. Thus, emotional influences and attention have clear effects on motoneuron excitation in humans.

PERIPHERAL MECHANISMS IN MUSCLE PAIN SYNDROMES OF PSYCHOSOCIAL ORIGIN

Although central neural mechanisms participate in the modulation of pain perception, it is likely that the muscle pain syndromes somehow originate in the periphery, at least in their nonchronic forms. Pain from the muscle is mediated through fine myelinated (group III) and unmyelinated (group IV) nerve fibres terminating as free nerve endings within the muscle. These nerve fibres are activated by noxious chemical (bradykinin, potassium) or mechanical stimuli. Some noxious chemicals (e.g. bradykinin) have a secondary effect by stimulating the release of prostaglandines and neuropeptides (substance-P, calcitonin gene-related peptide) which facilitate the response of nociceptors to the primary stimuli. Thus, if a painful condition is maintained, it usually gets worse with time.

Disturbances of skeletal muscle that activate nociceptors include trauma, mechanical overload, ischemia, myositis with inflammation, and changes in muscle tone (Mense, 1993). Trauma, eccentric contractions, and myositis are not likely to initiate CTD in office work. Ischemia may seem unlikely to cause CTD in work situations with biomechanically well-adjusted workplaces and a median load below 5 per cent maximal voluntary contraction (MVC) in the trapezius, when many workers develop trapezius myalgia (Figure 5.2). However, resting intramuscular pressure in trapezius muscles with fibrosis is much higher than a normal trapezius (Hagert and Christenson, 1990) and oxygen tension is reduced in trapezius muscles with work-related myalgia (Larsson *et al.*, 1990), indicating that ischemia may still be a problem. Another point of uncertainty concerns the capillary circulation in the muscle. The microcirculation is very inhomogeneous in muscle at rest (Iversen *et al.*, 1989). This inhomogeneity usually disappears in working muscle, but the capillary circulation at low static loads has not been examined. Local ischemia under these conditions can therefore not be excluded.

Ischemia is even more likely in painful conditions of shoulder muscles such as the supraspinatus, where intramuscular pressure generally is high due to the enclosure of the muscle in a compartment between the scapula and a tense fascia. Intramuscular pressure in supraspinatus is high enough to restrict blood flow under moderate arm abductions and elevations (Järvholm *et al.*, 1988).

A moderate increase in muscle tone due to mental or psychosocial stress is usually not considered a contributor to muscle pain (Mense, 1993). However, pain due to occupational exposure develops over periods of months and years, and the pathophysiological mechanisms underlying occupational pain symptoms can therefore not be studied with confidence as an acute phenomenon. If a moderate increase in muscle tone should contribute to muscle pain, this may be related to prolonged activation of low-threshold motor units. Such activation results in hypertrophy, potassium release into the interstitial space, metabolic depletion, and elevation of the intracellular concentration of calcium. A sustained increase in free calcium causes mithochondrial calcium overload and stimulates phospholipase activity with a subsequent increase in free radicals and lipid peroxidation (Edwards, 1988). Increased fibre size, reduced energy content and increased occurrence of 'ragged-red' fibers (fibers with a positive reaction to NADH-tetrazolium reductase) have been reported in work-related trapezius myalgia (Larsson *et al.*, 1988; Lindman *et al.*, 1991). 'Ragged-red' fibers have a mithocondrial dysfunction and are always type I. An increased concentration of intracellular and extracellular free radicals is demonstrated in heavy exercise and is associated with low- frequency fatigue (Reid *et al.*, 1992a; b).

These physiological responses will happen in muscle fibres with a prolonged activity pattern regardless of the overall activity level in the muscle. The responses have pathophysiological potential, but we do not yet know whether they are relevant in the development of muscle pain syndromes.

IS OVEREXERTION OF LOW-THRESHOLD MOTOR UNITS A CAUSAL FACTOR IN SOME MUSCLE PAIN SYNDROMES?

A hypothesis of a pathophysiological mechanism in some forms of CTD, where single motor units are overexerted in an otherwise quiescent muscle, is attractive. The difficulty in establishing a dose–effect relation at low muscle activity levels, and muscle pain syndromes developing in work situations with a median load level of only a few per cent MVC can be understood in terms of this hypothesis. The hypothesis is feasible according to the Henneman size principle (Henneman *et al.*, 1965), stating that the recruitment order of motor units is orderly, with small motor units recruited first in voluntary contractions (Milner-Brown *et al.*, 1973).

We have introduced an analysis to quantify the occurrence of short periods with minimal EMG activity ('EMG gaps'), in an attempt to quantify continuous, low-level muscle activity (Veiersted *et al.*, 1990). The aim of the analysis is to detect periods of inactivity of sufficient duration to indicate disruption in the activity pattern of low-threshold motor units. An EMG level of 0.5 per cent EMG_{max} (~ 5 μV) was selected as the lowest level that could reliably be detected above noise level (1.5 μV) in our EMG recording system. The time resolution was 0.2s, able to detect a train of impulses at a frequency of 5 Hz or higher. The lowest rate of sustained activity in single motor units is 8–10 Hz. The EMG gap analysis should therefore be sensitive to prolonged muscle activity. However, some low-threshold motor units are active even at the low activity level of 0.5 per cent MVC. Individual motor units may have inactive periods at higher activity levels. Thus, the sensitivity of the gap analysis can be questioned. Analyses with thresholds at higher load levels are correspondingly less sensitive (Takala and Viikari-Juntura, 1991; Aarås, 1993).

The EMG gap analysis distinguished future patients from those remaining healthy in the longitudinal study of workers performing light, repetitive work tasks (see Figure 5.5; Veiersted *et al.*, 1993), but did not correlate with pain symptoms in the cross-sectional study of office workers and workers with light manual work (Jensen *et al.*, 1993). In a case-control study the gap analysis distinguished between manual workers, but not office workers with and without muscle pain syndromes (Vasseljen and Westgaard, 1995). The total gap time and the number of long gaps (>0.6 s) correlated with pain symptoms in the cross-sectional study for the office workers ($r^2 = 0.16$ and 0.10, respectively), but not for the workers with light repetitive work (Jensen *et al.*, 1993). Thus, the EMG gap analysis gave a positive result in the best controlled study, but the result was only partially confirmed in the other

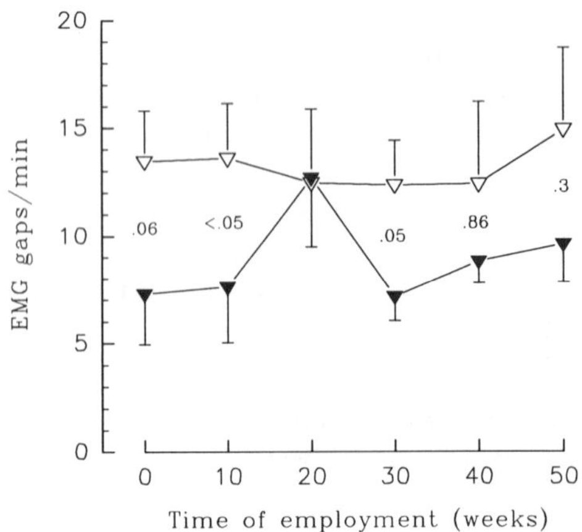

Figure 5.5 EMG gap analysis of workers developing acute trapezius myalgia (▼) and workers remaining healthy (▽). P-values as in Figure 5.2B. From Veiersted *et al.*, 1993.

studies. The discrepancy may be due to worker selection in the cross-sectional studies (healthy worker effects?), uncontrolled differences between groups, or chance.

In the longitudinal study there was a significantly higher tension level during forced rest pauses (machine stops) for the future patients than for those remaining healthy (Veiersted, 1993). Higher tension levels have also been observed among workers with pain symptoms during forced rest pauses (calibration of position sensors) in a group with manual work, but not in office work (Vasseljen and Westgaard, 1995). These findings can be interpreted as supportive of a hypothesis of continuous activation of low-threshold motor units. Subjects with work-related myalgia also show elevated activity during the relaxation phase in an isokinetic test with repeated contraction–relaxation cycles (Elert *et al.*, 1992). Thus, there is some evidence in favor of prolonged activation of low-threshold trapezius motor units in trapezius myalgia.

In another series of experiments we have looked at associations between musculoskeletal complaints in the shoulder and neck, and activity patterns during the reaction–time test and a muscle coordination test (Westgaard and Bjørklund, 1987). The rationale for these experiments is that subjects with pain symptoms may shown 'hyperactivity' during forced conditions, either associated to mental load or to arm movement. A problem with these tests is that we do not know the ecological validity of the test, i.e. whether the conditions we create represent conditions at work that promote muscle activity. These experiments must therefore be considered preliminary. In the cross-sectional study there was a strong correlation between the EMG response in a combination of the reaction–time test and the passive trapezius in the muscle coordination test, and the EMG gaps in the vocational recording (Westgaard *et al.*, 1993b). Office workers reporting psychosocial problems responded with significantly higher muscle tension in the reaction–time test than those without such problems. There was also a tendency of increased muscle activity in the reaction–time test and for the passive trapezius in the muscle coordination test for office workers with musculoskeletal complaints in the last 12 months, compared to those free of such complaints.

Despite some interesting results, the overall conclusion of these experiments is balanced toward the negative. This may be because the hypothesis of overexertion of low-threshold motor units is not correct. Alternatively the sensitivity and validity of the attempted measurements can be questioned, or a pathophysiological mechanism relating to overexertion of low-threshold motor units is only one of several mechanisms operating. It is particularly thought-provoking that groups distinguished on the basis of reported psychosocial problems and reporting a high level of musculoskeletal pain, cannot be distinguished on the basis of physiological measurement of muscle activity (i.e. supporting Figure 5.1C). Finally, it must be emphasized that the hypothesis of prolonged activation of low-threshold motor units in non-voluntary muscle activity is advanced only to explain the development of muscle pain at very low tension levels. Other pathophysiological mechanisms related to muscle activation certainly are important at higher load levels.

GENERAL DISCUSSION

We are probably dealing with a multifactorial etiology in CTDs. In particular we need to develop theories to explain increased risk at very low muscle activity levels.

The hypothesis of pathogenesis tied to hyperactivity of low-threshold muscle fibers is not new. It is implicit in many hypotheses of peripheral mechanisms in muscle pain syndromes (e.g. tension headache), due to the low tension levels observed in patients with these problems. The hypothesis has also been stated in relation to fibromyalgia (Henriksson, 1988). As such, CTDs relating to psychosocial factors are just adding to the list of muscle pain syndromes with a proposed similar etiology. A possible advantage as a newcomer to this collection of syndromes with a possible psychosocial origin, is that it may be easier to identify harmful exposure conditions and by that obtain a better understanding of exposure dose–effect relationships.

Leaving aside the problem of proving or disproving the hypothesis, how can a potential harmful effect of continuous muscle activation be counteracted? We may assume that a reduction of relevant psychological or psychosocial strain will reduce such activation. From the field of neurophysiology we know that dynamic movement causes inhibition of antagonists and thereby disrupts continuous activity patterns. Such 'natural' activity patterns are largely eliminated with the reduction of muscle usage in sedentary occupations ('postural fixity'). An important design criteria in the creation of new jobs may in the future be to increase the variation and even the level of force exertions, thereby causing more phasic activity patterns also in low-threshold motor units.

REFERENCES

AARÅS, A. 1993 Relationship between trapezius load and the incidence of musculoskeletal illness in the neck and shoulder, in NIELSEN, R. and JORGENSEN, K. (Eds), *Advances in Industrial Ergonomics and Safety V*, pp. 121–4, London: Taylor & Francis.

ALSTERMARK, B., KIMMEL, H. and TANTISIRA, B. 1987 Monosynaptic raphespinal and reticulospinal projection to forelimb motoneurons in cats, *Neuroscience Letters*, **74**, 286–90.

BARBEAU, H. and BÉDARD, P. 1981 Similar motor effect of 5-HT and TRH in rats following chronical spinal transection and 5,7-dihydroxytryptamine injection, *Neuropharmacology*, **20**, 477–81.

BRUNIA, C. H. M. and BOELHOUWER, A. J. W. 1988 Reflexes as a tool: a window in the central nervous system, in ACKLES, P. K., JENNINGS, J. R. and COLES, M. G. H. (Eds), *Advances in Psychophysiology*, Vol. 3, pp. 1–67, Greenwich, CT: JAI Press.

DOSTROVSKY, J. O., HU, J. W., SESSLE, B. J. and SUMINO, R. 1982 Stimulation sites in periaqueductal grey, nucleus raphe magnus and adjacent regions effective in suppressing oral–facial reflexes, *Brain Research*, **252**, 287–97.

DOSTROVSKY, J. O., SHAH, Y. and GRAY, B. G. 1983 Descending inhibitory influences from periaqueductal gray, nucleus raphe magnus, and adjacent recticular formation, II: Effects on medullary dorsal horn nociceptive and nonnociceptive neurons, *Journal of Neurophysiology*, **49**, 948–60.

EASON, R. G. and WHITE, C. T. 1961 Muscular tension, effort, and tracking difficulty: Studies of parameters which affect tension level and performance efficiency, *Perceptual and Motor Skills*, **12**, 331–72.

EDWARDS, R. H. T. 1988 Hypotheses of peripheral and central mechanisms underlying occupational muscle pain and injury, *European Journal of Applied Physiology and Occupational Physiology*, **57**, 275–81.

EKEN, T., HULTBORN, H. and KIEHN, O. 1989 Possible functions of transmitter-controlled plateau potentials in α motoneurones, in ALLUM, J. H. J. and HULLIGER, M. (Eds), *Progress in Brain Research*, **80**, pp. 257–67, Amsterdam: Elsevier.

Elert, J. E., Rantapää-Dahlqvist, S. B., Henriksson-Larsén, K., Lorentzon, R. and Gerdlé, B. U. C. 1992 Muscle performance, electromyography and fibre type composition in fibromyalgia and work-related myalgia, *Scandinavian Journal of Rheumatology*, **21**, 28–34.

Flor, H. and Turk, D. C. 1989 Psychophysiology of chronic pain: Do chronic pain patients exhibit symptom-specific psychological responses? *Psychological Bulletin*, **105**, 215–59.

Goldstein, I. B. 1972 Electromyography: A measure of skeletal muscle response, in Greenfield, N. S. and Sternback, R. A. (Eds), *Handbook of Psychophysiology*, pp. 329–62, New York: Holt, Rinehart & Winston.

Hagert, C.-G. and Christenson, J. T. 1990 Hyperpressure in the trapezius muscle associated with fibrosis, *Acta Orthopedica Scandinavia*, **61**, 263–5.

Hansen, S., Svensson, L. Hökfelt, T. and Everitt, B. J., 1983 5-Hydroxytryptamine-thyrotropin releasing hormone interactions in the spinal cord: Effect of parameters of sexual behavior in the male rat, *Neuroscience Letters*, **42**, 299–304.

Henneman, E., Somjen, G. and Carpenter, D. O. 1965 Functional significance of cell size in spinal motoneurons, *Journal of Neurophysiology*, **28**, 560–80.

Holmes, T. H. and Wolff, H. G. 1952 Life situations, emotions, and backache, *Psychosomatic Medicine*, **14**, 18–33.

Holstege, G. 1991 Descending motor pathways and the spinal motor system: Limbic and non-limbic components, in Holstege, G. (Ed.), *Role of the Forebrain in Sensation and Behavior*, pp. 307–421, *Progress in Brain Research*, **87**, Amsterdam: Elsevier.

Hounsgaard, J., Hultborn, H., Jespersen, B. and Kiehn, O. 1984 Intrinsic membrane properties causing a bistable behaviour of α-motoneurones, *Experimental Brain Research*, **55**, 391–4.

Hounsgaard, J. and Kiehn, O. 1985 Ca^{++} dependent bistability induced by serotonin in spinal motoneurons, *Experimental Brain Research*, **57**, 422–5.

Iversen, P. O., Standa, M. and Nicolaysen, G. 1989 Marked regional heterogeneity in blood flow within a single skeletal muscle at rest and during exercise hyperaemia in the rabbit, *Acta Physiologica Scandinavia*, **136**, 17–28.

Jacobs, B. L. 1986 Single unit activity of locus coeruleus neurons in behaving animals, *Progress in Neurobiology*, **27**, 183–94.

Jacobson, E. 1927 Action currents from muscular contractions during conscious processes, *Science*, **66**, 403.

Jacobson, E. 1930 Electrical measurements of neuromuscular states during mental activities, I: Imagination of movement involving skeletal muscle, *American Journal of Physiology*, **91**, 567–608.

Järvholm, U., Palmerud, G., Styf, J., Herberts, P. and Kadefors, R. 1988 Intramuscular pressure in the supraspinatus muscle, *Journal of Orthopaedic Research*, **6**, 230–8.

Jensen, C., Nilsen, K., Hansen, K. and Westgaard, R. H. 1993 Trapezius muscle load as a risk indicator for occupational shoulder–neck complaints, *International Archives of Occupational Environmental Health*, **64**, 415–23.

Kamwendo, K., Linton, S. J. and Moritz, U. 1991 Neck and shoulder disorders in medical secretaries, Part I: Pain prevalence and risk factors, *Scandinavian Journal of Rehabilitation Medicine*, **23**, 127-33.

Larsson, S.-E., Bengtsson, A., Bodegård, L., Henriksson, K. G. and Larsson, J. 1988 Muscle changes in work-related chronic myalgia, *Acta Orthopedica Scandinavia*, **59**, 552–6.

Larsson, S.-E., Bodegård, L., Henriksson, K. G. and Öberg, P. Å. 1990 Chronic trapezius myalgia: Morphology and blood flow studied in 17 patients, *Acta Orthopedica Scandinavia*, **61**, 394–8.

Lindman, R., Hagberg, M., Ängqvist, K.-A., Söderlund, K., Hultman, E. and

THORNELL, L.-E. 1991 Changes in muscle morpohology in chronic trapezius myalgia, *Scandinavian Journal of Work, Environment and Health*, **17**, 347–55.

MALMO, R. B. 1965 Psychological gradients and behaviour, *Psychological Bulletin*, **64**, 225–34.

MALMO, R. B. 1975 *On Emotions, Needs, and our Archaic Brain*, New York: Holt, Rinehart & Winston.

MASON, P., STRASSMAN, A. and MACIEWICZ, R. 1985 Is the jaw-opening reflex a valid model of pain?, *Brain Research Reviews*, **10**, 137–46.

MENSE, S. 1993 Peripheral mechanisms of muscle nociception and local muscle pain, *Journal of Musculoskeletal Pain*, **1**, 133–70.

MERSKY, H. (Ed.) 1986 Classification of chronic pain: Description of chronic pain syndromes and definition of pain terms, *Pain* (Suppl. 3), S1–S226.

MILNER-BROWN, H. S., STEIN, R. B. and YEMM, R. 1973 The orderly recruitment of human motor units during voluntary isometric contractions, *Journal of Physiology*, **230**, 359–70.

MOKHA, S. S., MCMILLAN J. A. and IGGO, A. 1986 Pathways mediating descending control of spinal nociceptive transmission from the nuclei locus coeruleus (LC) and raphe magnus (NRM) in the cat, *Experimental Brain Research*, **61**, 597–606.

REID, M. B., HAACK, K. E., FRANCHEK, K. M., VALBERG, P. A., KOBZIK, L. and WEST, M. S. 1992 Reactive oxygen in skeletal muscle, I: Intracellular oxidant kinetics and fatigue in vitro, *Journal of Applied Physiology*, **73**, 1797–804.

REID, M. B., SHOJI, T., MOODY, M. R. and ENTMAN, M. L. 1992 Reactive oxygen in skeletal muscle, II: Extracellular release of free radicals, *Journal of Applied Physiology*, **73**, 1805–9.

RIMEHAUG, T. and SVEBAK, S. 1987 Psychogenic muscle tension: The significance of motivation and negative affect in perceptual–cognitive task performance, *International Journal of Psychophysiology*, **5**, 97–106.

SAINSBURY, P. and GIBSON, J. G. 1954 Symptoms of anxiety and tension and the accompanying physiology changes in the muscular system, *Journal of Neurology, Neurosurgery and Psychiatry*, **37**, 216–24.

SCHOENEN, J. 1993 Exteroceptive suppression of temporalis muscle activity in patients with chronic headache and in normal volunteers: Methodology, clinical and pathophysiological relevance, *Headache*, **33**, 3–17.

SCHOENEN, J., JAMART, B., GERARD, P., LENARDUZZI, P. and DELWAIDE, P. J. 1987 Exteroceptive suppression of temporalis muscle activity in chronic headache, *Neurology*, **37**, 1834–6.

SCHOENEN, J., RAUBUCHL, O. and SIANARD, J. 1991 Pharmacologic modulation of temporalis exteroceptive silent periods in healthy volunteers, *Cephalagia* (Suppl. 11), **11**, 16–17.

SESSLE, B. J. and HU, J. W. 1981 Raphe-induced suppression of the jaw-opening reflex and single neurons in the trigeminal subnucleus oralis, and influence of naloxone and subnucleus caudalis, *Pain*, **10**, 19–36.

TAKALA, E.-P. and VIIKARI-JUNTURA, E. 1991 Muscular activity in simulated light work among subjects with frequent neck–shoulder pain, *International Journal of Industrial Ergonomics*, **8**, 157–64.

ULFHAKE, B., ARVIDSSON, U., CULLHEIM, S., HÖKFELT, T., BRODIN, E., VERHOFSTAD, A. and VISSER, T. 1987 An ultrastructural study of 5-hydroxytryptamine-, thyrotropin-releasing hormone- and substance P- immunoreactive axonal buttons in the motor nucleus of spinal cord segments L7–S1 in the adult cat, *Neuroscience*, **23**, 917–29.

VASSELJEN, O. and WESTGAARD, R. H. 1995 A case-control study of trapezius muscle activity in office and manual workers with shoulder and neck pain and symptom-free controls, *International Archives of Occupational and Environmental Health*, **67**, 11–18.

VASSELJEN, O., WESTGAARD, R. H. and LARSEN, S. 1995 A case-control study of psychological and psychosocial risk factors for shoulder and neck pain at the work place, *International Archives of Occupational and Environmental Health*, **66**, 375–82.

VEIERSTED, K.B. 1993 Sustained muscle tension as a risk factor for trapezius myalgia, in NIELSEN, R. and JORGENSEN, K. (Eds), *Advances in Industrial Ergonomics and Safety V*, pp. 15–19, London: Taylor & Francis.

VEIERSTED, K. B. and WESTGAARD, R. H. 1994 Subjectively assessed occupational and individual parameters as risk factors for trapezius myalgia, *International Journal of Industrial Ergonomics*, **13**, 235–45.

VEIERSTED, K. B., WESTGAARD, R. H. and ANDERSEN, P. 1990 Pattern of muscle activity during sterotyped work and its relation to muscle pain, *International Archives of Occupational and Environmental Health*, **62**, 31–41.

VEIERSTED, K. B., WESTGAARD, R. H. and ANDERSEN, P. 1993 Electromyographic evaluation of muscular work pattern as a predictor of trapezius myalgia, *Scandinavian Journal of Work, Environment and Health*, **19**, 284–90.

WÆRSTED, M., BJØRKLUND, R. A. and WESTGAARD R. H. 1991 Shoulder muscle tension induced by two VDU-based tasks of different complexity, *Ergonomics*, **34**, 137–50.

WÆRSTED, M., BJØRKLUND, R. A. and WESTGAARD, R. H. 1994 The effect of motivation on shoulder muscle tension in attention-demanding tasks, *Ergonomics*, **37**, 363–76.

WÆRSTED, M., EKEN, T. and WESTGAARD, R. H. 1993 Psychogenic motor unit activity: A possible muscle injury mechanism studied in a healthy subject, *Journal of Musculoskeletal Pain*, **1**, 185–90.

WALLASCH, T.-M. and GÖBEL, H. 1993 Exteroceptive suppression of temporalis muscle activity: Findings in headache, *Cephalagia*, **13**, 11–14.

WALLASCH, T.-M., NIEMANN, U., KROPP, P. and WEINSCHÜTZ, T. 1993 Exteroceptive silent periods of temporalis muscle activity: Correlation with neuropsychological findings, *Headache*, **33**, 121–4.

WALLASCH, T.-M., REINECKE, M. and LANGOHR, H.-D. 1991 EMG analysis of the late exteroceptive suppression period of temporal muscle activity in episodic and chronic tension-type headaches, *Cephalagia*, **11**, 109–12.

WESTGAARD, R. H. and BJØRKLUND, R. 1987 Generation of muscle tension additional to postural muscle load, *Ergonomics*, **30**, 911–23.

WESTGAARD, R. H. and JANSEN, T. 1992a Individual and work related factors associated with symptoms of musculoskeletal complaints, I: A quantitative registration system, *British Journal of Industrial Medicine*, **49**, 147–53.

WESTGAARD, R. H. and JANSEN, T. 1992b Individual and work-related factors associated with symptoms of musculoskeletal complaints, II: Different risk factors among sewing machine operators, *British Journal of Industrial Medicine*, **49**, 154–62.

WESTGAARD, R. H., JENSEN, C. and HANSEN, K. 1993a Individual and work-related risk factors associated with symptoms of musculoskeletal complaints, *International Archives of Occupational Environmental Health*, **64**, 405–13.

WESTGAARD, R. H., JENSEN, C. and NILSEN, K. 1993b Muscle coordination and choice–reaction time tests as indicators of occupational muscle load and shoulder–neck complaints, *European Journal of Applied Physiology and Occupational Physiology*, **67**, 106–14.

WINKEL, J. and WESTGAARD, R. H. 1992 Occupational and individual risk factors for shoulder-neck complaints Part II: The scientific basis (literature review) for the guide, *International Journal of Industrial Ergonomics*, **10**, 85–104.

CHAPTER SIX

Pathophysiology of cumulative trauma disorders

Some Possible Humoral and Nervous System Mechanisms

SIDNEY J. BLAIR

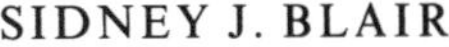

It has become evident that psychosocial factors appear to play a role in the development of cumulative trauma disorders (CTDs) (Berg *et al.*, 1991; NIOSH, 1990). The purpose of this paper is to discuss the pathophysiology of CTDs and to suggest that target organs could be sensitized and respond to various substances such as neuropeptides and neurotransmitters in an excessive way, in the presence of psychosocial stress. The various disorders of tissues will be described; the suggested manner in which the responses in these tissues may be modified by these substances will be elucidated.

SOFT TISSUE CHANGES ASSOCIATED WITH CTD

Some of the soft tissue and joint disorders include muscular disorders, tenosynovitis, synovitis, and peripheral nerve compressions (Armstrong *et al.*, 1987). Much is unknown about the relationship between specific stresses and cellular or tissue changes which underlie the different clinical conditions. In addition, some of the mechanisms described below may be interrelated and operational in more than one clinical condition. A common pathway appears to be the application of repetitive submaximal loads without allowing tissue to return to its resting state, or the too rapid application of load (Dobyns, 1991; Pitner, 1990).

Muscle pain (Hagberg, 1987; Sjogaard, 1990) and fatigue are the most common symptoms of CTDs. Muscular pain frequently follows acute trauma or muscular overexertion, or may also develop in a delayed manner from unaccustomed exercise or static loading. The precise mechanism for this pain is not yet established. Direct tissue injury, metabolic insufficiency secondary to lactic acid accumulation, or a local ischemic[1] state are all suspected mechanisms. With regard to the latter, muscle fibers undergo decrease in blood flow as a consequence of the increased tissue pressure associated with the muscle contraction. Another possible inciting event on the intracellular level has come to light through recent investigations of calcium release from the sarcoplasmic reticulum[2] (Hagberg, 1987; Imbriglia and Boland, 1984; Sjogaard, 1990). As cytosol-free calcium is increased, damage to the muscle cells can develop from the liberated free calcium. Mechanistic connections are not yet established, but a decrease in ATP[3] for pumping calcium and potassium ions across the membrane may occur with prolonged submaximal muscle tension and could be a link in the intracellular processes.

Synovitis of the tendon sheaths of the wrist and carpal tunnel are also frequently associated with repetitive loading. In a controlled study, Fuchs *et al.* (1991) identified obliteration of vessel lumens and edema[4] with minimal cellular involvement in tenosynovial biopses of patients undergoing operation for carpal tunnel syndrome. Schuind *et al.* (1990), studying similar histological specimens in carpal tunnel syndrome patients, found fibrous hyperplasia, increased amounts of collagen fiber, and localized necrotic areas. Based on these findings and review of related studies, these authors concluded that 'edema probably plays a major role in the pathogenesis of the disease (e.g. carpal tunnel syndrome), aggravating the swelling of the synovium, and therefore aggravating the friction in the carpal tunnel.' Schuind *et al.* were further of the opinion that their histological findings were typical of connective tissue undergoing degeneration following repeated mechanical stress. Castelli *et al.* (1980), studying cadaveric median nerve specimens, noted synovial membrane hyperplasia, arteriole and venous hypertrophy, endothelial reduplication, and increased epineural density in segments of the nerve which they postulated would be under greater mechanical stress.

Gelberman *et al.* (1981) identified a marked increase in canal pressure in carpal tunnel syndrome using the wick catheter in both flexion and extension. Szabo and Gelberman (1987) performed similar studies, finding increased pressure in the canal with flexion and extension of the wrist in carpal tunnel syndrome patients. More importantly, they noted prolonged pressure elevation and recovery times in the post-exercise period with carpal tunnel syndrome (CTS) patients as compared with the normal controls. Other investigators (Dahlin and Lundborg 1990; Carragee and Hentz, 1988), have found that low-level compression on peripheral nerves caused an impairment of microcirculation with subsequent increased oxygen depletion and leakage of fluids and proteins. This led to elevation of endoneural pressure, edema, and intraneural fibrosis.

Modulation of These Effects by the Nervous and Immune System

Next, a description of selected nervous system and immune system mechanisms will be presented with an explanation of how they might be activated subsequent to trauma and repetitive motion. Emphasis on these selected mechanisms stems largely from a need to better understand those challenging clinical cases characterized by persistent symptoms and ongoing problems.

Painful and nonpainful stimuli will cause discharge of sympathetic fibers,[5] releasing adrenergic chemicals which affect joints, muscle spindles, primary C-fibers, and the muscle itself (Levine, 1985; Levine *et al.*, 1988). In the joints, the postganglionic sympathetic fibers will discharge norepinephrine which will affect smooth muscle and secretory, lymphoid, and inflammatory cells. This is turn liberates proinflammatory agents such as prostaglandins. The C-fiber nociceptor[6] can be activated by various substances such as histamine, prostaglandin, substance P, neurokinin A, and calcitonin gene-related peptide; some of these substances also appear capable of activating immune cells.

These various factors appear to interact in ways that create complex and cyclical effects. For instance, these substances can exhibit 'reverse effects' on blood vessels (Heiby, 1988) causing either vasconstriction or vasodilatation and increasing capillary permeability (Hargreaves, 1990). As Payan (1992) reported, capillary permeability allows extravasation[7] of additional neuroactive and vasoactive substances such as bradykinin and serotonin. (See Figure 6.1.) These substances, if continually released, will cause the nerve endings to become increasingly sensitive, lowering their threshold to stimulation. This process, involving a lowered threshold and in which spontaneous pain can occur, is called sensitization. (See Figure 6.2.) Schaible and Schmidt (1986) showed that the nociceptors of joints and other synovial structures can become sensitized during inflammation.

With excessive C-fiber stimulation, there will be elaboration of various neuropeptides, such as substance P (Levine *et al.*, 1986; Levine *et al.*, 1988), which enhances histamine, prostaglandin and leukotriene release from mast cells. The release of substance P from the central dorsal horn can stimulate anterior horn cells and cause prolonged depolarization of those cells. With repetitive stimulation, the wide-dynamic-range neurons in the dorsal horn can be sensitized and will demonstrate an increased firing rate resulting in widespread pain.

We (Kijowski *et al.*, 1994) have recently studied the role of neuropeptides in the pathogenesis of CTDs at Loyola University Medical Center. The objective of this study was to investigate the role of several neuropeptides in the pathogenesis of CTDs of the upper extremity. The majority of the patients showed increased plasma

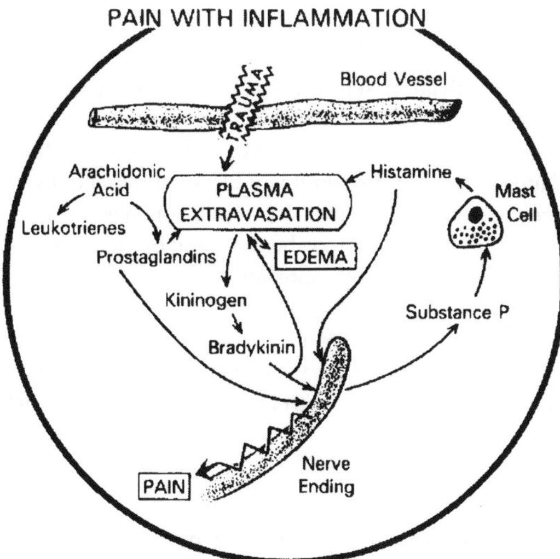

Figure 6.1 Schema of the positive-feedback relationship that develops during the course of inflammation secondary to sports-related injuries. (Reproduced, with permission, from K. M. Hargreaves, E. S. Troullos and R. A. Dionne, 1987, pharmacologic rationale for the treatment of acute pain, *Dent. Clin. North Am.* **31**, 675–94.)

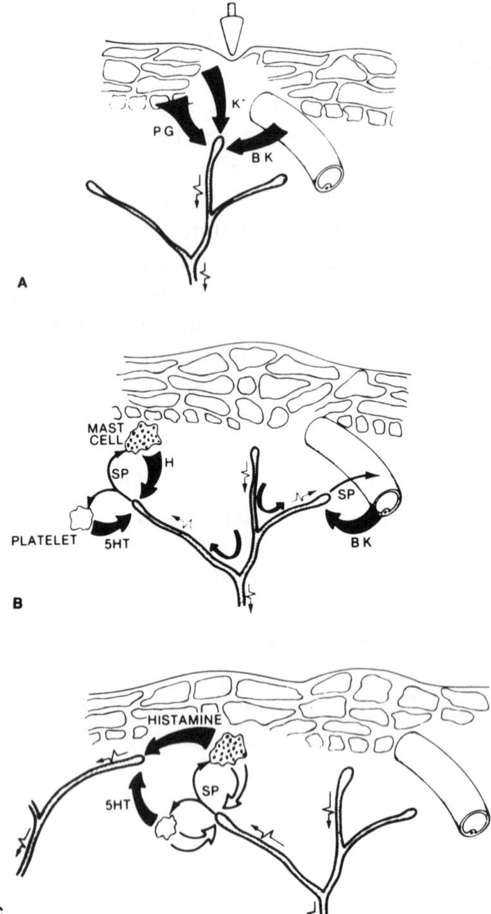

Figure 6.2 Events leading to activation, sensitization, and spread of sensitization of primary afferent nociceptor terminals. A. Direct activation by intense pressure and consequent cell damage. Cell damage leads to release of potassium (K +) and to synthesis of prostaglandins (PG) and bradykinin (BK). Prostaglandins increase the sensitivity of the terminal to bradykinin and other pain-producing substances. B. Secondary activation. Impulses generated in the stimulated terminal propagate not only to the spinal cord but into other terminal branches, where they induce the release of peptides including substance P (SP). Substance P causes vasodilation and neurogenic edema with further accumulation of bradykinin. Substance P also causes the release of histamine (H) from mast cells and serotonin (5HT) from platelets. C. Histamine and serotonin levels rise in the extracellular space, secondarily sensitizing nearby nociceptors. These leads to a gradual spread of hyperalgesia and/or tenderness. (Reproduced with permission of McGraw-Hill from Fields (1987).)

levels of bradykinin and calcitonin gene-related peptide, while one-half showed elevated levels of vasoactive intestinal peptide and neuropeptide Y (Kijowski *et al.*, 1994). If these substances are continually released they may cause nerve endings to display increased sensitivity to stimuli. It is hypothesized that, if an inflammatory mechanism is operative in some CTDs, these vasoactive peptides may be operative in those mechanisms.

The discipline of psychoneuroimmunology (Ader *et al.*, 1991) has demonstrated that there is a close interrelationship between the autonomic nervous system and the immune system. There is reason to suspect that stress factors may affect parts of the central nervous system which affect humoral factors possessing neuro-immunologic activity. These and other humoral factors may influence the transmission, modulation, and perception of pain. However, there is tremendous complexity to the scientific task of linking such psychological and emotional factors with biological mechanisms, clinical disease, and patient symptoms. It is well beyond the scope of this chapter to even outline the full scope of such a task or the science relevant to it.

IMPLICATIONS

Surgery for carpal tunnel syndrome will frequently cause exacerbation of pain in the tendon sheaths in the first carpo-metacarpal and the pisotriquetral joints, in the wrist and hand. There is also likely to be increased sensitivity of the skin in the region of the surgery. If these structures were mildly involved prior to surgery, the pain and swelling in these joints may be exacerbated. The shoulder may also respond with increased pain and limitation of motion. The recent use of endoscopic procedures, in which there is a smaller incision and less tissue trauma, may decrease some of these symptoms. Many surgical and nonsurgical patients have an excessive sympathetic response with pain, swelling, and thermoregulatory changes. These symptoms appear to resemble the condition called reflex sympathetic dystrophy (Veldman *et al.*, 1993).[8]

These clinical observations and some of the foregoing neuroimmunological discussion point to an inflammatory component in the pre- and post-surgical process, and in the decreased ability of these patients to exercise or perform repetitive activities. Steroids may be indicated for their anti-inflammatory effect. Early sympathetic nerve blocks and steroids may be particularly appropriate when a persistent pain syndrome has clinical features suggesting sympathetically maintained or sympathetically mediated pain. Similarly, the presence of edema and pain are indications for intervention in the patient's activities. While expert physical therapy with supervised reactivation is considered a mainstay in the treatment of sympathetically maintained pain syndromes, inordinate amounts of physical therapy or physical activity may exacerbate symptoms and adversely affect the underlying condition. With better understanding of these mechanisms and concerns, better modes of treatment should be developed, especially for the subset of CTD cases that do not respond readily to current conventional approaches.

NOTES

The author wishes to acknowledge help in the editing of this paper from one of his patients, Robert Piersanti, and his friend Walter A. Heiby, author of *The Reverse Effect*. The author also wishes to acknowledge Susan Shewczyk for her skillful technical assistance.

1 Ischemic refers to a relative deficiency of blood and the oxygen that it carries.

2 Sarcoplasmic reticulum is a structure within muscle cells.

3 ATP is adenosine triphosphate, an important compound in which the energy of a muscle is 'stored.'

4 Edema refers to fluid accumulation which can result in swelling (and increased pressure if the swelling occurs in a relatively closed compartment such as the carpal tunnel).

5 The sympathetic nervous system is part of the autonomic (as distinguished from voluntary) nervous system. Its influence is widespread throughout the body and is primarily exerted through the release of epinephrine (also known as adrenalin) into local tissues through the nerve endings of sympathetic fibers.

6 C-fibers are the most common type of peripheral nerves which carry 'pain messages' to the central nervous system. Nociceptor is a nerve receptor that is preferentially sensitive to stimuli that are noxious or would become noxious if prolonged (Merskey, 1986).

7 Extravasation is roughly equivalent to 'leaking out.'

8 Reflex sympathetic dystrophy (RSD), is a complex and somewhat puzzling disorder. The term 'sympathetically maintained pain' has been used (by some) in recent years to include not only classic RSD, but also to describe a broader range of cases displaying limited or borderline features of RSD. These cases, which some would argue are less typical versions of the classic, widely acknowledged, and full manifested forms of RSD, are subject to much wider difference of opinion.

REFERENCES

ADER, R., FELTEN, D. L. and COHEN, N. (Eds) 1991 *Psychoneuroimmunology*, San Diego, CA: Academic Press.

ARMSTRONG, T. J., FINE, L. J., GOLDSTEIN, S. A., LIFSHITZ, Y. R. and SILVERSTEIN, B. A. 1987 Ergonomic considerations in hand and wrist tendinitis, *Journal of Hand Surgery*, **12A**(2), 830–7.

BERG, M., ARNETZ, R. E., LIDEN, S., ENEROTH, P. and KALLNER, D. 1992 Technostress: psychophysiological study of employees with VDU-associated skin complaints, *JOM*, **34**(7).

CARRAGEE, E. J. and HENTZ V. R. 1988 Repetitive trauma and nerve compression, *Orthop. Clin. North Am.*, **19**(1), 157–64.

CASTELLI, W. A, EVANS, F. G., DIAZ-PEREZ, R. and ARMSTRONG, T. J. 1980 Intraneural connective tissue proliferation of the median nerve in the carpal tunnel arch, *Physical Medicine and Rehabilitation*, **61**, 418–22.

DAHLIN, L. B. and LUNDBORG, G. 1990 The neurone and its response to peripheral nerve compression, *Journal of Hand Surgery*, **15B**, 5–10.

DOBYNS, J. H. 1991 Cumulative trauma disorders of the upper limb, *Hand Clin.* **7**(3), 587–95.

FIELDS, H. L. 1987 *Pain*, New York: McGraw-Hill.

FRANKENHAEUSER, M. 1979 Psychoneuroendocrine approaches to the study of emotion as related to stress and coping, *Current Theory and Research in Motivation*, **26**, 123–62.

FUCHS, P. C., NATHAN, P. A. and MYERS, L. D. 1991 Synovial histology in carpal tunnel syndrome, *Journal of Hand Surgery*, **16A**, 753–8.

GELBERMAN, R. H., HERGENROEDER, P. T. and HARGENS, A. R. 1981 The carpal tunnel syndrome: A study of carpal canal pressures, *Bone Joint Surgery*, **63**, 380–3.

HAGBERG, M. 1987 Shoulder pain-pathogenesis, in HADLER, N. M. (Ed.), *Clinical Concepts in Regional Musculoskeletal Illness*, pp. 191–200, Orlando, FL: Grune & Stratton.

HARGREAVES, K. M. 1990 Mechanisms of pain sensation, in LEADBETTER, W. D. (Ed.), *Sports-Induced Inflammation: Clinical and Basic Science Concepts*, pp. 383–92, Park Ridge, IL: American Academy of Orthopedic Surgeons.

HEIBY, WALTER, H. 1988 *The Reverse Effect*, 1st Edn, pp. 55–81, Deerfield, IL: Medi-Science Publishers.

IMBRIGLIA, J. E. and BOLAND, D. M. 1984 An exercise-induced compartment syndrome of the dorsal forean: A case report, *Journal of Hand Surgery*, **9A**, 142–3.

KIJOWSKI, R., HOPPENSTEADT, D., CHINTHAGADA, M., CHEJFEU, M., FAREED, J. and BLAIR, S. 1994 Studies on the role of neuropeptides in the pathogenesis of cumulative trauma disorders, *J. Federation of American Societies for Experimental Biology*, **8**(4), 682.

LEVINE, J. D. 1985 Reflex neuroseptic inflammation, *Journal of Neuroscience*, **5**(5), 1380–5.

LEVINE, J. D., CODERRE, T. J. and HELMS, C. 1988 Beta-adrenergic mechanisms in experimental arthritis, *Proc. Natl. Acad. Sci. USA*, **85**, 4553–6.

LEVINE, J. D., FIELDS, H. and BASBAUM, A. 1993 Peptides and the primary afferent nociceptor, *Journal of Neuroscience*, **13**(6), 2273–86.

LEVINE, J. D., LAM, D. and TAIWO, Y. O. 1986 Hyperalgesic properties of 15-lipoxygenase products of arachidonic acid, *Proc. Natl. Acad. Sci. USA*, **83**, 5331–4.

LUNDBORG, G., MEYERS, R. and POWELL, H. 1983 Nerve compressions and increased fluid pressure: A 'miniature compartment syndrome,' *Journal of Neurosurgery and Psychiatry*, **46**, 119–24.

MERSKEY, H. 1986 Classification of chronic pain: Descriptions of chronic pain syndromes and definitions of pain terms, *Pain*, Suppl. 3, S215–S221.

NIOSH 1990 Health Hazard Evaluation Report, US West Communications, Phoenix, AZ, Minneapolis, MN, Denver, CO, Cincinnati, OH, US Department of Health and Human Services, Public Health Service Centers for Disease Control, *National Information for Safety and Health*, **89**, 299–2230.

PAYAN, D. G. 1992 The role of neuropeptides in EALLIN, S. I., GOLDSTEIN, I. M. and SNYDERMAN, R. (Eds), *Inflammation: Basic Principles, and Clinical Correlates*, 2nd Edn, New York: Raven Press.

PITNER, M. A. 1990 Pathophysiology of overuse injuries in the hand and wrist, *Hand Clin.*, **6**(3), 355–63.

SCHAIBLE, H. G. and SCHMIDT, R. F. 1986 Discharge characteristics of receptors with fine afferents from normal and inflamed joints: Influence of analgesics and prostaglandins, *Agents Actions*, **19**(Supp.), 99–117.

SCHUIND, F., VENTURA, M. and PASTEELS, J. L. 1990 Idiopathic carpal tunnel syndrome: Histologic study of flexor tendon synovium, *Journal of Hand Surgery*, **15A**, 497–503.

SJOGAARD, G. 1990 *Work-Induced Muscle Fatigue and its Relation to Muscle Pain*, Copenhagen: National Institute of Occupational Health.

STERNBERG, F. M. (Moderator), CHORUSUS, G. P., WILDER, R. L. and GOLD, P. W. (Discussants) 1992 NIH Conference: The stress response and regulation of inflammatory disease, *Annals of Internal Medicine*, **117**(10), 854–84.

SZABO, R. M. and GELBERMAN, R. H. 1987 The pathophysiology of nerve entrapment syndromes, *Journal of Hand Surgery*, **12A**(5) 880–4.

VELDMAN, H. J. M., REYNEN, H. M., ARNTZ, I. F. and GORIS, R. J. A. 1993 Signs of symptoms of reflex sympathetic dystrophy: Prospective study of 829 patients, *Lancet*, **342**, 1012–16.

CHAPTER SEVEN

Psychosocial factors and musculoskeletal disorders

Summary and Implications of Three NIOSH Health Hazard Evaluations of Video Display Terminal Work

JOSEPH J. HURRELL JR., BRUCE P. BERNARD, THOMAS R. HALES, STEPHEN L. SAUTER and EDWARD J. HOEKSTRA

INTRODUCTION

The National Institute for Occupational Safety and Health (NIOSH) has had a long-standing interest in the potential health effects of work with video display terminals (VDTs). Musculoskeletal disorders, in particular, have been of special concern (NIOSH, 1991). From the beginning, it was suspected that work-related psychosocial factors contribute to the development of musculoskeletal disorders associated with VDT work. As a consequence, an assessment of psychosocial factors was incorporated into the study designs of three recent NIOSH Health Hazard Evaluations (HHEs) which assessed musculoskeletal disorders and their related risk factors among employees utilizing VDTs. While these three studies differed in numerous ways, a common aspect of each was a relatively broad-based assessment of job stress factors, often called job stressors, felt to have some potential involvement in the etiology of the musculoskeletal disorders. Using similar, and in some cases identical, multi-item measures, these studies assessed the potential contribution of such stressors as perceived job pressure, workload, workload variability, cognitive demands, job control, job security, hostility from clients, and electronic monitoring to musculoskeletal disorders. This chapter provides a summary of these three HHEs.

TELECOMMUNICATIONS STUDY I

In 1992, the American Federation of Government Employees (AFGE) request an evaluation of work-related upper-extremity (UE) musculoskeletal disorders among teleservice representatives at Social Security Administration Teleservice Centers (TSCs) nationwide (Hoekstra *et al.*, 1994). The request was made as a result of concerns regarding what appeared to be excess levels of such disorders among employees performing this type of work. The job of teleservice representative involves responding to toll-free calls for assistance and requires both keyboard data entry and computer and manual searches for information. Telephone lines are staffed from 7 a.m. to 7 p.m. and computer systems automatically route incoming calls to the next available representative. Representatives typically have less than one second between calls. Throughout the day, a computer system monitors the number and length of calls taken by the representatives. Calls are also monitored by a supervisor for accuracy of information provided to the customer.

To address AFGE's concerns, a cross-sectional survey study was conducted at 2 of the 37 total TSCs. The two centers selected for study (Boston and Fort Lauderdale) were thought to be typical of other centers throughout the United States with respect to the type of equipment used and the demographics of the employees. The study focused on UE musculoskeletal disorders, which were assessed using self-report symptom questionnaires. In addition, the questionnaire solicited information on worker demographics, individuals factors (extant medical conditions, and nonwork activities), and job stressors. The physical workstations were assessed by the NIOSH study team using checklists of workstation configurations. Of the 114 eligible teleservice representatives employed at the facilities, all 108 at work on the days of the investigation completed the self-administered survey questionnaire (100 per cent participation). The mean age of the study participants was 42 years; 64 per cent were female. The mean seniority on the current job was 4.7 years.

Five types of UE musculoskeletal disorders were defined for analysis based upon self-reports of frequency, duration, and intensity of symptoms and absence of prior injury. These were: neck, shoulder, elbow, hand–wrist, and back disorders. For each of the body areas, a disorder was considered present if any symptoms (pain, numbness, tingling, aching, stiffness, or burning) in the affected part occurred within the preceding year and all of the following applied: (1) there was no preceding acute, nonoccupational injury (such as dislocation, fracture, or tendon tear); (2) symptoms began after starting the current job; (3) symptoms lasted for more than one week or occurred at least once a month within the past year; (4) symptoms were reported as 'moderate' (the midpoint) or worse on a five-point intensity scale. Sixty-eight per cent of the participants reported symptoms that met the case definition for at least one of the five disorders considered: neck, shoulder, elbow, hand–wrist, or back disorders. The prevalence was: neck – 44 per cent, shoulder – 35 per cent, elbow – 20 per cent, hand–wrist – 30 per cent, and back – 33 per cent.

Multiple logistic regression models were built to identify risk factors for the five musculoskeletal disorders. This technique determines the degree of association between predictor variables and outcome variables. A model was built for each of the five outcome variables. Numerous individual and job variables were found to be predictive of the five musculoskeletal outcome measures in the final regression models. Of relevance here, two job stressors were found to be significantly associated with musculoskeletal disorders. Workload variability (or surges in workload) was found to be associated with neck disorders, while job control was found to be inversely associated with back disorders. Workload variability was also found to be associated with self-reported physical and mental exhaustion.

TELECOMMUNICATIONS STUDY II

In 1989, NIOSH received a joint HHE request from the Communications Workers of America and US West Communications to examine the effects of VDT work on musculoskeletal disorders among Directory Assistance Operators (DAOs). To address this concern, a cross-sectional study of 533 telecommunications workers (including DAOs and workers from four additional job classifications) from three different metropolitan areas in the United States was undertaken (Hales *et al.*, 1992).

This investigation focused on the UE musculoskeletal system which, as in the teleservice representatives study reported above, was assessed using a symptom questionnaire. However, unlike the study reported above, this study also included a physical examination. Ninety per cent of the 573 selected employees participated in the study. The mean age of the participants was 38 years, and the mean tenure in current job was 6 years. Seventy-eight per cent of the participants were female.

Two types of musculoskeletal outcomes were considered: (1) potential work-related UE *disorders* defined by physical examination *and* by questionnaire (based on self-reports of frequency, duration, and intensity of symptoms and absence of prior injury), and (2) UE musculoskeletal *symptoms* defined by (the same) questionnaire alone (based upon a cumulative score of symptom frequency, duration, and intensity).

Twenty-two per cent of participants met the case definition for potential work-related UE *disorders*. Probable tendon-related disorders were the most common (15 per cent of cases). Probable nerve entrapment syndromes represented less than 5 per cent of cases. The hand–wrist was the UE area most affected (12 per cent of participants), followed by the neck area (9 per cent), elbow area (7 per cent), and shoulder (6 per cent).

Relationships between workplace factors and UE *disorders* were examined using multiple logistic regression. Separate models were generated for each of the four UE areas (neck, shoulder, elbow, hand–wrists). Relationships between workplace factors and the magnitude of UE *symptoms* were examined using multiple linear regression. Separate models were generated for each of the same four UE areas.

A number of individual and job variables were found to be predictive of the two types of musculoskeletal outcomes in the final regressions models. However, most of the significant predictors had only modest elevations in odds ratios, or explained only modest amounts of the variance in the outcome measures. Of particular interest, job stressor variables denoting intensified workload (e.g. increasing work pressure, high levels of information processing, demands and workload variability) were associated with increased UE *disorders* (particularly neck *disorders*). All three of these stressors were also significantly associated with UE *symptoms*. (Alternatively, self-reports of overtime work and increasing hours of VDT work were associated with decreased UE *symptoms*.) UE *symptoms* were also found to be buffered by increased social support from co-workers and supervisors.

Five of the 11 variables measuring workers' perceptions of the effects of electronic performance monitoring were found to be related to increased UE *symptoms*. However, no significant relationships were found between these measures and UE *disorders*. UE *symptoms* were most common among workers who perceived the monitoring system to adversely affect social and supervisory relationships, and to cause increased workload and reduced motivation.

Information to estimate the total keystrokes per day was available for 174 (71 per cent) of the DAOs. Increasing total keystrokes per day was not associated with either UE *disorders* or *symptoms*. However, the low number of keystrokes performed per day by DAOs (mean = 15,950 or 35 per minute) and the low variability of keystrokes among the participants limit the ability to generalize these results to other VDT workers such as data entry operators who may perform many times this number of keystrokes per day.

Analyses of postural and workstation design factors were precluded by methodological limitation including high intercorrelation among the predictor variables, limited variability in several predictors, and the fact that DAOs were not assigned to specific workstations (thus reducing the reliability of exposure measurements).

NEWSPAPER STUDY

In 1989, the *Los Angeles Times* newspaper submitted a request to NIOSH for assistance in evaluating UE musculoskeletal disorders among employees performing VDT work at two facilities (Bernard *et al.*, 1993). The editorial staff of the newspaper speculated that the introduction of VDTs and a keyboard specifically designed for use in the editorial department may have been responsible for an increase in musculoskeletal disorders. To assess the nature and distribution of employee UE symptoms, and possible causal factors, four departments (Circulation, Classified Advertising, Accounting and Finance, and Editorial) were selected for study.

Phase I

In the first phase of this two phase study, UE symptoms were evaluated using a self-administered questionnaire, and cases of UE disorders were defined, as in the first telecommunications study reported above, by questionnaire alone (i.e. using frequency, duration, and intensity of symptoms in the affected area, and absence of previous injury). As in the two studies discussed above, the questionnaire was used to obtain information on worker demographics and individual factors, job tasks, and job stress. As in the previous studies, physical ergonomic aspects of the workstation and workplace were assessed; however, circumstances (ongoing workstation and office redesign) precluded the reliable use of these data as risk factors for UE disorders.

Ninety-three per cent of the 1,050 eligible employees participated in this phase of the study. The mean age of participants was 39 years and the mean seniority on the current job was 11 years. Fifty-six per cent of the participants were female. Forty-one per cent of participants reported symptoms meeting the case definition for at least one UE disorder. Neck symptoms (26 per cent) were the most frequently reported, followed by hand–wrist symptoms (22 per cent), shoulder symptoms (17 per cent), and elbow symptoms (10 per cent). Employees in the Editorial Department had the lowest prevalence of UE disorders (38 per cent) for the four departments studied.

Multiple logistic regression models were built to identify risk factors for UE symptoms in the neck, shoulder, and hand–wrist. As in the DAO study reported above, variables corresponding to perceived increased workload demands (e.g. increased time working under deadline, increased job pressure) were found to be associated with increased neck, shoulder, or hand–wrist symptoms. A dose–effect relationship was found between time spent working at the VDT and reporting of hand–wrist symptoms. As in the DAO study, these effects were buffered by higher levels of supervisory support.

In the overall logistic models, which included individuals from all departments, the job stress factors were less powerful predictors of disorders compared to job tasks and demographic variables. However, in departments with higher concentration of clerical and data-entry VDT operators, job stressors were more important predictors of neck, shoulder, and hand–wrist disorders. In contrast, there were no significant job stressor predictors in the regression models for hand–wrist disorders in the Editorial Department where jobs involve higher job control, worker participation, and a variety of tasks. To investigate this discrepancy, job stress scores were examined across departments. Results indicated that consistently more favorable conditions were reported by workers in the Editorial Department (although workload demands were high) compared to those in the Circulation Department where jobs were characterized by more clerical tasks. These results suggest that the reduced salience of job stressors as predictors among the editorial staff may be due to reduced exposure to stressful conditions.

Phase 2

In the second phase of this investigation, a case-control study was conducted to determine whether the risk factors for hand–wrist disorders identified in Phase 1 could be confirmed using a more restrictive case definition. Randomly selected cases who fulfilled the criteria for a hand–wrist disorder on the Phase 1 questionnaire were compared to controls with respect to results of physical examination of the hands and wrists and nerve conduction velocity (NCV) testing.

One hundred and thirty participants were randomly selected from the hand–wrist cases identified via questionnaire in the first phase of the study. Likewise, 99 participants reporting no UE symptoms were randomly selected as controls. Upon physical examination, 53 per cent of cases and 12 per cent of controls had one or more positive hand–wrist findings. As in the DAO's study, tendon-related cases were the most common (over 46 per cent of cases).

As in the first phase of the study, multiple logistic regression models were constructed to identify risk factors associated with the more restrictive hand–wrist case definition which involved both positive physical findings and the questionnaire criteria. The results were consistent with Phase I findings in that both female gender and increased time spent typing at the VDT were among the important predictors of disorders. Both a perceived increase in hours spent typing during the last year and a perceived change in overall workload during the past year were found to be significantly associated with increased disorders.

CONCLUSIONS

Overall, the results of these three studies add to the growing body of evidence linking psychosocial factors, in this case job stress factors, to musculoskeletal disorders among office workers who use VDTs. In particular, these studies suggest that perceived work pressure and variability in workload are salient predictors of UE disorders (particularly neck disorders). The causal mechanisms linking the psychosocial environment at work to musculoskeletal disorders is clearly not well understood (see Chapter 1 of this volume). However, several possible mechanisms can be postulated. The perception of stressful conditions (i.e. job stressors) may increase the awareness (and possibility of over reporting) of musculoskeletal symptoms or may affect perceptions regarding their cause (i.e. increased attribution to the workplace). Alternatively and/or additionally, stressful job conditions may be associated with more physically (i.e. biomechanically) demanding situations or may produce increased muscle tension and consequent biomechanical strain caused by stress-induced static muscle loads (Aronsson *et al.*, 1992). This increased static load may be especially prominent in the neck and shoulder girdle muscles (Arndt, 1987).

All three studies reported here suffer from a number of inherent weaknesses. Cross-sectional studies cannot determine whether self-reported working conditions are causally related to musculoskeletal outcomes nor the direction of causation. In each study there was also the potential for a problem with 'survivor bias,' that is, not including people who left their jobs because of the problems of interest (i.e. job stressors, musculoskeletal disorders). The possibility for statistically significant associations due to chance alone (i.e. Type I error) must be considered, given the large number of analyses performed. Finally, these studies did not assess the impact of nonwork-related variables and their possible association with musculoskeletal disorders. For example such factors as childcare, home responsibilities, or recreational activities, which were not addressed, may have some impact on the occurrence of musculoskeletal symptoms and disorders.

The three studies discussed in this chapter were conducted as HHEs and were therefore each aimed at answering specific practical questions posed to NIOSH by the HHE requestors. For example, were there excess musculoskeletal problems at the particular worksites studied, what were the causes of musculoskeletal disorders at the worksite, and what could be recommended to reduce the risk of developing such problems? The studies were clearly not meant to address definitively the role of psychosocial factors in the development of musculoskeletal disorders and they clearly underscore methodological difficulties that interfere with advancement in this area. Yet, despite the limited scope of these studies and their inherent weaknesses, they consistently point to workload and variance in workload as factors that are associated with musculoskeletal disorders.

As alluded to above, a major problem in linking job stress factors to musculoskeletal disorders is the reliance on retrospective studies to the near exclusion of longitudinal or prospective and follow-up designs. Second, while the studies reported here used similar measures, there is a general need for researchers to use more standardized methods for assessing psychosocial risk factors on the job (see Hurrell *et al.*, 1988) and musculoskeletal symptoms and disorders. There is also clearly a need for use of collateral measures for assessing working conditions. These measures should go far beyond self-reports of job incumbents and include assessments by co-workers and managers and objective measures which might be obtained through job or ergonomic analyses. Representative sampling procedures and replications are clearly needed to ensure that the findings will have general application. For example, the use of multiple worksites or industries in the investigation of a particular occupation is desirable. Finally, increased use of advanced statistical methods, such as structural analysis, to improve the understanding of causal mechanisms and pathways is required.

REFERENCES

ARNDT, R. H. 1987 Work pace, stress and cumulative trauma disorders, *Journal of Hand Surgery*, **12**, 866–71.

ARONSSON, G., BERGQVIST, U. and ALERS, A. 1992 *Work Reorganization and Musculoskeletal Discomfort in VDT Work*, Stockholm: Arbetarskyddverket.

BERNARD, B., SAUTER, S. L., PETERSEN, M., FINE, L. and HALES, T. 1993 *HETA Report 90-013-2277*, Los Angeles, CA: Los Angeles Times; Cincinnati, OH: National Institute for Occupational Safety and Health.

HALES, T., SAUTER, S., PETERSEN, M., PUTZ-ANDERSON, V., FINE, L., OCHS, T., SCHLEIFER, L. and BERNARD, B. 1992 *HETA Report 89-299-2239*, US West Communications Phoenix, Arizona Minneapolis, Minnesota Denver, Colorado. Cincinnati, OH: National Institute for Occupational Safety and Health.

HOEKSTRA, E. J., HURRELL, J. J., JR. and SWANSON, N. G. 1994 *HETA Report 92-0382-2450*, Social Security Administration Teleservice Centers Boston, Massachusetts Fort Lauderdale, Florida. Cincinnati, Ohio: National Institute for Occupational Safety and Health.

HURRELL, J. J., JR., MURPHY, L. R., SAUTER, S. L. and COOPER, C. L. 1988 *Occupational Stress: Issues and Developments*, New York: Taylor & Francis.

NATIONAL INSTITUTE FOR OCCUPATIONAL SAFETY AND HEALTH 1991 NIOSH publications on video display terminals (revised). Cincinnati, OH: DTMD.

PART TWO

Issues for Management, Prevention, and Further Research

CHAPTER EIGHT

A psychosocial view of cumulative trauma disorders

Implications for Occupational Health and Prevention

S. D. MOON

Cumulative trauma disorder (CTD) has become the most common, costly, and disabling category of occupational illness in the United States, affecting a wide spectrum of business and industry (USDL, 1994).[1] Musculoskeletal pain and related disability creates massive human and financial cost for society, whether its origins are personal, work-related, or somewhere in between (IOM, 1991; Magni, 1993). Much remains unsettled regarding distribution of this cost (Walsh, 1991) and the associated responsibility for prevention (Millar, 1988). In the United States, these unsettled issues lie squarely amidst a larger societal dialogue about distributing illness costs and health-care controls among individuals, government, and employers (Deyo *et al.*, 1991; Salmon, 1990).

The size and notoriety of the CTD problem creates a powerful demand for prevention policy response. Some argue that responding through broad regulation of the workplace lacks a sufficient scientific basis (Sandler, 1993). Increasing research of occupational CTD should rapidly expand that scientific basis and resulting regulatory precision. However, the CTD phenomenon may be inseparable from its sociocultural context (see Chapter 9 of this volume). Although biomedical science traditionally defines the limits of disease and injury, society defines illness and influences the response to it (Eisenberg, 1977; Tarlov, 1988; Waxler, 1981). Tension between these roles continually challenges paradigms of disease and illness.[2] Where illness diverges from traditional standards of measurable disease or where the boundaries of either are shifting, biomedicine is prodded to look deeper and reconsider its standards. In that setting, nonbiomedical explanations (e.g. psychosocial influences) also receive more consideration.

Occupational CTD is partly defined by prior exposure to noninstantaneous biomechanical stressors. These stressors appear linked to the manifestation of CTD in clearly important ways. Clinically, the timing between these stressors and subsequent symptoms is often compelling. These links have been long suspected and anecdotally described for numerous occupations (Putz-Andersen, 1988; Ramazzinni, 1713). Various associations have been epidemiologically characterized (see Andersson, 1981; Dimberg *et al.*, 1989; English *et al.*, 1995; Hagberg *et al.*, 1992;

Hales, 1994; Stock, 1991). Cross-sectional data is often based on subjective symptom reports, sometimes enhanced with clinical exams (i.e. Silverstein *et al.*, 1987). Some studies (mostly with carpal tunnel syndrome or osteoarthritic conditions) have also incorporated objective outcome measures other than physical exam, yielding 'positive' (Barnhart *et al.*, 1991; Osorio *et al.*, 1994; Stenlund *et al.*, 1992; Stetson *et al.*, 1993), 'negative' (Schottland *et al.*, 1991), and controversial or inconclusive (Hadler, 1978; Nathan *et al.*, 1988; Nathan, 1992) findings in terms of supporting causal links to work. Using a unique CTD study design, Moore and Garg (1994) demonstrated a positive association between biomechanical risk factors and clinically determined CTDs other than carpal tunnel syndrome (CTS), although no statistically significant association with CTS was demonstrated. Pathophysiological explanations for certain CTD conditions have been suggested (Armstrong *et al.*, 1984; Parniapour *et al.*, 1990; Pitner, 1990; Schuind *et al.*, 1990); other studies have cast doubt on specific aspects of commonly suspected mechanisms (Fuchs *et al.*, 1991). 'Overuse syndromes' in sports medicine provide a non-occupational parallel for some clinical syndromes and conceptual models relating to the occupational arena (Pitner, 1990).

However, many uncertainties remain. In some work settings, biomechanical stressors may strongly predict an excess of CTD diagnoses. In other settings, biomechanics alone does not seem to explain the observed CTD phenomenon. Other causes have been suggested and explored (Cannon *et al.*, 1981; de Krom *et al.*, 1990; Nathan, 1990; Vessey *et al.*, 1990; Werner *et al.*, 1994), including psychosocial factors (Bernard *et al.*, 1993; Faucett and Rempel, 1994; Hales *et al.*, 1992; Leino, 1989; World Health Organization, 1989; see also Chapters 1, 4, 5, and 7 of this volume). Cause and cure for the CTD problem remains controversial and complex, especially in the office environment. The issue provokes questions that existing epidemiologic data and basic science cannot yet answer. It highlights weaknesses in traditional case definitions, outcome measures, exposure assessments, and causation concepts for musculoskeletal pain disorders (Cunningham and Kelsey, 1984). For instance, should the defining threshold for CTD be dysfunction, pain/discomfort, or damage? Is there a verifiable continuum between the three? What are safe or hazardous levels of exposure to biomechanical stressors? Should CTD resolution be measured by absence of pain or by correction of measurable damage or dysfunction? (Moon, 1993b).

The CTD phenomenon fundamentally challenges paradigms by which society defines, adjudicates, and tries to reduce pain and suffering reflected in a host of musculoskeletal problems. For many work settings, and especially the office environment, CTD has demanded a rapid awakening to new complexities of occupational health and safety. The meaning and significance of CTD varies considerably with the perspective and role of the person, agency, or study using the term. This chapter seeks to bridge these perspectives by addressing selected dilemmas and opportunities. The pitfalls are many, starting with terminology.

WHAT IS A PSYCHOSOCIAL FACTOR?

Those who have not a thorough insight into both the signification and purpose of words will be under chances, amounting almost to certainty, of reasoning or inferring incorrectly.

John Stuart Mill

The purpose of words is to convey ideas. When the ideas are grasped, the words are forgotten. Where can I find a man who has forgotten words? He is the one I would like to talk to.

Chuang Tzu

'Psychosocial' is simply defined as pertaining to mental or psychological as well as social aspects (Taylor, 1988; Mish, 1991). The term conveys a variety of meanings, sometimes unclearly specified, across different sources. Sauter and Swanson (Chapter 1 of volume) expand on the definition and bring needed clarification. Commonly recognized psychosocial factors include nonphysical aspects of the work environment or social milieu, often as reflected in expressed thoughts, feelings, perceptions, attitudes, and other behaviors. These factors can be loosely viewed in three categories, which clearly overlap and interrelate:

1. *Objective work environment* Factors relatively inherent to the workplace itself and *somewhat* objectifiable, as distinguishable from related effects, perceptions, and reactions in affected workers: i.e. job demands and controls, monotonous work, time pressure, lack of job clarity, etc. (Bongers *et al.*, 1993).
2. *Responses to inquiry* These focus more upon worker perceptions that are dependent upon or sensitive to workplace characteristics: i.e. 'job satisfaction' (Bigos, 1991), 'Do you regard your work as interesting and stimulating?'
3. *Measures of pre-existing and presumably personal characteristics* These reflect features that are more inherent, stable, and viewed as individually variable: i.e. personality type, coping styles, attitudes toward health, social class, psychological dysfunction (Bongers *et al.*, 1993).

Some chapters in this book address potential influences that, strictly speaking, are not primarily and purely psychosocial. For instance, workstyle (see Chapter 11 of this volume) may reflect *interaction* between individual characteristics and the objective or perceived characteristics of the work environment. Other behavior patterns may partly result from psychological or social factors, but arguably reflect economic and cultural influences as well. For example, 'pain behaviors' (Brena and Chapman, 1981) may reflect interaction between psychological characteristics, cultural context, and feedback from the social milieu. In that vein, certain behaviors might be viewed as important *avenues* through which the interaction of these multiple factors could be expressed. Taken as a whole, several contributions to this volume suggest a complex interactive web between primary workplace psychosocial factors, their avenues of expression, and the larger economic and cultural milieu. Operational definitions of 'psychosocial influences' may thus depend on the expansiveness of one's mechanistic hypotheses (see Chapters 1, 3, 4, 9, 12, and 14 of this volume).

As this and other chapters will make clear, the relative importance assigned to certain nonbiophysical (e.g. psychosocial or quasi-psychosocial) factors depends greatly on the 'stage' of the CTD problem being considered. Primary prevention and most CTD research tends to focus on objective workplace characteristics and employee perceptions of the workplace. Fine (1994) notes the epidemiologic difficulties of doing otherwise. The study of tertiary (e.g. disability) prevention and chronic musculoskeletal pain frequently expands the focus to *individual* psychosocial factors (Colligan *et al.*, 1988; Leavitt, 1990; Polatin *et al.*, 1989) and influences from outside the work environment (Derebery and Tullis, 1983; Stutts and Kasdan, 1993).

The structures and dynamics of compensating health-care providers and Workers' Compensation claimants may conceivably affect critical perceptions and behaviors, although the influences themselves are largely rooted in culture, politics, and economics (Butler, 1983; Hadler, 1989; Lundeen, 1989; Mendelson 1993; Oshfeldt, 1993; Worrall, 1983).

WHAT IS CTD?

As complexity rises, precise statements lose meaning and meaningful statements lose precision.

P. McNeill and Frieberger, *Fuzzy Logic*

Exploring this topic requires alertness to different meanings conveyed by the CTD label, which is widely recognized but biomedically imprecise. Sharply divergent impressions about occupational CTD may partly be due to differences in the observed mix of clinical conditions or populations and settings in which they occur. The following descriptions of 'CTD' reflect some of its qualities, criteria, or implications.

An Etiologic Hypothesis that Creates an Umbrella

Several terms largely synonymous with CTD are in common usage; these include repetitive strain injury, repetitive motion illness, occupational overuse, or overexertion syndromes. Each conveys an important element of an etiological hypothesis and creates an umbrella, covering a variety of traditional medical diagnoses and clinical presentations. This hypothesis, its underlying assumptions, and related methods of investigation are increasingly incorporated, but remain controversial (Freeman, 1990; Hadler, 1990; Nathan, 1992).

A List of Diagnostic and/or Injury Codes

Some lists of CTD diagnoses are derived from published reports of suspected or demonstrated associations, based on clinical observations or (predominantly) cross-sectional studies (Putz-Anderson, 1988). Some researchers and authors create specific lists with mixtures of selected three- and four-digit International Classification of Disease (ICD) codes (see Hales, 1994; Park *et al.*, 1992); others define similar groups of physician diagnoses considered 'soft-tissue disorders' (i.e. English *et al.*, 1995). One CTD case definition in a Workers' Compensation claims study required both specific diagnoses (tenosynovitis, bursitis, neuritis, and ganglion) and a documented judgment that injury occurred over a prolonged period through overexertion, as opposed to impact (Tanaka *et al.*, 1988).

A Continuum of Severity and Irreversibility

Browne *et al.* (1984) suggested that the symptoms of 'repetition strain injuries' could be categorized in four stages; with physical signs, persistent symptoms when off work, possible sleep disturbance, and greater chronicity occurring only in latter stages. Chaffin (1991) describes a similar four-stage progression in the occupational CTD and suggests biomechanically based prevention strategies between each stage. The Nirschl Pain Phase Scale ranks the manifestations of 'overuse syndrome' into seven progressively severe categories (O'Connor *et al.*, 1994; Wilder *et al.*, 1993). Although Nirschl's scale arose in a sports medicine context related to musculotendinous problems, it adds conceptual support to the commonly echoed and compelling assertion that early intervention is critical to CTD outcome.

A Potentially Multifactorial Problem

Individuals who present with musculoskeletal pain or paresthesia associated with work activity may display more than one CTD diagnosis type. These diagnoses may simply coexist or be related in various ways. One may precede and directly precipitate the other (e.g. flexor tendonitis and carpal tunnel syndrome). They may coexist and lower the threshold for the manifestation of each other (e.g. cervical root disorders and distal compression neuropathies – see Dahlin and Lundborg, 1990). Pain symptoms may develop in previously asymptomatic areas due to increased or awkward compensatory patterns of use. Non-CTD diagnoses may interact to increase susceptibility, delay recovery, or increase severity of CTDs (e.g. diabetes, obesity, tobacco use, and circulatory problems). Such non-CTD diagnoses (e.g. diabetes) may provide an 'alternative' (e.g. nonwork-related) causal explanation. The legal perspective sometimes forces a distinction as to whether such conditions are 'alternative' and predominant *causes* versus the basis of increased *susceptibility* to primary causation by work (Moon, 1993a, 1993c; Vessey *et al.*, 1990).

When symptoms persist or the clinical findings are nonspecific and imprecise, an intensified search for explanations may reveal 'abnormalities' which can neither be conclusively accepted nor excluded as causes for the presenting clinical problem (e.g. X-ray evidence of degenerative changes in the cervical spine in the setting of arm pain). Through these and other mechanisms, an individual presenting with suspected CTD can acquire multiple diagnoses due to different physicians' opinions or as the manifestations evolve. Some professionals view some types of CTD as a dysfunctional 'anatomic unit'. This unit conceptually includes the entire muscle-tendon unit, its bony attachments, and the surrounding neurovascular environment – plus the biomechanical effects of distant but functionally related musculoskeletal elements (see MacKinnon and Novak, 1995).

In short, the realities of clinical practice force the reduction of sometimes complex pain problems into primary diagnostic categories. Studies of diagnostic consistency between examiners are virtually nonexistent for most musculoskeletal problems. Thus, one examiner's 'tendonitis' may differ from another's and the resulting aggregate data sources may fail to reflect underlying variables that are important in causation and outcome.

Anatomically Diverse Problems with Differing Levels of Objective Verifiability

With respect to the upper extremity, Cherniak (1994) suggests three categories:

- anatomically defined and pathophysiologically quantifiable (i.e. carpal tunnel syndrome);

- anatomically defined and semi-quantifiable (i.e. tendonitis);
- anatomically nonspecific (upper-extremity pain syndromes in some office-work outbreaks).

In practice, there is ample room for controversy about what constitutes quantifiability and anatomic specificity in a particular pain syndrome. Such decisions probably vary with experience, examination techniques, interpretation of the patient's responses to examination, beliefs about pathophysiology, and judgments as to what findings on physical exam are significantly abnormal. For example, almost 90 per cent of cases in an Australian study of office workers exhibited 'tender points' insufficient in number to support the diagnosis of 'fibrositis' (by definition, an anatomically diffuse condition). Its authors (Miller and Topliss, 1988) did not interpret those tender points as supporting a *regional* myofascial pain syndrome or '*localized* fibromyalgia' diagnosis. Other practitioners would probably have disagreed (Granges and Littlejohn, 1993; Travell and Simons, 1983). There appears to be a recent trend towards physician acceptance of *generalized* fibrositis (fibromyalgia) as an entity (Wolfe *et al.*, 1990). *Local or regional* myofascial pain is a different (though arguably related) entity, which is more commonly suspected or identified by some practitioners in a CTD context. The inclusion of various forms of myofascial pain under the CTD umbrella remains controversial (Whorton *et al.*, 1992); but the issue of work-related myofascial pain encapsulates some crucial problems. This entity showcases certain legal, scientific, and practical difficulties presented by the CTD concept, especially when the CTD falls into the 'anatomically nonspecific' category. These difficulties include distinction between pain, dysfunction, and damage; reliability of case definitions for testing the CTD hypothesis; and determination of the point where the postulated effects of cumulative trauma have resolved even if pain persists.

A Disability Process

Disability is part and parcel of CTD in a special sense. Sudden (non-CTD) musculoskeletal injury may result from accidental, atypical, and presumably nonrecurring causes. However, the ergonomic risk factors for CTD are defined as *inherent* to the job and presumably capable of causing further harm unless modified. Each CTD case thus invokes the question of 'disability', albeit temporary and/or limited to specific work activities or demands.

A Legally Defined Portion of all Relations between Work and Activity-related Pain Syndromes

Different types of work–pain interactions create different responsibilities for the employer. These roughly reduce to three categories which are progressively inclusive, as depicted in Figure 8.1.

A. CTD which meets applicable Workers' Compensation standards.

B. OSHA-recordable CTD.[3]

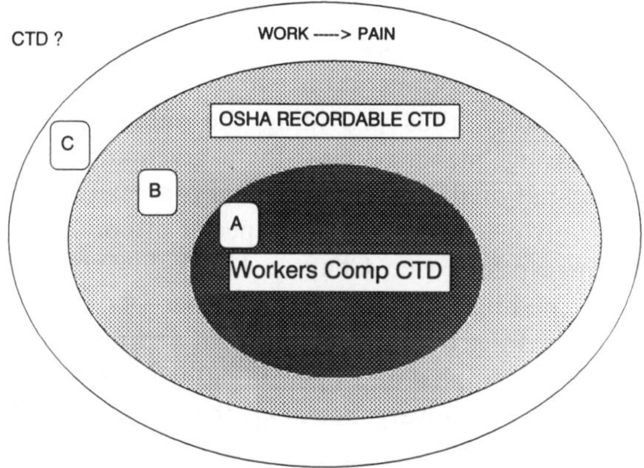

Figure 8.1 Work and pain: subsets and implications (Moon).

C. Neurological or musculoskeletal pain problems which create barriers to job performance, which increase health or safety risks, or whose symptoms are provoked by work.

The entire set of work–pain interactions (A, B, and C) impacts a workforce and its employer, and deserves attention for numerous important reasons (see Chapter 15 of this volume). Among the more recent reasons, the Americans with Disabilities Act (ADA) requires nondiscrimination and reasonable accommodation in virtually all aspects of hiring and employment for qualified disabled individuals. Public health prevention efforts and regulatory influences are largely responsible for consolidating and defining the occupational CTD concept (DHHS, 1990; Millar, 1988). Strictly speaking, circles A and B define the limits of occupational CTD. However, these boundaries are scientifically controversial and practically unsettled, particularly with respect to Workers' Compensation (Freeman, 1990). Legal concepts and standards of proof regarding causation sometimes differ substantially from medical or scientific perspectives (Danner and Sagall, 1977). Work-relatedness determinations may be greatly influenced by Workers' Compensation precedent or statutory language in a particular jurisdiction (Larson, 1992), and by prevailing perceptions and practices in the medical community and beyond (Hadler, 1992).

Most studies of CTD, particularly those that fail to control for potential confounding factors or ignore the temporal relations between symptom onset and initiation of work exposure, cannot reliably distinguish between two subtly different situations:

1. Work causes tissue damage (or verifiable, significant physiologic dysfunction) which produces symptoms
   versus
2. Symptoms develop from pre-existing, possibly dormant, independently emerging, or otherwise undefined health conditions which are not work-induced 'damage' – *and* work is the setting in which these *symptoms* increase, become subject to greater awareness, or create limitation in one's activities.

This distinction is of interest for research, legal, and prevention purposes. It is also a fundamental conceptual basis of controversy (see Hadler, 1992). However, making this distinction is clinically difficult and may seem irrelevant to many, especially to patients who hurt more with their work.

Health-care providers' perceptions about work-relatedness effectively create the numerators in some studies, thus providing the sufficient and potentially self-fulfilling basis for assessing 'increased risk' for a given occupation.[4] While this is also true for other occupational illness, the critical process of assessing causation in CTD is sufficiently controversial to warrant special attention to factors that may influence physician perceptions (see Chapter 13 of this volume) and the related behaviors of diagnostic coding and billing (see Chapter 14 of this volume).

Therefore, 'CTD' may differ by time, region, legal and regulatory context, and the method by which CTD is sampled and operationally defined. In clinical practice, a CTD designation depends on convergence of (1) the employee's behavior of presenting symptoms to a health-care system; (2) perception of the physician or other evaluator that a job includes relevant 'ergonomic hazards', and (3) the identification of clinical findings which the examiner perceives as consistent with the CTD designation (Moon, 1992).

The interactions between these three spheres create seven subcategories.[5] Each worker's circumstance would theoretically fall into one of the 'zones' described in Table 8.1 and depicted in Figure 8.2. In concept, a population's distribution across these categories may explain some of the observed differences in CTD rates between work groups with similar tasks in different settings. This distribution may also influence resource allocations among prevention and management strategies for workplace pain problems.

A Marker of Ergonomic Deficiency or Disharmony

As a practical matter, the conceptual link between CTD and ergonomics is widely accepted in workplaces, medical care, and regulatory policy. An occupational CTD designation requires that a physical ergonomic problem, hazard, or misfit be

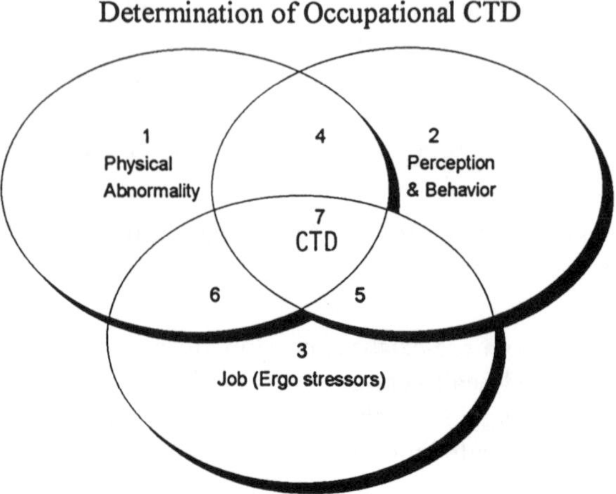

Figure 8.2 CTD determination (Moon, 1992).

Table 8.1 Work, pain and CDT: zones of relationship (Moon).

Zone	Physical abnormality	Ergonomic stressors	Critical perceptions or behaviors	Example
1	Present	Not significant	No symptoms presented for diagnosis or case finding.	Managerial employee with abnormal nerve conduction, ganglion cyst, bony x-ray changes, etc. Symptoms absent or not concerning.
2	Absent, undetected, insufficient, unrelated	Not significant	Symptoms presented. Correlation with physical findings and ergonomic stressors judged insufficient for CTD status.	Office worker with varied tasks who has diffuse musculoskeletal pain in multiple sites, normal x-rays, and no other findings; may disagree with denial of CTD status.
3	Absent, undetected, insufficient, or unrelated	Present, arguably 'hazardous'	No symptoms presented (or judged insufficient in light of anatomic location and physical findings).	Full-time data entry worker comfortably keying at high speed with non-adjustable and poorly designed work station, subject to electronic monitoring.
4	Present, detected, and related to symptoms	Insignificant (or variable) relationship to symptoms without causal link to underlying *condition*	Symptoms and physical findings are perceived and classified as a personal medical diagnosis.	1) Office worker with rheumatoid arthritis or 2) new office worker with pre-existing osteoarthritis of both hands, symptoms worse at end of shift. Objective signs of disease not progressive and symptoms return to baseline on days off.
5	Absent, undetected, insufficient, or unrelated	Do not cause or aggravate condition, but may provoke symptoms	Symptoms presented and judged to have some relationship to work. Nature of relationship and clinical findings lead to judgment this is not an occupational CTD.	Keyboard operator with muscular neck pain, worse at end of shift. Clinical findings suggest muscular pain with no other abnormalities. Symptoms resolve with simple work modifications.
6	Present	Significant 'cause' of physical abnormality	Symptoms not reported or revealed.	Outdoor worker performing highly forceful, repetitive, and awkward wrist motions in cold. Chooses not to report tendonitis symptoms.
7	Present	Present	Symptoms reported. CTD status affirmed by physician and accepted by patient, reflecting their perceptions about causation in this situation.	Wrist tendonitis in long-time data entry worker with no personal risk factors; high-speed, day-long data entry with extreme wrist posture, etc. Symptoms closely correlate with work.

demonstrated or suspected. This chapter, and much of this volume, suggests that some merit exists in conceptually equating 'CTD' with 'ergonomic illness' (Hansen, 1993). However, effective action based on that causal notion probably requires an expansion beyond a purely biomechanical view of ergonomics to include a broader range of elements that create disharmony in the fit between work and worker.

HOW IS A CTD MEASURED?

As discussed above, CTD cases are not typically identified by direct, objective measurement of the biological effect (i.e. damage) of the 'microtrauma' suspected of causing them. Leaving aside the problems with inferring a link to specific sources of microtrauma, there are major limitations to measuring damage or dysfunction in CTD cases. Neurodiagnostic studies (e.g. nerve conduction tests) represent an important exception, despite their less than perfect correlation with clinical assessment of compression neuropathies, such as carpal tunnel syndrome (Franzblau and Blitz, 1993). Moreover, the majority of CTDs are not compression neuropathies (Hales, 1994). More reliable and accessible objective measures of pathology would immensely benefit CTD prevention, surveillance, clinical management, and research; but there is a further problem. Even where objective abnormalities are found, the relation between pathology and symptoms is often unclear (Hagberg and Wegman, 1987; Waddell, 1987). In short, purely objective means of confirming most CTD diagnoses are largely unavailable. Clinical evaluation remains essential; and its process probably warrants scrutiny, given the critical function it serves.

The current level of reliance on the report of pain and paresthesia in clinical CTD evaluation may diminish with increased capacity to measure early biological effects of microtrauma in individuals. Current CTD prevention, assessment, and management appears to be guided in large measure by the perception and interpretation of pain (by workers/patients); and of behaviors by which pain is communicated, tested, and acknowledged (by workers/patients and physicians/evaluators).[6] The clinical evaluation process, even with anatomically specific CTD presentations, requires inference about the nature, degree, and cause of damage or dysfunction. These inferences are highly dependent upon communications between patient and physician, especially when pain is the issue. Simply noting the vulnerability of this 'dialogue' to the influence of external psychosocial factors is important but inadequate. This transaction itself – expression of pain and its clinical interpretation – is inherently psychosocial; and it represents a crucial 'dialogue'. As Engel (1988) emphasizes in a somewhat broader context, 'As an integral component of the process whereby the clinician gains knowledge of the patient's condition, it is thus clear that dialogue is truly foundational to scientific work in the clinical realm.'

The study and treatment of pain has achieved increasing recognition as an important discipline. Keefe and Egert (Chapter 10 of this volume) and Fordyce (Chapter 12) relate some psychological and behavioral facets of this discipline to the CTD phenomenon. Growing interest has been reflected in publications addressing pain theory and research (Fields, 1987; Wall and Melzack, 1989); standardized classification and nomenclature (Merskey, 1986); educational guidelines for physicians (IASP, 1991); and clinical guidelines organized by pain syndrome types (Bonica, 1990), or specifically focused on the injured worker with hand or arm pain

(Chaplin, 1991). A consensus publication addresses clinical, behavioral, and public policy perspectives on pain and disability (IOM, 1987). A recent legal treatise summarizes problems with determining compensation based on pain (Pryor, 1991). Risking oversimplification, several important themes can be distilled from such sources:

1. Pain is not a simple sensation, but a complex sensory and emotional experience.
2. Chronic pain and acute pain differ fundamentally. This should be reflected in their evaluation and management.
3. Central neurophysiologic pain pathways reflect both sensory–discriminative (location, quality) and affective–motivational (meaning) components of pain.
4. Current knowledge of pain neurophysiology suggests many complexities and many unanswered questions.
5. Absence of detected damage does not justify a blanket assumption that reported pain is less real or less severe.

THE ERGONOMIC INTERFACE

You have seen him spout; then declare what this spout is; can you can tell water from air? My dear sir, in this world it is not so easy to settle these plain things.

Hermann Melville, describing the whale's spout in *Moby Dick*

The preceding section suggests that the value of using 'CTD' as an outcome entity is tempered by difficulties in measuring, describing, and understanding the diverse and complex circumstances that lie beneath the CTD rubric. The exposure side of the exposure–outcome equation warrants similar scrutiny. CTDs are a mixed breed in that they 'share common requisites with both injury and illness surveillance' (Baker *et al.*, 1988; Silverstein *et al.*, 1986). The complexity of occupational 'exposure' to biomechanical hazards should not be underestimated. The 'ergonomic interface' includes multiple biomechanical risk factors whose cumulative biological effects are suspect causes for CTD. Large gaps remain in understanding the amounts of such 'exposures' which are either hazardous or safe (Gerr *et al.*, 1991). What remains unexplained or controversial may partly be due to inadequate characterization of these stressors and difficulties in quantifying them. However, a trap may lie in conceptualizing these stressors as completely external to the worker.

Although all occupational exposure occurs through an interface between the environment and the worker, the ergonomic interface differs significantly from a typical industrial hygiene model. Hazardous exposure to chemical substances is a function of quantitative levels in the work environment.[7] Ergonomic 'exposure' occurs across an interface largely *defined by human activity*. Physical exertion, contact, movement, or static positioning typically create the physical exposure,[8] especially in office settings which lack vibrational and cold exposure. The fixed constraints and predictable demands of some work environments can profoundly influence how these physical actions translate into hazardous exposure. However, as several chapters in this volume suggest, factors other than the physical work environment modify physical actions and may affect the resulting perception of sensory feedback relating to those actions (see Chapters 5 and 11 of this volume). These and other factors may influence the individual's capacity, opportunity, or motivation to alter the exposure interface in response to such feedback (see Chapters 2 and 3 of this volume).

Individual variation occupies a special role in the ergonomic interface, such that certain characteristics (i.e. height, grip size), capacities (i.e. strength), and workstyle are intrinsic elements of the exposure equation (see Chapter 11 of this volume). Personal factors affect susceptibility to some occupational illness and injury (Werner *et al.*, 1994). In some CTD studies, such factors may rival if not outweigh the identified physical work demands (Loslevor and Ranaivosoa, 1993; Nathan, 1993a, 1994). Ranges in employee susceptibility must be accommodated and included in the scope of protective workplace guidelines. These goals are appropriately addressed by fitting the job to the worker's characteristics and capacities, a time-honored occupational prevention principle which is central to ergonomics (Nordin and Frankel, 1987; Pheasant, 1991). When critical elements in this balance are nonphysical, the fitting process receives comparatively little guidance from scientific, regulatory, legal, or social standards.

ETHICAL CONCERNS

This chapter reflects a 'biopsychosocial' slant. Even at its simplest, such an approach to CTD predicts complex research issues and hurdles to practical application; but ethical issues may be the greatest concern. The central ethical concern is the danger of blaming workers for the CTD phenomenon. Raising the psychosocial issue at all may be risky. It may be impossible to prevent the focus from drifting toward the individual. Explorations of individual variations in psychosocial or behavioral characteristics present a dual risk: the nonphysical may be discounted, and individual variations may invite blame rather than accommodation (see Chapter 13 of this volume; Tesh, 1988). Current regulations and legal principles provide some protection against overt discrimination and create incentives for employers to fit the workplace to a diverse workforce. The ADA requires reasonable accommodation. OSHA standards require that employers provide a workplace free of recognized hazards. Workers' compensation principles require employers to take responsibility for the worker 'as is,' complete with pre-existing conditions and susceptibilities. Notwithstanding those protections, a 'personological,' worker-blaming perspective remains a danger.

Explorations of workstyle, economic incentives, and cognitive–behavioral interventions (*particularly if extended into the primary and secondary prevention arena*) also risk blaming the worker (see Chapters 10, 11, 12, and 14 of this volume). These risks may be justified in part by another dilemma, which itself has important ethical overtones and crucial implications – the relationship between control and responsibility in the workplace. Themes of control and responsibility pervade the occupational psychosocial literature. They also surface routinely during analysis of the ergonomic interface and the development of strategies to improve it. A worker's control of the ergonomic interface may depend not only on education and involvement, but on responsibility and empowerment (see Chapter 15 of this volume). Translating those requirements into the psychosocial arena enters relatively uncharted waters.

Certain behaviors, often linked to enhanced somatic perceptions, are frequently encouraged in ergonomics education and training programs (e.g. stretching exercises, rest breaks, postural awareness, and early reporting of pain). Work rules and policies may formalize the responsibility to act on these recommendations. Certain personal characteristics may conceivably increase CTD risk and be modifiable through behavior (Nathan, 1993a). Employer efforts to control this worker-based aspect of the ergonomic interface are typically limited to voluntary wellness programs. In theory, when worker-based factors significantly influence the CTD risk, this knowledge may provide opportunity for individuals to exert control on their ergonomic interface (Toivanen *et al.*, 1993). Simply sharing such information may not raise ethical concerns, but related issues of responsibility may be provocative and controversial (DeJoy and Southern, 1993; Gerr and Letz, 1992).

DYNAMICS OF DISABILITY: CYBERNETIC AND COMPLEX

Disablement is at one and the same time a condition of the body and an aspect of social identity – a process set in motion by somatic causes but given definition and meaning by society. It is preeminently a social state.

Robert Murphy, *The Body Silent*

... the question is how to assure benefits for all who need them, while avoiding a policy so generous that it imposes an unacceptable fiscal burden .... Because the experience of pain is different for each person, how is it possible to assess pain and determine a severity beyond which one should not be expected to work? This the crux of the problem.

IOM Committee on Chronic Pain, Disability, and Chronic Illness Behavior, *Pain and Disability*[9]

Median disability time due to CTD (repetitive motion disorders) has now surpassed that from any other occupation illness (USDL, 1994). 'Overexertion injuries' (including occupational back pain) have previously been estimated to disable 60,000 workers permanently and 4,300,000 temporarily per year. This is in contrast to 600,000 annual disabilities from 'impact injuries' at work (Chaffin, 1991). Tracking of long-term disability outcomes with upper-extremity CTD is limited, but at least one study suggests a significant three-year persistence of symptoms and functional disturbance (Kemmlert *et al.*, 1993).

The traditional conceptual framework describing the stages of disability starts with pathology-producing impairment, which produces limitation, which produces disability (IOM, 1991). Prevention strategies echo this linear framework: primary prevention of pathology, secondary prevention of impairment and limitation, and tertiary prevention of disability. Pragmatically, these four 'stages' with their three links must be verified to satisfy requirements of legal and administrative systems which sanction disability. This model fits some subsets and cases of CTD. In these, the pathology is demonstrable and/or the clinical syndrome is distinct. The impairment, limitation, and disability are biomedically predictable (or preventable with timely intervention) and are in accord with demonstrable pathology.

In many other cases, the biomedical thread extending from pathology to disability seems tenuous in contrast to other factors. Some of this may be due to medical science's current inability to detect physical pathology adequately and then correlate it with pain symptoms which create disability. However, experience with pain-related disability argues for considering factors that lie beyond strict biomedical science (i.e. Haldeman, 1990; Leavitt, 1990; Pryor, 1991; Stutts and Kasdan, 1993). Most observed associations between disability and nonbiomedical factors are cross-sectional, which obviously limits conclusions about cause and effect. However, such factors predict disability outcome in some studies of work-related back pain (Greenwood, 1990; Bigos, 1991). Upper-extremity disability predictors have received much less attention to date. Cheadle *et al.* (1994) recently reported associations between some nonbiomedical factors and work-related disability, including those cases with carpal tunnel syndrome diagnoses. In the same population, Adams *et al.* (1994) reviewed outcome of carpal tunnel syndrome (CTS) surgery, found no relationship to preoperative severity, and concluded that 'disability following surgery for occupational CTS may be related to other medical, psychosocial, administrative, legal, or work-related factors not evaluated in this study.' Another study of overexertion injuries, *not* limited to spinal pain, suggests that social support at work predicted more favorable perception of future work capacity (Kemmlert *et al.*, 1993). Morgan *et al.* (1994) found their patients disabled with chronic work-related upper-extremity disorders differed from those working by sharing more indeterminate findings; and reporting more pain, anger with employer, fear of pain, involvement in litigation, indeterminate physical findings, number of upper-extremity surgeries, and inability to identify a precipitating injury. No significant differences were noted in symptom duration, job description, or time on the job. Upper-extremity CTD research has not progressed to evaluating correlations between pathology, impairment, and disability. The more mature study of such links in lower back pain suggests relatively low correlations (Waddell, 1987). The resulting calls for a broader biopsychosocial model of back pain disability should probably apply to other occupational pain problems, including CTD (Nachemson, 1983).

An Institute of Medicine panel (IOM, 1991) proposed a general disability model which acknowledges the interaction between contextual and personal factors that influence progression to disability, but remains an essentially linear depiction of the disability process. (see Figure 8.3.) CTD disability assessment routinely points out limitations in conceptual models and associated bureaucratic responses. CTD disability is extremely *relative* to specific work demands and its development or prevention frequently depends on *feedback* (between job, worker, physician, etc.). In this context, the spectrum of 'disability' ranges from total inability to work, even with job modifications, to minor degrees of relative incapacity or reduced effectiveness. Work incapacity is not 'all-or-none,' nor is it static. This concept is intertwined with the widely accepted value of early return to modified work after 'injury' (Himmelstein and Pransky, 1994; Moon *et al.*, forthcoming).

The central philosophy of ergonomics offers a de-medicalized view of the work disability continuum. At heart, ergonomics seeks to match job demands to worker capabilities (Hales, 1994). 'When job demands overwhelm an employee's mental or physical capacity, his or her health, comfort, and productivity may be adversely affected' (Eastman Kodak, 1983). Day to day, workers balance their capacities, motivations, and coping skills against the demands, constraints, and opportunities of the job. When imbalance occurs, timely adjustment (a cybernetic response by the work organization) may prevent progression to total work incapacity (see Chapter 2 of this volume).[10]

The type or extent of objective pathology may not be the *triggering* or *critical* element in the CTD disability process (see Chapter 12 of this volume). Similar conclusions have been drawn with respect to a related phenomenon, medical absenteeism (Bartone, 1989; Hoverstad and Kjolstad, 1991; Clegg *et al.*, 1987; Levi, 1984). In a sense, this viewpoint recognizes the importance of imbalance in both biological

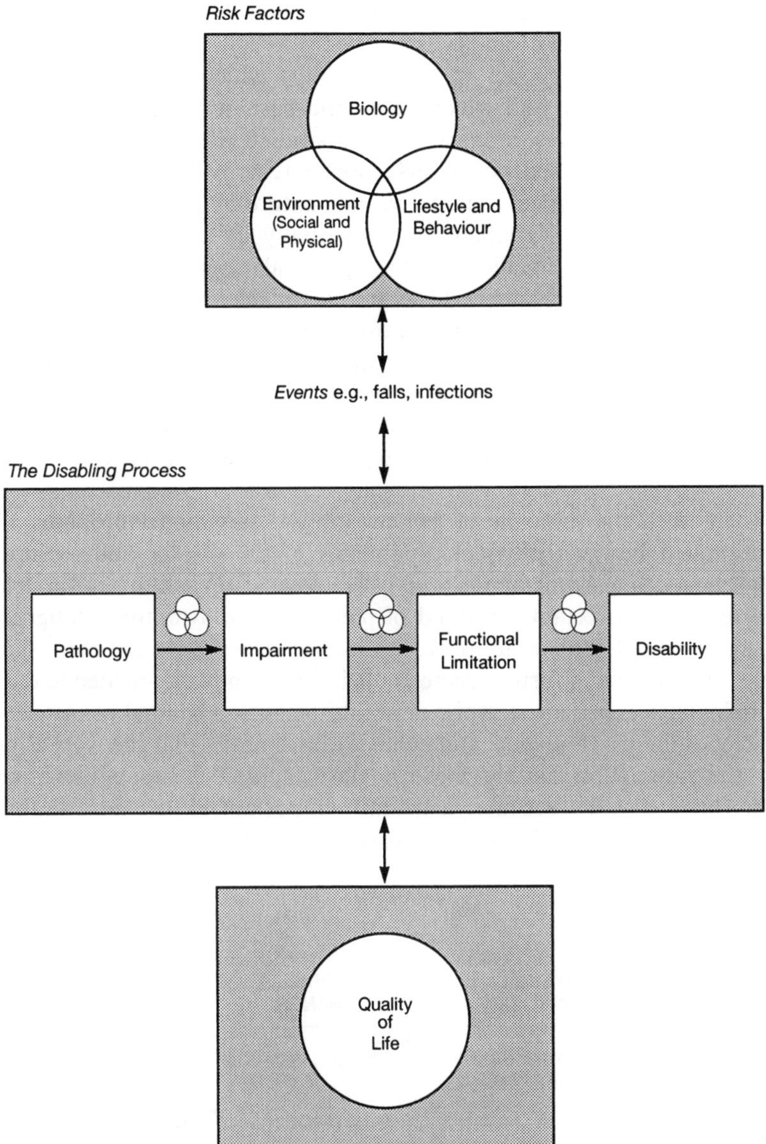

Figure 8.3 Disability model, reprinted with permission, from *Disability in America: Toward a National Agenda for Prevention*. Copyright 1991 by the National Academy of Sciences. Courtesy National Academy of Sciences Press, Washington, DC.

and psychosocial aspects of the ergonomic interface.[11] It is speculative whether and to what degree external reinforcers or inhibitors might influence the form of illness by which this imbalance manifests and is transformed into a diagnosis. At minimum, such *potential* influences exist. They appear in patterns of somatization which are learned, culturally reinforced, and normal (Kirmayer, 1984); in the somatic bias which is arguably inherent to most medical encounters (Young, 1989); in other aspects of the physician–patient dynamic (Clair, 1993; Waitzkin, 1991); and in characteristics of insurance and disability coverage.[12]

One multidimensional model of work disability which reflects some of the perspectives described above and which forms the basis for evaluation and rehabilitation for work disability secondary to occupational musculoskeletal disorders is illustrated in Figure 8.4 (Feuerstein, 1991; Feuerstein, 1993). The Rochester Model of Work Disability emphasizes the multivariate nature of this problem and identifies four broad categories of variables that potentially affect work disability and/or facilitate work re-entry (medical status, physical capabilities, work demands, psychological/behavioral resources). The first factor relates to the impact of medical status on the workers' neurologic, musculoskeletal, and cardiovascular systems. Specifically, the model proposes that medical status can affect the capacity of the neurological, musculoskeletal, and cardiovascular systems to meet the biologic demands of work. This impairment in medical status typically does not account for the majority of variance in work disability suggesting the need to identify other factors as well.

Consistent with the principle of 'person–job fit,' this model proposes a second factor: mismatch between physical capabilities of the worker and required work demands (biomechanical, metabolic, and psychological). When this mismatch or discrepancy results in a certain threshold of pain, physical symptoms, fatigue, and/or distress, an increased probability of work absence is likely. As the pain, symptoms, and distress continue and further decrements in function (work-related and activities of daily living) are experienced, work disability persists. The final component of the model includes the psychological and behavioral resources that the worker brings to bear on the interaction among medical status, physical capabilities, and work demands. These variables become particularly important as the work disability persists; however, it is proposed that these 'psychosocial' factors can also play a signifi-

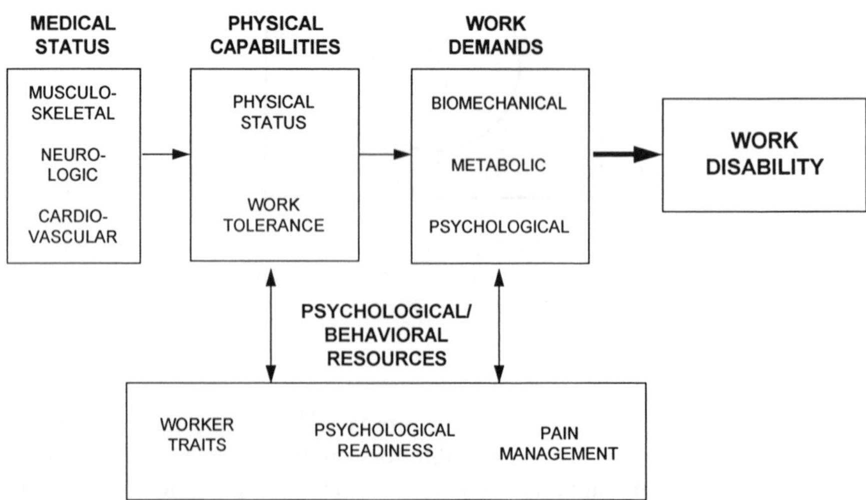

Figure 8.4 The Rochester Model of Work Disability (Feuerstein, 1993). (Reproduced with permission of Plenum Publishing Corporation.)

cant role in the early phases of work absence/work disability. These variables are divided into worker traits or characteristics such as ability to work as a team member, productivity, workstyle (see Chapter 11 of this volume), psychological readiness to work (e.g. expectations regarding ability to work, ability to perform certain physical functions, family, co-worker and supervisor support, levels of anxiety, dysphoria, anger), and ability to manage pain or other persistent or recurrent neurological or musculoskeletal symptoms. The Rochester Model of Work Disability appears to address some essential factors affecting work disability by considering medical, workplace, and psychological variables. It provided the basis for a rehabilitation program targeted at chronic work disability secondary to a range of occupational upper-extremity disorders (Feuerstein *et al.*, 1993) and an occupational medicine research clinic specializing in work-related upper-extremity disorders (Himmelstein *et al.*, 1994).

This section earlier raised the issue of minor work incapacity or reduced effectiveness that can precede a formal diagnosis. The pre-diagnosis CTD disability dynamic has received little attention from a medical perspective, although several models address processes that may lead to symptoms (see Chapters 1, 3, and 4 of this volume). Edwards (1992) has proposed a Cybernetic Model of Stress, Coping and Well-being in Organizations which is presented here *not* as a CTD model, but for its conceptual relevance to the pre-diagnosis arena.

This model, depicted in Figure 8.5, hinges on a mismatch (discrepancy) between perceptions and desires which is perpetually alterable through *feedback*. The model is manifestly *de-medicalized* in that the outcome is '*well-being*' (defined as psychological and physical health of the employee). Finally, it describes an ongoing '*coping*'

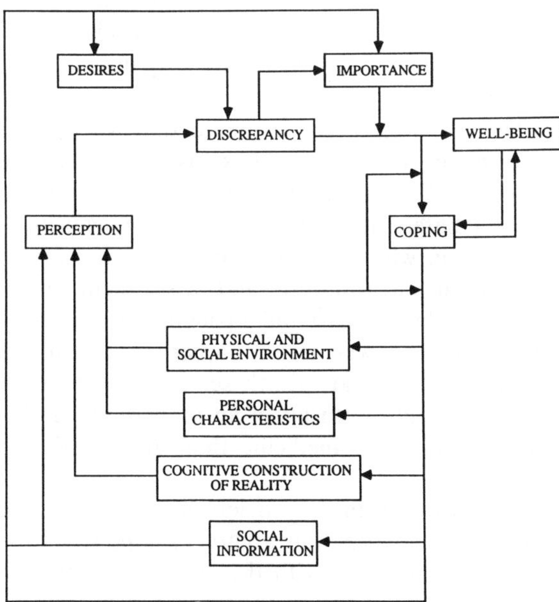

Figure 8.5 A Cybernetic Model of Stress, Coping, and Well-being in Organizations (courtesy of the *Academy of Management Review* and Jeff Edwards, PhD, School of Business Administration, University of Michigan).

dynamic (selection and implementation of strategies) which can ultimately influence both sides of the mismatch/discrepancy. Perceptions and desires are not equivalent to demands and capabilities; but the mismatch concept is analogous. Again, this model addresses stress, not CTD. Stress may represent a crucial mechanistic link between psychosocial influences and CTD. However, this model is *not* referenced in that vein, but for its depiction of hypothetical mechanisms through which individuals and their organizations respond to preserve well-being. A similar focus on well-being through cybernetic mechanisms that facilitate coping may be valuable in addressing pre-diagnosis CTD 'disability;' but only if coping is *not* viewed as silent suffering and stoicism, but in its more active sense of 'contending ... on even terms or with success' (Morris, 1969).

IS MEDICALIZATION RISKY?

The medical label may protect the patient ... only to submit him to interminable instruction, treatment, and discrimination, which are inflicted on him for his professionally presumed benefit.

I. Illich, *Medical Nemesis*

Disability prevention ideally starts with recognition and intervention at the early signs of disease that cause disability. In most ergonomics programs, early reporting of pain is a key element which is widely and justifiably endorsed. From a clinical perspective, it often seems critical to good outcome. Proactive *surveys* of pain levels in a workplace are also frequently advised as part of surveillance. This advice often generates concern that increased attention to discomfort and pain may not be completely desirable; that such may lead to excessive 'medicalization' of people's experiences, perceptions, and problems – in essence creating illness (see Chapter 12 of this volume; Hadler, 1990).

Allman *et al.* (1993) cite Kleinman's estimate that '70–90 per cent of all self-recognized episodes of sickness are managed exclusively outside the perimeter of the formal health care system.' They suggest that 'doctors' offices would be overwhelmed if people immediately acted on the symptoms causing them discomfort'. That decision to act (and in what manner) presumably has multiple determinants, including judgments about 'attribution' and assessment of consequences (see Chapter 3 of this volume; Pennebaker and Epstein, 1983). Economic forces potentially operate at this point as well (see Chapter 14 of this volume; Ellis and McGuire, 1990).[13] The concern that 'health services can be damaging as well as helpful' (Armstrong, 1989) might even affect an individual's decision, although this issue has been more a critique of medicine than an investigated determinant of care-seeking (Illich, 1976).

The expanding medicalization in this society has been described as a threat to individual autonomy, independence, and ability to cope (Illich, 1976; Zola, 1972). Given the complexities of pain along with the diversity of incentives that surround occupational disability, concern about encouraging pain reporting and resulting medicalization is understandable. These concerns may ring especially true for clinicians with experience managing chronic pain problems. As an IOM committee notes, illness behavior related to the experience of pain 'usually does not proceed

... from one well-defined stage to another. Rather, there are likely to be bidirectional interactions between four elements – symptom perception, symptom interpretation, symptom expression, and coping behaviors' (IOM, 1987). However, naive extrapolation from the chronic pain arena should be avoided, particularly regarding assumptions that social and cultural reinforcers of *chronic* pain behavior are influential in the early stages of CTD. Still, the power of sociocultural messages deserves recognition and respect, particularly with the complex phenomenon of pain (see Chapters 3, 12, and 13 of this volume; Pryor, 1991). Physicians (and others) send important messages to their own patients (Kirmayer, 1984; Young, 1989), but may also contribute to the societal message heard by other patients, future patients, and the working well person.

From a scientific perspective, unanswered questions persist regarding distinctions and relationships between (a) endorsement of subjective pain/discomfort in response to workplace inquiry, (b) the behavior of presenting such symptoms in a medical context, and (c) the identification of disease at various levels of anatomic specificity and objective verifiability. Cherniak (1994) appropriately cautions against assuming that proactive sampling for pain/discomfort can predict anatomically specific CTD cases. The practical value of ergonomic adjustments in response to discomfort seems intuitive and certainly has broad anecdotal support. A crucial dilemma arises when such adjustments cannot proceed without medicalization and diagnosis, which then justify formal work accommodations.

ROLE OF THE 'PHYSICIAN': EVALUATOR OF HEALTH STATUS, PROVIDER OF HEALTH CARE[14]

There are two handicaps to the practice of medicine .... The first is the eternal charlatanism *of the patient who is full of* fake *diseases and phantom agonies. The second is the basic incompetence of the human mind, medical or otherwise, to observe without prejudice, acquire information without becoming too smug to use it intelligently, and most of all, to apply its wisdom without vanity.*

Ben Hecht[15]

Hecht's harsh and provocative quote lends a backdrop for directly addressing a great concern in undertaking the psychosocial factor–CTD topic: the potential for creating impressions that some CTD pain is only 'in the mind' or that CTD patients are malingering. *Neither* is implied here. Barsky (1981) reviews numerous studies suggesting that 'many persons who visit doctors are without serious medical disease,' that 'less than half the identified problems of ambulatory patients are clear somatic diagnoses,' and that 'other nonbiomedical factors must be important in explaining why they have gone to a doctor.' These are Hecht's 'fake' diseases, but does their prevalence say more about the patient or the system? The conceptual separation of mind and body is deeply embedded in medical thinking (Engel, 1988). Kuhn (1970) notes that 'paradigms gain status to the extent that they are successful in solving problems, and they lose status as paradoxes multiply.' Hecht's depiction of 'charlatanism' may mean the patient's problem, as presented and understood, simply matches poorly to the physician's paradigm. Biomedicine is often successful in explaining and resolving pain problems. Where biomedicine fails, sharply dichotomizing the problem into mind versus body provides an explanation for that failure which is often more convenient than justifiable.

'Malingering' describes the typically untestable hypothesis that a patient is consciously faking symptoms. The behavior of some patients probably does respond to the complex and conflicting incentives inherent in the experience of being symptomatic with a Workers' Compensation ailment. Divergence of patient behavior from biomedically based expectations has fostered the concepts of secondary gain, abnormal illness behavior, compensation neurosis, conditioned and learned pain behaviors, and symptom magnification. None equates to true malingering, but these concepts can be misinterpreted as a measure of motivation, an entity similar to pain in that it is critical but *immeasurable*. Assessing and judging another person's motivations is a value-laden endeavor, which draws on culture-based assumptions and is subject to bias of undefined extent.

Still, society looks to physicians to discern validity of subjective complaints. In the current era of cost scrutiny and concern about insurance fraud, the issue predictably arises in some CTD cases, and smolders beneath some perspectives on the entire CTD phenomenon. The question has received much attention in occupational back pain, but less so with upper-extremity disorders (Stutts and Kasdan, 1993). A consensus group convened by the Social Security Commission (Foley *et al.*, 1987) concluded that the incidence of actual malingering was probably very low in Social Security Disability claimants with musculoskeletal pain.[16] Distinct from conscious malingering are the issues of multiple (and often conflicting) incentives that accompany occupational pain disability; and issues of variation in people's coping strategies and capacities (Mechanic, 1962). Making judgments about the impact of those incentives or about the relative validity of symptoms becomes a thorny and uncertain task (see Chapter 12 of this volume; Moon *et al.*, forthcoming).

The second handicap described by Hecht reflects the inherent conservatism of scientific medicine and the arrogance that critics see in some of its practitioners. A step further, this handicap highlights what society requires of the physician: decision and action in the face of uncertainty. Yesterday's uncertainties sometimes yield to today's science, perhaps shifting a 'phantom agony,' as Hecht described it, to a category perceived as more legitimate.[17] Science alone, however, does not drive this evolution. This chapter's introduction alludes to progressive modification of disease and illness concepts through tension between society and biomedicine. The crux of this dynamic lies in the physician–patient relationship, where some reconciliation must occur between the sometimes 'discrepant agendas' of physicians and patients. The crux focuses more sharply when physicians act as evaluators, certifiers of the legitimately sick, or agents 'of social control geared to promoting and sustaining a work ethic in the population' (Allman *et al.*, 1993; Waitzkin, 1991).

Certifying illness or disability can be straightforward with anatomically specific CTD conditions, where impaired function seems consistent with demonstrable pathology, etc. However, many cases are not straightforward. Roemmich (1961) identified a common dilemma. Speaking of the Social Security Disability Insurance program, he stated: 'Most diseases we encounter ... prevent work because they produce in man an uncomfortable sensation when he works. These sensations are dyspnea, pain, fatigue, or a combination .... There are no biological techniques which can measure dyspnea, pain or fatigue.'[18]

Required to act, but limited by the uncertainties of judging another person's pain expressions, physicians presumably cope and respond in different ways. Uncertainty may create 'fear of personal inadequacy and failure' for the physician (Gerrity *et al.*, 1992). Allman *et al.* (1993) further suggest that, when time pressures limit critical thinking and attention to individual uniqueness, 'stereotypical thinking will most likely occur.' Some physicians order tests, the extent and nature of which vary with a number of factors, including physician specialty and geographic location of the physician (Cherkin *et al.*, 1994). Some comfortably equate absence of demonstrated, objective signs of damage or impairment with no significant disease. Some may liberalize their criteria for inferring that damage or physical dysfunction exists. Each physician probably responds in all these ways to some extent, presumably influenced by training, peer pressure, experience, emerging scientific thought, societal pressures, and other factors. The Institute of Medicine (IOM) Committee on Pain and Disability notes the various forces that are believed to influence physician judgments in the area of disability evaluation and recommends research in this area (IOM, 1987).

To the degree that it involves 'personal troubles' with 'roots in social issues beyond medicine,' Waitzkin (1989) argues that 'the technical structure of the medical encounter ... masks a deeper structure that may have little to do with the conscious thoughts of professionals about what they are saying and doing.' He finds these encounters tend to exclude and discourage statements or actions by physicians to address or change the 'contextual source' of the patient's difficulties.[19] Waitzkin contends that these encounters reinforce the definition of health as ability to work. He contends that they also support the current social order and exert social control. He emphasizes that micro-level interpersonal medical encounters are significantly shaped by macro-level structures in society, including capitalistic ideologies about economic productivity (Waitzkin and Britt, 1989).[20] Presumably, physicians vary in their responsiveness to such macro-level influences depending on their personal philosophies and incentives (McKinlay and Stoeckle, 1990). Clinical productivity, malpractice avoidance, and patient satisfaction are other incentives that influence physician behavior (Cockerman, 1993; Ritchey, 1993).

Lack of *social* support, at work and otherwise, surfaces repeatedly in association with CTD incidence and outcome (Bigos *et al.*, 1991; Kemmlert *et al.*, 1993). Describing his Psychosocial Resource Model, Clair (1993) notes that formal support *from physicians* mediates potentially harmful consequences of psychosocial stressors. He enumerates 'humanistic communication qualities' of information giving, reciprocity, affect, and personalization as empirically desirable physician attributes. This supportive function represents another way in which physicians act as agents of society; a more benign-appearing role than 'promoter of work ethic,' though a social control mechanism none the less. Whether providing support, advocating for change in 'contextual sources,' or systematically ignoring contextual sources of troubles, the physician exerts effect on a dynamic critical to all individuals: *coping*. Successful coping (contending on equal terms or with success) is probably dependent on multiple factors and is subject to many determinants; some relating to the individual, some to the workplace, some to sociocultural context, and some to the physician's efforts and attitude.

Tension may develop between three roles that physicians play: (1) independent evaluator, (2) supporter of coping, and (3) patient advocate. Apart from advocating for the patient's ultimate well-being, however envisioned, the physician may also advocate for illness/disability status; for restrictions on work demands; or for access to work even though some risk of harm (from that work) is suspected. Waitzkin

(1989) notes that 'the micropolitics of medical encounters limits doctors' capacity to respond to patients' contextual difficulties.' While this may well be true, the CTD phenomenon *has* prodded and empowered physicians to indirectly address contextual sources of their patients' problems. Recommending modifications in work environments and work demands of individuals exerts an aggregate and eventual effect on contextual sources of their problems.

Can physicians go further to *directly* address the psychosocial context of individuals? Individual work recommendations carry different medicolegal significance than do ergonomic changes for primary prevention in a workforce. Individual work restrictions sanction an illness or 'disability' status for an individual. The following dynamic has become widely acceptable. Patient presents a problem and its physical symptoms. Problem is medicalized and symbolized as a physical diagnosis. Employer accepts recommendations to modify physical work demands or workplace characteristics (as the implied cause for the original problem).

What happens if any link in this chain loses its 'physical' label? Are workplaces ready to formally implement medical restrictions overtly directed to the psychosocial environment – based on a CTD type of diagnostic label? Further, what danger or discredit does the patient face in disclosing contextual sources of troubles that are of a psychosocial or motivational nature? (see Chapter 13 of this volume.) Once the problem becomes a diagnosis and enters the Workers' Compensation arena, it is no longer confidentially protected from administrators of the Workers' Compensation benefit. How vigorous and explicit should the physician be in addressing and documenting contextual sources of a psychosocial nature? Presentation of a physical pain problem implies a sort of license for the physician to explore potential physical causes. Pushing into the nonphysical arena may generate resistance, perhaps violating a tacit social contract.

From the sociomedical perspective described above, the medical encounter is highly subject to larger sociocultural influence. Through it, physicians function as agents of society, exerting control *and* providing support. Their actions promote certain behaviors, create perceptions in society, and have economic impact for individuals and employers. In addition to providing biomedical treatment, the physician functions as evaluator, supporter of coping, gatekeeper, advocate for entitlements, and a source of recommended work accommodations.

TRANSITIONAL IMPLICATIONS FOR OCCUPATIONAL HEALTH

Occupational health professionals must sometimes balance the three 'physician' roles described above – a typically challenging task. However, they have special access to promote primary prevention and to provide consultation for organizational decision-makers. Neither task is simple. Employers may be understandably reluctant to step back from a purely legalistic view of responsibility in relation to CTD. Adjustments in responsibility and control over the ergonomic interface often requires significant evolution in corporate cultures, workplaces, and workforces (see Chapter 15 of this volume, Green and Baker, 1991, Warner *et al.*, 1988). Enthusiasm for such evolution may be tempered by the bare-knuckled questions: *whose* costs (employer, individual, or society) and *when*? Even when supported by compelling rationale and promises of eventual cost-savings and productivity enhancement, prevention remains a 'long-term proposition and often runs counter to short-term profit objectives of the firm.' Its capacity to enhance productivity falls short of the 'easiest and quickest way to do so: downsizing' (Walsh, 1991).

More realistic determination of total costs may nudge employers toward seizing greater responsibility – not less (French, 1990; Oxenburgh, 1991). Walsh (1991) notes: 'perhaps if companies would, or could, account more fully for their human capital costs associated with erosion in the vitality and capacity of a labor force, the indirect costs of illness (physical and mental) would loom larger than they do.' Linking CTD prevention with the promotion of job satisfaction is accumulating increasing conceptual support (Bigos *et al.*, 1991; see Chapter 15 of this volume). For some employers, the CTD phenomenon may justify efforts to include 'exposures' and individual capacities relating to both mind and body in the ergonomics equation. Likewise, many organizations will take some responsibility for *all* interactions between musculoskeletal pain and work, especially those that affect productivity and worker satisfaction. A broad view of activity-related pain in the workplace addresses the full spectrum of discomfort/pain: work-related or not and medically treated or not.

Less constrained by demands of medical and legal systems, primary prevention efforts may be less required to dichotomize responsibility, to split (or ignore) mind problems versus body problems, or to reduce the complexities of human experience into a numerical diagnosis code. The coordination of primary with secondary and tertiary prevention deserves extra thought (see Chapter 19 of this volume). Biomedical paradigms and physician roles, despite their limitations, inevitably dominate the response to diagnostically labelled occupational pain problems. Wholesale adoption of these paradigms in primary prevention of office-related pain problems may amplify those limitations and miss opportunity. Shifting from an 'illness' to a 'wellness' model for prevention requires health professionals to make significant adjustments in style and role.

Such conceptual expansions challenge sharp distinctions between disease, illness and wellness, especially for pain problems that are interrelated with work in complex or poorly definable ways. Such expansions raise difficult questions about workers' compensation, disability benefits, and other entitlements. Implementing such concepts risks disrupting traditional matrices of responsibility and control. This complicates efforts to apportion blame, but may better recognize the reality of individual problems and promote effective solutions. It requires employees to assume more responsibility for their 'ergonomic interfaces' while becoming empowered to affect their work milieu (see Wallerstein and Weinger, 1992). It requires organizations to address their internal conflicting incentives and treat occupational health as a system-wide issue, necessary to long-term survival (see Chapters 14 and 15 of this volume).

CONCLUSION

Gradual biomechanical insult causes pain, biomedical dysfunction, and sometimes damage, the distinctions being subject to much interpretive controversy in office-related CTDs. Pain serves as a presumptive surrogate for damage, but it serves that role imperfectly. Pain demands recognition. It acts as one of the commonest 'calling cards' through which illness is sanctioned, laden with the presumption that it represents *physical* disease especially if persistent and severe. Absence of clear-cut biomedical diagnosis does *not* rule out *bona fide* physically based pain. Identification of 'objective markers' of disease or symptom patterns depends somewhat on the physician's skill, diagnostic enthusiasm, and belief system, as well as limitations of scientific technology.

Pain is ultimately irrefutable, but fundamentally subjective; a 'complex sensory and emotional experience.' Its perception, expression, and long-term implications are, by all indications, subject to multiple nonbiomedical influences. Similar influences probably affect the insult or discomfort generated at the ergonomic interface. Such factors probably affect recognition of sensations or early symptoms; the perceived opportunity or motivation to adjust responsively; and the meaning attached to the experience of 'symptoms.' When this dynamic reaches to the medical encounter, patient and physician bring perceptions, constraints, and agendas into a critical 'dialogue.' This encounter is the fundamental mechanism through which an anatomically and symptomatically diverse spectrum of ailments is sorted, some being designated as occupational CTDs. This encounter is typically definitive, producing the diagnosis which becomes the basis for comparison between populations and the most universally acceptable measure of the problem. Sources of variance in the outcome of this medical encounter deserve attention.

The affected individual makes the distinction between pain and discomfort, and largely determines the point at which pain warrants medical attention and when it is sufficiently reduced for work return. Society expects physicians to interpret, verify, or reject the legitimacy of such judgments. In doing so, the clinician must act in the face of uncertainty, assessing cause and capacity in terms that translate into existing legal and bureaucratic frameworks. Complexity pervades the CTD issue – from causation assessment to diagnostic process and disability dynamics. Physicians treat and support. They also evaluate, judge, and recommend. All these actions have impact in the workplace and the community.

Though biomedically imprecise, the CTD label crystallizes some crucial legal, regulatory, and economic implications of pain problems and work. These far-reaching implications provoke highly diverse perspectives which sometimes appear mutually disallowing. Cross-perspective discord often arises when addressing CTD through traditional biomedical and legalistic models; or through strategies designed purely for injury prevention or disease surveillance. Interjection of psychosocial and sociocultural constructs runs the risks of confusing causal attribution; of being irrelevant in biomechanically determined and biomedically distinct cases; of discounting valid individual problems; and of diverting attention from legitimate biomechanical risks. However, CTD may represent the leading edge of a paradigm shift in society's understanding of work, health, productivity, and their interrelationships. Considered at that level, incorporating the psychosocial component is inevitable. Resolution of this issue is unlikely in the short-term, but gradual evolution may be promoted through dialogue between various professional disciplines and other parties in society. The following questions illustrate the need for diverse input, given the overlap and interaction between needs and goals of scientific research and policy-making.

1. Which psychosocial factors are open to consideration? If limited to those controlled by the workplace, should they be considered hazardous in the same sense and at similar levels as biomechanical stressors? Given the dangers and drawbacks of personological explanations (see Chapters 3 and 13 of this volume), is any expansion justifiable into psychosocial elements under the potential control

of individuals? If so, what responsibilities are implied and how can the risks to worker confidentiality and credibility be managed?

2. What are common *deterrents* to assessing psychosocial factors in the work environment and taking action to 'improve' those factors? What changes would neutralize those deterrents? What expansions to current measures of cost and productivity would be appropriate to reflect the postulated benefits?
3. Can guidelines be developed regarding subjective discomfort/pain levels which individuals are allowed or expected to tolerate at work? How might these vary in (1) applying ADA requirements regarding access to work, (2) proactive screening for pain in the workplace, and (3) the frequent divergence between chronic pain severity and 'pathology' measurable by reliable conventional means?
4. How should prevention efforts be distributed among the targets of discomfort, pain, objective dysfunction, damage, or disability? To what degree do these factors progressively predict each other?
5. Is there an effective alternative to continued reliance on physician judgment as the linchpin in causation and work capacity decisions? What methods are available (and acceptable) to evaluate underlying external factors affecting such judgments?

NOTES

1 Occupational *illness* does not include occupational lower back pain, which is classified as an occupational injury for the purposes of Occupational Safety and Health Administration (OSHA) recording. Whether occupational back pain is a product of cumulative trauma or should be considered a CTD for other purposes is a separate issue.

2 For example, some aspects of the CTD phenomenon challenge biomedical constructs which (1) sharply separate disease/damage from health/normal function and (2) imply a progressive, mechanistic chain of causation for those musculoskeletal pain disorders not arising from instantaneous, violent injury forces.

3 These recording requirements appear to mandate CTD classification for diagnosed disorders which are not *wholly* attributable to nonwork causes if they fit certain criteria regarding duration, job exposure, relationship of symptoms to work, etc. (Duvall, 1993; USDL, 1988; OSHR, 1991). OSHA Guidelines (USDL, 1990) state: 'in terms of recordability for OSHA recordkeeping regulations, BLS guidelines state that, unless a CTD illness was caused solely by a non-work-related event or exposure off-premises, it is presumed to be work-related.' However, Hansen (1993) notes that some interpretations of OSHA 200 log recordability of CTD as an occupational illness may be arbitrary. He further advocates shifting from the CTD concept to that of 'ergonomic illnesses ... diagnoses of gradual onset for which ergonomic exposure increases relative risk.'

4 The most commonly necessary (though usually not sufficient) Workers' Compensation criterion for CTD is 'increased risk.' Simply put, does the job create a greater risk for the specific CTD in question than the risk of the general public (or working public)? Epidemiologic evidence, if available, may be brought to light in cases that are highly contested. However, sufficient proof is frequently limited to a physician's opinion that, more likely than not, the risk is increased. Circle A (Workers' Compensation) in Figure 8.1 entails substantially different employer/insurer responsibilities compared to circle B (OSHA-200 log recordable). The differential between these categories in various settings is largely unreported. Experience suggests that it may be significantly influenced by situational conditions including the insurer's claims management style (see Carragee and Hentz,

1988), the company's culture, and other factors surrounding the employer–employee relationship (see Chapter 15 of this volume).

5 In the model depicted in Figure 8.2, perceptions and behavior of *both* worker/patient and physician/evaluator are operative. This can create controversy regarding qualification for the CTD category. The examples given are probably more reflective of one jurisdiction's Workers' Compensation standards than of OSHA recording requirements. Also, the distinction between identifiable versus identified abnormalities is complex in musculoskeletal pain disorders. Clinically, this distinction depends upon the intensity of the search for abnormalities and upon differing beliefs as to which findings, in what degree, are abnormal and relevant to the complaint.

6 This is unavoidably so. Many types of CTD syndromes present with relatively consistent, characteristic symptom complexes and physical findings so that reports of pain (spontaneous, activity-related or examiner-provoked) are essential to the diagnostic process. Further, symptoms may arguably precede objective findings in some CTD conditions; at least symptoms may occur at a degree of some pathological process (e.g. nerve compression) below that objectively measurable by commonly used techniques (for example, see Szabo *et al.*, 1984a and 1984b). Although not rigorously tested, the value of early CTD intervention is widely supported and difficult to dispute from a pragmatic perspective.

7 Various worker characteristics and behaviors modify chemical exposure across a biological interface and alter the effect. The worker is not a completely passive recipient of the toxic chemical, but quantitative environmental levels remain principal benchmarks and primary prevention targets.

8 Personal actions can alter absorptions and other determinants of toxicity with chemical exposure, but personal actions are *integral* to 'ergonomic exposures'.

9 'Chronic' is underlined for emphasis to raise caution against extrapolating from the chronic pain arena to the early treatment arena where some would argue that no level of increased pain due to work is acceptable (and more would agree that any *increased* pain/discomfort must be acceptable to the patient).

10 A similar cybernetic quality in organizations may represent a central mechanism by which job stress is controlled (Edwards, 1992). Reflecting the themes of balance and organizational responsiveness, Johansson and Aronsson (1991) recommend 'identification of resources for control and coping with job demands' as a primary target for future psychosocial research along with investigation for 'an appropriate balance between job demands and resources for control.'

11 To some degree, this mirrors one concept of stress which is 'understood in the sense of an unbalanced relation between individual and environment' (Leino, 1989). Hypothetically, this imbalance can presumably manifest in different ways, including stress-related symptoms such as tension, anxiety, fatigue, or depression which carry a more *psychological* connotation; or in a more ostensibly *physical* form such as headache, gastrointestinal, cardiovascular, or musculoskeletal symptoms.

12 Although the situation is evolving, Workers' Compensation claims of a 'mental–mental' (a psychological problem from a nonphysical cause) or 'physical–mental' (a physical problem from a nonphysical cause) nature have been administratively disallowed in some jurisdictions and subject to rigorous scrutiny in others (Warshaw, 1988). Outside the Workers' Compensation arena, medical and disability insurance tends to limit benefits more for 'mental and nervous' conditions as compared to diagnoses considered 'physical.'

13 Both of these references describe 'moral hazard,' a well-recognized term in economics and the insurance industry. This arguably unfortunate term runs considerable risk for provoking misunderstanding and resistance outside these communities. However, it cuts directly to some issues regarding the dynamics of benefits utilization which may be unavoidable in a comprehensive assessment of the CTD phenomenon.

14 Aspects of the physician role are increasingly filled by professionals other than medical doctors (McKinlay and Stoeckle, 1990), so the term 'physician' is meant broadly.
15 My italics in Hecht's quote.
16 This clinician's personal impression (and bias) is that pure malingering (conscious presentation of nonexistent symptoms) is uncommon in our large and diverse population of workers with upper-extremity activity-related pain.
17 A clinical exam on an identical patient may have been described as revealing 'no objective findings' 20 years ago; 'subjective, diffuse soft-tissue tenderness' 10 years ago; and 'myofascial pain syndrome' or 'fibromyalgia' today. The same diversity of conclusions regarding the same patient is not uncommon among contemporaneous practitioners.
18 The measurement of fatigue correlates in specific muscles may be a slight exception to Dr Roemmich's 1961 assessment.
19 Waitzkin (1989) uses the example of a depressed patient whose period of allotted disability (after a heart attack) is expiring just as his union intends to go on strike (presumably affording the patient less financial security than if he were still certified for disability). The physician–patient encounter 'medicalizes' the problem. It produces antidepressant and tranquilizer prescriptions, assurance that work is good for mental health, and encouragement to return to work, but does not address the critical, initiating contextual issue: uncertain employment.
20 In many work settings, production pressure is highly intertwined with the CTD issue. It arguably represents a 'contextual source' underlying (1) biomechanical stressors (high repetition), (2) some psychosocial factors, and (3) employers' reluctance to adopt an ergonomically preferable, but economically threatening work modification.

REFERENCES

Adams, M. L., Franklin, G. M. and Barnhart, S. 1994 Outcome of carpal tunnel surgery in Washington State workers compensation, *American Journal of Industrial Medicine*, **25**, 527–36.

Allman, R. M., Yoels, W. C. and Clair, J. M. 1993 Reconciling the agendas of physicians and patients, in Clair, I. M. and Allman, R. M. (Eds), *Sociomedical Perspectives in Patient Care*, pp. 29–46, Lexington, KY: University Press of Kentucky.

Andersson, G. B. 1981 Epidemiologic aspects on low-back pain in industry, *Spine*, **6**, 53–60.

Armstrong, D. 1989 Evaluating health care, in *An Outline of Sociology as Applied to Medicine*, pp. 108–17, Boston: Wright.

Armstrong, T., Castelli, W. A., Evnas, F. G. and Diaz-Perez, R. 1984 Some histological changes in the carpal tunnel contents and their biomechanical implications, *Journal of Occupational Medicine*, **26**, 197–201.

Baker, E. L., Melius, J. M. and Millar, J. D. 1988 Surveillance of occupational illness and injury in the United States: Current perspectives and future directions, *Journal of Public Health Policy*, Summer, 198–221.

Barnhart, S., *et al.* 1991 Carpal tunnel syndrome among ski manufacturing workers, *Scandinavian Journal of Work Environment and Health*, **17**, 46–52.

Barsky, A. J. 1981 Hidden reasons some patients visit doctors, *Annals of Internal Medicine* **94**(1), 492–8.

Bartone, P. T. 1989 Predictors of stress-related illness in city bus drivers, *Journal of Occupational Medicine* **31**(8), 657–63.

Bernard, B., Sauter, S., Petersen, M., Fine, L. and Hales, T. 1993 *Health Hazard Evaluation Report, Lost Angeles Times*, (HETA No. 90-013-2277), National Institute for Occupational Safety and Health, Center for Disease Control and Prevention.

Bigos, S. J., *et al.* 1991 A prospective study of work perceptions and psychosocial factors affecting the report of back injury, *Spine*, **16**(1), 1–6.

BONGERS, P. M., DE WINTER, C. R., KOMPIER, M. A. and HILDEBRANCLT, V. 1993 Psychosocial factors at work and musculoskeletal disease, *Scandinavian Journal of Work, Environment and Health*, **19**(5), 297–312.

BONICA, J. D. (Ed.) 1990 *The Management of Pain*, 2nd Edn, Philadelphia, PA: Lea & Febiger.

BRENA, S. and CHAPMAN, S. 1981 The 'learned pain syndrome,' *Postgraduate Medicine*, **69**, 53–62.

BROWNE, C. D., NOLAN, B. M. and FAITHFULL, D. K. 1984 Occupational repetition strain injuries: Guidelines for diagnosis and management, *Medical Journal of Australia*, **140**, 329–32.

BUTLER, R. J. 1983 Wage and injury rate response to shifting levels of worker's compensation, in WORRALL, J. D. (Ed.), *Safety and the Workplace: Incentives and Disincentives in Workers' Compensation*, pp. 61–86, Ithaca: ILR Press.

CANNON, L. J., BERNACKI, E. J. and WALTER, S. D. 1981 Personal and occupational factors associated with carpal tunnel syndrome, *Journal of Occupational Medicine*, **23**, 255–8.

CARRAGEE, E. J. and HENTZ, V. R. 1988 Repetitive trauma and nerve compression, *Orthopedic Clinics North America*, **19**, 157–64.

CHAFFIN, D. B. 1991 Biomechanical basis for prevention of overexertion and impact trauma in industry, in GREEN, G. M. and BAKER, F. (Eds), *Work, Health and Productivity*, pp. 100–12, New York: Oxford University Press.

CHAPLIN, E. R. 1991 Chronic pain and the injured worker: A sociobiological problem, in KASDAN, M. L. (Ed.), *Occupational Hand and Upper Extremity Injuries and Diseases*, pp. 13–45.

CHEADLE, A., FRANKLIN, G., WOLFHAGEN, C., SAVARINO, J., LIU, P. Y. and WEAVER, S. C. 1994 Factors influencing the duration of work-related disability: A population-based study of Washington State workers' compensation, *American Journal of Public Health*, **84**(2), 190–6.

CHERKIN, D. C., DEYO, R. A., WHEELER, K. and CIOL, M. A. 1994 Physician variation in diagnostic testing for low back pain: Who you see is what you get, *Arthritis and Rheumatism*, **37**(1), 15–22.

CHERNIAK, M. 1994 Upper extremity disorders, in ROSENSTOCK, L. and CULLEN, M. R. (Eds), *Textbook of Clinical Occupational and Environmental Medicine*, pp. 376–88, Philadelphia, PA: Saunders.

CLAIR, J. M. 1993 The application of social science to medical practice, in CLAIR, J. M. and ALLMAN, R. M. (Eds), *Sociomedical Perspectives in Patient Care*, Lexington, KY: University Press of Kentucky.

CLEGG, C., WALL, T. and KEMP, N. 1987 Women on the assembly line: A comparison of main and interactive explanations of job satisfaction, absence and mental health, *Journal of Occupational Psychology*, **60**, 273–87.

COCKERMAN, W. C. 1993 The changing pattern of physician–patient interaction, in CLAIR, J. M. and ALLMAN, R. M. (Eds), *Sociomedical Perspectives in Patient Care*, pp. 47–57, Lexington, KY: University Press of Kentucky.

COLLIGAN, M. J., *et al.* 1988 Psychological indicators of recovery from back pain, in AGHAZADEH, F. (Ed.), *Trends in Ergonomics/Human Factors*, Amsterdam: North-Holland/Elsevier.

CUNNINGHAM, L. S. and KELSEY, J. L. 1984 Epidemiology of musculoskeletal impairments and associated disability, *American Journal of Public Health*, **74**, 574–9.

DAHLIN, L. B. and LUNDBORG, G. 1990 The neurone and its response to peripheral nerve compression, *Journal of Hand Surgery*, **15B**, 5–10.

DANNER, D. and SAGALL, E. L. 1977 Medicolegal causation: A source of professional misunderstanding, *American Journal of Law and Medicine*, **3**(3), 304–8.

DE KROM, M. C., KESTER, A. D., KNIPSCHILD, P. G. and SPAANS, F. 1990 Risk factors for carpal tunnel syndrome, *American Journal of Epidemiology*, **132**(6), 1102–10.

DeJoy, D. M. and Southern, D. J. 1993 An integrative perspective on work-site health promotion, *Journal of Occupational Medicine*, **35**, 1221–30.

Derebery, V. J. and Tullis, W. H. 1983 Delayed recovery in the patient with a work compensable injury, *Journal of Occupational Medicine*, **25**, 829–35.

Deyo, R. A., Cherkin, D., Conrad, D. and Volinn, E. 1991 Cost, controversy, crisis: Low back pain and the health of the public, *Annual Review of Public Health*, **12**, 141–56.

DHHS 1990 *Healthy People 2000: National Health Promotion and Disease Prevention Objectives*, Washington, DC: Department of Health and Human Services, Public Health Service.

Dimberg, L., Olafsson, A., Stefansson, E., Aagaard, H., Oden, A., Andersson, G. B., Hansson, T. and Hagert, C. G. 1989 The correlation between work environment and the occurrence of cervicobrachial symptoms, *Journal of Occupational Medicine*, **31**(5), 447–53.

Duvall, M. 1993 Digest of official interpretations of the bureau of labor statistic record-keeping guidelines for occupational injuries and illnesses, *Occupational Safety and Health Reporter*, February, 1716–17.

Eastman Kodak 1983 *Ergonomic Design For People at Work*, Vol. 1, New York: Van Nostrand Reinhold.

Edwards, J. R. 1992 A cybernetic theory of stress, coping, and well-being in organizations, *Academy of Management Review*, **17**, 238–74.

Eisenberg, L. 1977 Disease and illness: distinctions between professional and popular ideas of sickness, *Culture, Medicine and Psychiatry*, **1**, 9–23.

Ellis, R. L. and McGuire, T. G. 1990 Optimal payment systems for health services, *Journal of Health Economics*, **9**, 375–96.

Engel, G. L. 1988 How much longer must medicine's science be bound by a seventeeth century world view?, in White, K. L. (Ed.), *The Task of Medicine: Dialogue at Wickenburg*, pp. 113–36, Menlo Park, CA: Kaiser Foundation.

English, C. J., Maclaren, W. M., Court-Broson, C., Hughes, S. P., Porter, R. W., Wallace, W. A., Graves, R. J., Pettrick, A. J. and Soutar, C. A. 1995 Relations between upper limb soft tissue disorders and repetitive movements at work, *American Journal of Industrial Medicine*, **27**(1), 75–90.

Faucett, J. and Rempel, D. 1994 VDT-related musculoskeletal symptoms: Interactions between work posture and psychosocial work factors, *American Journal of Industrial Medicine*, **26**, 597–612.

Feuerstein, M. 1991 A multidisciplinary approach to the prevention, evaluation, and management of work disability, *Journal of Occupational Rehabilitation*, **1**, 5–12.

Feuerstein, M. 1993 Musculoskeletal injuries: Causes and effects, *Rehabilitation Management*, **6**, 30–5.

Feuerstein, M., Callan-Harris, S., Hickey, P., Dyer, P., Armbruster, W. and Carosella, A. M. 1993 Multidisciplinary rehabilitation of chronic work-related upper extremity disorders: Long-term effects, *Journal of Occupational Medicine*, **35**(4), 396–403.

Fields, H. L. (Ed.) 1987 *Pain*, New York: McGraw-Hill.

Fine, L. J. 1994 Why we should consider both physical and psychosocial factors, Presentation to Fourth International Conference of the Institute of Occupational Health, Milan, October.

Foley, K., *et al.* 1987 *Report of the Commission on the Evaluation of Pain*, Social Security Administration Pub. #64-031, Washington, DC: US Govt Printing Office.

Franklin, G. M., *et al.* 1991 Occupational carpal tunnel syndrome in Washington State, 1984–1988, *American Journal of Public Health*, **81**(6), 741–6.

Franzblau, A. and Blitz, S. 1993 Medical screening of office workers for upper extremity cumulative trauma disorders, *Archive of Environmental Health*, **48**, 164–9.

FREEMAN, R. F. 1990 Going aroung and around with CTDs: A look at the legal issues, *Occupational Safety and Health Reporter*, June 13, 63–7.

FRENCH, M. T. 1990 Estimating the full cost of workplace injuries, *American Journal of Public Health*, **80**, 1118–19.

FUCHS, P. C., NATHAN, P. A. and MYERS, L. D. 1991 Synovial histology in carpal tunnel syndrome, *Journal of Hand Surgery*, **16A**, 753–8.

GERR, F. and LETZ, R. 1992 Risk factors for carpal tunnel syndrome in industry: Blaming the victim?, letter; comment, *Journal of Occupational Medicine*, **34**, 1117–19.

GERR, F., LETZ, R. and LANDRIGAN, P. J. 1991 Upper-extremity musculoskeletal disorders of occupational origin, *Annual Review of Public Health*, **12**, 543–66.

GERRITY, M. S., *et al.* 1992 Uncertainty and professional work: Perceptions of physicians in clinical practice, *American Journal of Sociology*, **97**, 1022–51.

GRANGES, G. and LITTLEJOHN, G. 1993 Postural and mechanical factors in localized and generalized fibromyalgia/fibrositis syndrome, in VAEROY, H. and MERSKEY, H. (Eds), *Progress in Fibromyalgia and Myofascial Pain*, pp. 329–48, Amsterdam: Elsevier.

GREEN, G. M. and BAKER, F. 1991 Conclusions and issues for future work, in GREEN, G. M. and BAKER, F. (Eds), *Work, Health and Productivity*, pp. 277–92, New York: Oxford University Press.

GREENWOOD, J. G. 1990 Early intervention in low back disability among coal miners in West Virginia: Negative findings, *Journal of Occupational Medicine*, **32**, 1047–52.

HADLER, N. M. 1978 Hand structure and function in an industrial setting, *Arthritis and Rheumatism*, **21**, 210–20.

HADLER, N. M. 1989 Disabling backache in France, Switzerland, and The Netherlands; Contrasting sociopolitical constraints on clinical judgment, *Journal of Occupational Medicine*, **10**, 823–31.

HADLER, N. M. 1990 Cumulative trauma disorders: An iatrogenic concept, Editorial, *Journal of Occupational Medicine*, **32**, 38–41.

HADLER, N. M. 1992 Arm pain in the workplace: A small area analysis, *Journal of Occupational Medicine*, **34**(2), 113–19.

HAGBERG, M., MORGENSTERN, H. and KELSH, M. 1992 Impact of occupations and job tasks on the prevalence of carpal tunnel syndrome, *Scandinavian Journal of Work, Environment and Health*, **18**, 337–45.

HAGBERG, M. and WEGMAN, D. H. 1987 Prevalence rates and odds ratios of shoulder neck diseases in different occupational groups, *British Journal of Industrial Medicine*, **44**, 602–10.

HALDEMAN, S. 1990 Presidential address, North American Spine Society: Failure of the pathology model to predict back pain, *Spine*, **15**, 718–24.

HALES, T. 1994 Ergonomic hazards and upper-extremity musculoskeletal disorders, in WALD, P. H. and STAVE, G. M. (Eds), *Physical and Biological Hazards of the Workplace*, pp. 13–41, New York: Van Nostrand Reinhold.

HALES, T., SAUTER, S., PETERSEN, M., PUTZ-ANDERSON, V., FINE, L., OCHS, T., SCHLEIFER, L. and BERNARD, B. 1992 *Health Hazard Evaluation Report, US West Communications* (HETA No. 89-299-2230), National Institute for Occupational Safety and Health, Center for Disease Control and Prevention.

HANSEN, J. 1993 OSHA regulation of ergonomic health, *Journal of Occupational Medicine*, **35**, 42–6.

HIMMELSTEIN, J., DRONEY, T., PRANSKY, G., MORGAN, W. and FEURESTEIN, M. 1994 Development of a multidisciplinary research clinic for patients with work-related upper extermity disorders, *Journal of Ambulatory Care Management*, **17**(2), 34–43.

HIMMELSTEIN, J. and PRANSKY, G. 1994 The evolving health care marketplace: Implications for occupational outcome studies, Presentation at Treatment and Prevention of Upper Extremity Disorders: Challenges in Outcomes Research, Denver, October.

HOVERSTAD, T. and KJOLSTAD, S. 1991 Use of focus groups to study absenteeism due to illness, *Journal of Occupational Medicine*, **33**(10), 1046–54.

IASP TASK FORCE ON PROFFESSIONAL EDUCATION 1991 in FIELDS, H. (Ed.), *Core Curriculum for Professional Education in Pain*, Seattle: International Association for the Study of Pain Publications.

ILLICH, I. 1976 *Medical Nemesis: The Expropriation of Health*, New York: Pantheon.

IOM (INSTITUTE OF MEDICINE) COMMITTEE ON PAIN, DISABILITY, AND CHRONIC ILLNESS BEHAVIOR 1987 in OSTERWEIS, M., KLEINMAN, A. and MECHANIC, D. (Eds), *Pain and Disability: Clinical, Behavioral, and Public Policy Perspectives*, Washington, DC: National Academy Press.

IOM (INSTITUTE OF MEDICINE) COMMITTEE ON NATIONAL AGENDA FOR THE PREVENTION OF DISABILITY 1991 Magnitude and dimensions of disability in the United States, in TARLOV, A. *Disability in America*, Washington, DC: National Academy Press.

JOHANSSON, G. and ARONSSON, G. 1991 Psychosocial factors in the workplace, in GREEN, G. M. and BAKER, F. (Eds), *Work, Health and Productivity*, New York: Oxford University Press.

KEMMLERT, K., ORELIUS-DALLNER, M., KILBORN, A. and GAMBERALE, F. 1993 A three-year follow-up of 195 reported occupational overexertion injuries, *Scandinavian Journal of Rehabilitation Medicine*, **25**(1), 16–24.

KIRMAYER, L. 1984 Culture, affect, and somatization, *Transcultural Psychiatry Research Reviews*, **21**, 159–88, 237–62.

KNIGHT, K. K., GOETZEL, R. Z., FIELDING, J. E., EISEN, M., JACKSON, G. W., KAHN, T. Y., KENNY, G. M., LIADE, S. W. and DUANN, S. 1994 An evaluation of Duke University's LIVE FOR LIFE health promotion program on changes in worker absenteeism, *Journal of Occupational Medicine*, **36**(5), 533–6.

KUHN, T. S. 1970 *The Structure of Scientific Revolution*, 2nd Edn., Chicago: University of Chicago Press.

LARSON, A. 1992 Arising out of employment, in LARSON, A. (Ed.), *The Law of Workers' Compensation*, Vol. 1, pp. 3.1–3.8, New York: Matthew Bender.

LEAVITT, F. 1990 The role of psychological disturbance in extending disability time among compensable back injured industrial workers, *J. Psychosom. Res.*, **34**(4), 447–53.

LEINO, P. 1989 Symptoms of stress predict musculoskeletal disorders, *J. Epid. Comm. Health*, **43**(3), 293–300.

LEVI, L. 1984 Work, stress, and health, *Scandinavian Journal of Work, Environment and Health*, **10**, 495–500.

LOSLEVOR, P. and RANAIVOSOA, A. 1993 Biomechanical and epidemiological investigation of carpal tunnel syndrome at workplaces with high risk factors, *Ergonomics*, **36**, 537–54.

LUNDEEN, C. 1989 Factors affecting workers compensation claims activity, *Journal of Occupational Medicine*, **31**, 653–56.

MAGNI, G. 1993 The epidemiology of musculoskeletal pain, in VAEROY, H. and MERSKEY, H. (Eds), *Progress in Fibromyalgia and Myofascial Pain*, pp. 3–21, Amsterdam: Elsevier.

MACKINNON, S. and NOVAK, C. 1994 Clinical commentary: pathogenesis of cumulative trauma disorder, *Journal of Hand Surgery (Am)*, **19**, 873–83.

MCKINLAY, J. B. and STOECKLE, J. D. 1990 Corporatization and the social transformation of doctoring, in SALMON, E. J. (Ed.), *The Corporate Transformation of Health Care, Issues and Directions*, pp. 133–49, Amityville, NY: Baywood.

MECHANIC, D. 1962 The concept of illness behavior, *Journal of Chronic Diseases*, **15**, 189–94.

MENDELSON, G. 1993 Compensation and motivation in relation to musculoskeletal pain, in VAEROY, H. and MERSKEY, H. (Eds), *Progress in Fibromyalgia and Myofascial Pain*, pp. 101–12, Amsterdam: Elsevier.

MERSKEY, H. 1986 Classification of chronic pain: Descriptions of chronic pain syndromes and definitions of pain terms, *Pain*, Suppl. 3, S215–S221.

MILLAR, J. D. 1988 Summary of 'Proposed national strategies for the prevention of leading work-related diseases and injuries, part 1,' *American Journal of Industrial Medicine* **13**, 233–40.

MILLER, M. H. and TOPLISS, D. J. 1988 Chronic upper limb pain syndrome (repetition strain injury) in the Australian workforce: A systematic cross-sectional rheumatological study of 229 patients, *Journal of Rheumatology*, **15**, 1705–12.

MISH, F. C. (Ed.) 1991 *Webster's Ninth New Collegiate Dictionary*, Springfield, MA: Merriam-Webster.

MOON, S. D. 1992 Conservative management of cumulative trauma disorders of the upper extremity, Presentation at Effective Responses to the Cumulative Trauma Epidemic, Duke University Medical Center Conference, Wilmington, NC, June.

MOON, S. D. 1993a Causation analysis, Presentation at Annual Conference of American College of Occupational and Environmental Medicine, Atlanta, April.

MOON, S. D. 1993b Clinical assessment of cumulative trauma disorders, Presentation at Annual Conference of American College of Occupational and Environmental Medicine, Atlanta, April.

MOON, S. D. 1993c Management of workers with cumulative trauma disorders, Presentation at Annual Conference of American College of Occupational and Environmental Medicine, Atlanta, April.

MOON, S. D., BRIGHAM, C. and SYDNOR, M. (forthcoming) Cumulative trauma disorders: impairment and disability assessments, in DICKERSON, O. B. and ERDIL, M. E. (Eds), *Cumulative Trauma Disorders: Prevention, Evaluation, and Treatment*, New York: Van Nostrand Reinhold.

MOORE, J. S. and GARG, A. 1994 Upper extremity disorders in a pork processing plant: Relationships between job risk factors and morbidity, *American Industrial Hygiene Association*, **55**(8), 703–15.

MORGAN, W. J., *et al.* 1994 Chronic work-related upper extremity disorders: Variables affecting disability, Presentation to 49th Annual Meeting of the American Society for Surgery of the Hand, Cincinnati, October.

MORRIS, W. (Ed.) 1969 *The American Heritage Dictionary*, New York: American Hertiage.

NACHEMSON, A. 1983 Work for all: For those with low back pain as well, *Clinical Orthopaedics* **179**, 77–85.3.

NATHAN, P. A. 1990 Work-related carpal tunnel syndrome, *Journal of the American Medical Association*, **263**, 236–7.

NATHAN, P. A. 1992 Review of ergonomic studies of carpal tunnel syndrome, letter, *American Journal of Industrial Medicine*, **21**, 895–7.

NATHAN, P. A. 1993 Carpal tunnel syndrome and its relation to general physical condition, *Hand Clinics*, May.

NATHAN, P. A., MEADOWS, K. D. and DOYLE, L. S. 1988 Occupation as a risk factor for impaired sensory conduction of the median nerve at the carpal tunnel, *Journal of Hand Surgery*, **2**, 167–70.

NATHAN, P. A., TAGIKAWA, K., KENISTON, R. C., MEADOWS, K. D. and LOCKWOOD, R. S. 1994 Slowing of sensory conduction of the median nerve and carpal tunnel syndrome in Japanese and American workers, *Journal of Hand Surgery* (*Br*), **19**(1), 30–4.

NORDIN, M. and FRANKEL, V. H. 1987 Evaluation of the workplace: an introduction, *Clin. Ortho. Rel. Res.*, **221**, 85–8.

O,CONNOR, F. G., WILDER, R. P. and SOBEL, J. R. 1994 Overuse injuries of the elbow, *Journal of Back and Musculoskeletal Rehabilitation*, **4**, 17–30.

OSHFELDT, R. L. 1993 Contractual arrangements, financial incentives, and physician–patient relationships, in CLAIR, J. M. and ALLMAN, R. M. (Eds), *Sociomedical Per-*

spectives in Patient Care, Lexington, KY: University Press of Kentucky.

OSHR 1991 OSHA guidance clarifies recording criteria for hearing loss, cumulative trauma disorders, *Occupational Safety and Health Reporter*, **21**, 77–8.

OSORIO, A. M., AMES, R. G., JONES, J., CASTORINA, J., REMPEL, D., ESTRIN, W. and THOMPSON, D. 1994 Carpal tunnel syndrome among grocery store workers, *American Journal of Industrial Medicine*, **25**(2), 229–45.

OXENBURGH, M. 1991 How to evaluate the cost of sickness, injury, and absenteesim, in *Increasing Productivity and Profit through Health and Safety*, pp. 11–53, Chicago: CCH International.

PARK, R. M., NELSON, N. A., SILVERSTEIN, M. A. and MIRER, F. E. 1992 Use of medical insurance claims for surveillance of occupational disease, an analysis of cumulative trauma in the auto industry, *Journal of Occupational Medicine*, **34**(7), 731–7.

PARNIAPOUR, M., NORDIN, M., SKOVRON, M. L. and FRANKEL, V. H. 1990 Environmentally induced disorders of the musculoskeletal system, *Med. Clin. North Am.*, **74**(2), 347–59.

PENNEBAKER, J. W. and EPSTEIN, D. 1983 Implicit psychophysiology: Effects of common beliefs and idiosyncratic physiologic responses on symptom reporting, *Journal of Personality*, **51**, 468–96.

PHEASANT, S. (Ed.) 1991 *Ergonomics, Work and Health*, Gaithersburg, MD: Aspen.

PITNER, M. A. 1990 Pathophysiology of overuse injuries in the hand and wrist, *Hand Clinics*, **6**(3), 355–64.

POLATIN, P. B., GATCHEL, R. J., BARNES, D., MAYER, H., ARENS, C. and MAYER, T. C. 1989 A psychosociomedical prediction model of response to treatment by chronically disabled workers with low-back pain, *Spine*, **14**(9), 956–61.

PRYOR, E. S. 1991 Compensation and the ineradicable problems of pain, *George Wash Law Review*, **59**, 239–306.

PUTZ-ANDERSON, V. (Ed.) 1988 *Cumulative Trauma Disorders: A Manual for Musculoskeletal Diseases of the Upper Limbs*, New York: Taylor & Francis.

RAMAZZINNI, B. 1713 *De Morbis Artificum Diseases of Workers*, Trans. W. C. WRIGHT 1940 Chicago: University of Chicago Press.

RITCHEY, F. J. 1993 Fear of malpractice litigation, the risk management industry, and the clinical encounter, in CLAIR, J. M. and ALLMAN, R. M. (Eds), *Sociomedical Perspectives in Patient Care*, pp. 114–38, Lexington, KY: University Press of Kentucky.

ROEMMICH, W. 1961 Determination, evaluation, and rating of disabilities under the Social Security system, *Industrial Medicine and Surgery*, **30**, 60–3.

SALMON, J. W. 1990 Introduction and background, in SALMON, J. W. (Ed.), *The Corporate Transformation of Health Care, Issues and Directions*, pp. 5–18, Amityville, NY: Baywood.

SANDLER, H. M. 1993 Are we ready to regulate cumulative trauma disorders?, *Occupational Hazards*, June, 50–3.

SCHOTTLAND, J. R., KIRSCHBERG, G. J., FILLINGHAM, R., DAVIS, V. P. and HOGG, F. 1991 Median nerve latencies in poultry processing workers, *Journal of Occupational Medicine*, **33**(5), 627–31.

SCHUIND, F., VENTURA, M. and PASTEELS, J. L. 1990 Idiopathic carpal tunnel syndrome: Histologic study of flexor tendon synovium, *Journal of Hand Surgery*, **15A**, 497–503.

SILVERSTEIN, B. A., FINE, L. J. and ARMSTRONG, T. J. 1986 Carpal tunnel syndrome: Causes and prevention strategy, *Seminars in Occupational Medicine*, 213–21.

SILVERSTEIN, B. A., FINE, L. J. and ARMSTRONG, T. J. 1987 Occupational factors and carpal tunnel syndrome, *American Journal of Industrial Medicine*, **11**, 343–58.

STENLUND, B., GOLDIE, I. and MARIONS, O. 1992 Diminished space in the acromioclavicular joint in forced arm adduction as a radiographic sign of degeneration and osteoarthrosis *Skeletal Radiology*, **21**(8), 529–33.

STETSON, D. S., SILVERSTEIN, B. A., KEYSERLING, W. M., WOLFE, R. A. and ALBERS, J. W. 1993 Median sensory distal amplitude and latency: Comparisons between nonexposed managerial/professional employees and industrial workers, *American Journal of Industrial Medicine*, **24**(2), 175–89.

STOCK, S. R. 1991 Workplace ergonomic factors and the development of musculoskeletal disorders of the neck and upper limbs: A meta-analysis, *American Journal of Industrial Medicine*, **19**, 87–107.

STUTTS, J. T. and KASDAN, M. L. 1993 Disability: A new psychosocial perspective, *Journal of Occupational Medicine*, **35**(8), 825–7.

SZABO, R. M., GELBERMAN, R. H. and DIMICK, M. P. 1984a Sensibility testing in patients with carpal tunnel syndrome, *Journal of Bone Joint Surgery*, **66**, 60–4.

SZABO, R. M., GELBERMAN, R. H., WILLIAMSON, R. V., DELLAN, A. L., YANI, N. C. and DIMICK, M. P. 1984b Vibratory sensory testing in acute peripheral nerve compression, *Journal of Hand Surgery (Am)*, **9A**(1), 104–9.

TANAKA, S., SELIGMAN, P., HALPERIN, W., THUN, M., TIMBROOK, C. L. and WASIL, J. J. 1988 Use of workers' compensation claims data for surveillance of cumulative trauma disorders, *Journal of Occupational Medicine*, **30**(6), 488–92.

TARLOV, A. R. 1988 Patient and population perspective, in WHITE, K. L. (Ed.), *The Task of Medicine: Dialogue at Wickenburg*, pp. 30–46, Menlo Park, CA: Kaiser Foundation.

TAYLOR, E. J.) (Ed.) 1988 *Dorland's Illustrated Medical Dictionary*, 27th Edn., Philadelphia, PA: Saunders.

TESH, S. 1988 *Hidden Arguments*, New Brunswick: Rutgers.

TRAVELL, J. G. and SIMONS, D. G. 1983 *Myofascial Pain and Dysfunction: The Trigger Point Manual*, pp. 331–559, Baltimore, MD: Williams and Wilkins.

TOIVANEN, H., HELIN, P. and HANNINEN, O. 1993 Impact of regular relaxation training and psychosocial working factors on neck–shoulder tension and absenteeism in hospital cleaners, *Journal of Occupational Medicine*, **35**, 1123–30.

USDL (US DEPARTMENT OF LABOR) 1988 *Recordkeeping Guidelines for Occupational Injuries and Illnesses*, OMB Publication 1220-0029, USDL, Washington, DC: Bureau of Labor Statistics.

USDL (US DEPARTMENT OF LABOR) 1990 *OSHA Guidelines for Establishing Ergonomics Programs in Meatpacking Plants*, Washington, DC.

USDL (US DEPARTMENT OF LABOR) 1994 *Work Injuries and Illnesses by Selected Characteristics, 1992* USDL-94-213, Washington, DC.

VESSEY, M. P., VILLARD-MACKINTOSH, L. and YEATES, D. 1990 Epidemiology of carpal tunnel syndrome in women of childbearing age: Findings in a large cohort study, *International Journal of Epidemiology*, **19**(3), 655–9.

WADDELL, G. 1987 A new clinical model for the treatment of low back pain, *Spine*, **12**, 632–44.

WAITZKIN, H. B. 1989 A critical theory of medical discourse: Ideology, social control, and the processing of social context in medical encounters, *Journal of Health and Social Behavior*, **30**, 220–39.

WAITZKIN, H. B. 1991 *The Politics of Medical Encounters: How Patients and Doctors Deal with Social Problems*, New Haven: Yale University Press.

WAITZKIN, H. B. and BRITT, T. 1989 A critical theory of medical discourse: How patients and health professionals deal with social problems, *International Journal of Health Services*, **19**(4), 577–97.

WALL, P. D. and MELZACK, R. (Eds) 1989 *Textbook of Pain*, London: Churchill-Livingston.

WALLERSTEIN, N. and WEINGER, M. 1992 Health and safety education for worker empowerment, *American Journal of Industrial Medicine*, **22**, 619–35.

WALSH, D. C. 1991 Costs of illness in the workplace, in GREEN, G. M. and BAKER, F. (Eds), *Work, Health and Productivity*, pp. 217–40, New York: Oxford University Press.

WARNER, K. E., WICKIZER, T. M., WOLFE, R. A., SCHILDROTH, J. E. and SAMUELSON, M. H. 1988 Economic implications of workplace health promotion programs: Review of the literature *Journal of Occupational Medicine*, **30**(2), 106–12.

WARSHAW, L. J. 1988 Occupational stress *Occup Med: State of Art Rev*, **3**, 587–93.

WAXLER, N. E. 1981 The social labelling perspective on illness and medical practice, in EISENBERG, L. and KLEINMAN, A. (Eds), *The Relevance of Social Science for Medicine*, pp. 283–306, Boston: Reidel.

WERNER, R. A., ALBERS, J. W., FRANZBLAU, A. and ARMSTRONG, T. J. 1994 The relationship between body mass index and the diagnosis of carpal tunnel syndrome, *Muscle Nerve*, **17**(6), 632–6.

WHORTON, D. *et al.* 1992 Does fibromyalgia qualify as a work-related illness or injury?, in PERRY, G. (Ed.), Occupational Medicine Forum, *Journal of Occupational Medicine*, **34**, 968.

WILDER, R. P., NIRSCHL, R. P. and SOBEL, J. 1993 Elbow and forearm, in BUSCHBACHER, R. (Ed.), *Musculoskeletal Disorders: A Practical Guide for Diagnosis and Rehabilitation*, Ontario: Andover Medical Publishers.

WOLFE, F., SMYTHE, H. A., YUNUS, M. B., BENNETT, R. M., BOMBARDIER, C., GOLDENBERG, D. L., TUGWELL, P., CAMPBELL, S. M., ABELES, M. CLARK, P. *et al.* 1990 The American College of Rheumatology 1990 Criteria for the Classification of Fibromyalgia: Report of the Multicenter Criteria Committee, *Arthritis and Rheumtism*, **33**(2), 160–72.

WORLD HEALTH ORGANIZATION 1989 Work with visual display terminals: Psychosocial aspects and health, *Journal of Occupational Medicine*, **31**, 957–68.

WORRALL, J. D. 1983 Compensation costs, injury rates, and the labor market, in WORRALL, J. D. (Ed.), *Safety and the Workplace: Incentives and Disincentives in Workers' Compensation*, pp. 1–17, Ithaca: ILR Press.

YOUNG, K. 1989 Disembodiment: The phenomenology of the body in medical examinations, *Semiotica*, **73**, 43–66.

ZOLA, I. K. 1972 Medicine as institution of social control, *Sociological Review*, **20**, 487–504.

CHAPTER NINE

Some social and cultural anthropologic aspects of musculoskeletal disorders as exemplified by the Telecom Australia RSI epidemic

B. HOCKING

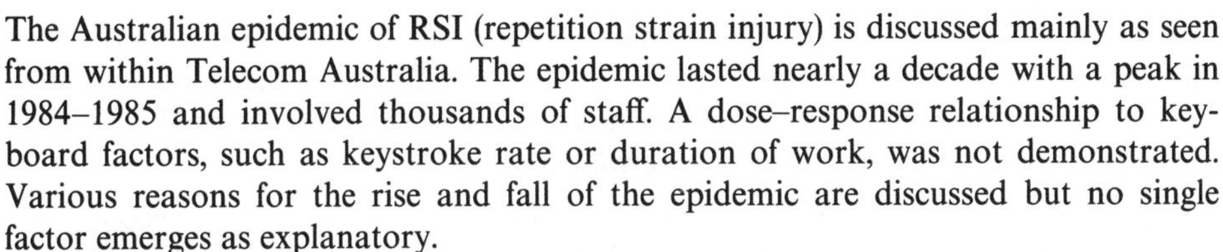

The Australian epidemic of RSI (repetition strain injury) is discussed mainly as seen from within Telecom Australia. The epidemic lasted nearly a decade with a peak in 1984–1985 and involved thousands of staff. A dose–response relationship to keyboard factors, such as keystroke rate or duration of work, was not demonstrated. Various reasons for the rise and fall of the epidemic are discussed but no single factor emerges as explanatory.

A model derived from medical anthropology is suggested which brings together multiple factors. The model is intended to enlarge our thinking about disease and the social processes that give rise to illness in normal people. The implications of the Australian experience for other countries is discussed including a strategy for management of such as epidemic at the community and workplace levels, as well as management of the affected individual.

The possible usefulness of the model for understanding some other nonlinear dose–response work-related conditions is raised.

This chapter develops a medical anthropological interpretation of the RSI epidemic that affected Telecom Australia staff. As a necessary precursor the epidemic is outlined and reasons for its rise and fall considered. But before proceeding please detour to the footnote on the author at the end of the chapter (p. 153).

THE EPIDEMIC

Computerization of work began in the Western world including Australia during the 1970s and office systems appeared widely in the late 1970s and early 1980s.

Various health concerns were raised about visual display terminal (VDT) work including radiation emissions, and effects on pregnancy and on vision, especially the development of cataracts. For example, the alleged effects on vision lead to a remarkable saga of changes in health standards by regulators in Australia (Hocking, 1985). However, musculoskeletal disorders were not a prominent health issue in the literature (Cakir *et al.*, 1979), although research had taken place on the muscle discomfort of telegraphists in Australia during the 1970s (Duncan and Ferguson, 1974). None the less, it should be noted that the RSI epidemic emerged in a setting of multiple concerns about the effects of VDT systems on health.

The epidemic in Telecom has been described in detail elsewhere (Hocking, 1987, 1989, 1993). Telecom Australia is a telecommunications utility which during the 1980s employed approximately 85 000 staff in a wide variety of occupations. The organization is wholly owned by the federal government. The staff are highly unionized and joint union–management health and safety committees were set up in the early 1980s. There is a beneficial workers' compensation scheme which covers costs of time lost from work plus related medical expenses and may convert to long-term payment in the event of permanent disability. Common-law (tort) action also may be taken against an employer if negligence is considered to have caused an accident. Medical care for all Australians is usually provided by general practitioners who are remunerated nearly equally under the national health service (Medicare) as for compensation cases (See Chapter 14 of this volume). Telecom, like most Australian organizations, does not provide general medical care for its staff.

In the early 1980s reports began to be received of staff working on VDTs developing painful arms. This condition became known as RSI and this term is used throughout the paper, although other diagnostic terms are mentioned below. The numbers of reports rose steadily to a peak in 1984–1985 of over 1000 lost-time accidents per year and then began to decline to near zero by 1989 (Figure 9.1).

Statistical features of the RSI epidemic were as follows:

- Some keyboard staff were much more affected than others. In Telecom telephonists were particularly affected (343 per 1000) compared to clerks (284 per 1000) or telegraphists (34 per 1000).
- The incidence of RSI cases was not correlated with keystroke rate. Telephonists who have low keystroke rates of around 1000 per hour had a high incidence (343 per 1000), whereas clerks and telegraphists with medium and high (over 12 000 per hour) keystroke rates had a lower incidence of 284 and 34 respectively. Thus keystroke was inversely related to incidence.
- Within the same occupational group some work locations had a high incidence of RSI and others a low incidence. The telephonists in Perth, Western Australia (WA) experienced 504 cases per 1000 staff, compared to Sydney, New South Wales (NSW) with 182 cases per 1000. A similar observation of variable incidence has been made in America by Hadler (1992).
- The incapacity associated with the condition was considerable. The average time lost per case was 24.4 days, but this also varied between states even in the same occupation. For telephonists in WA the average was 38.7 days compared to 21.3 days in Queensland.
- The incidence of RSI cases was not correlated with duration of keyboard work. Part-time telephonists suffered proportionately as much as full-time telephonists. In addition, younger telephonist staff were slightly more affected, and years of being a telephonist did not correlate with the onset of RSI.

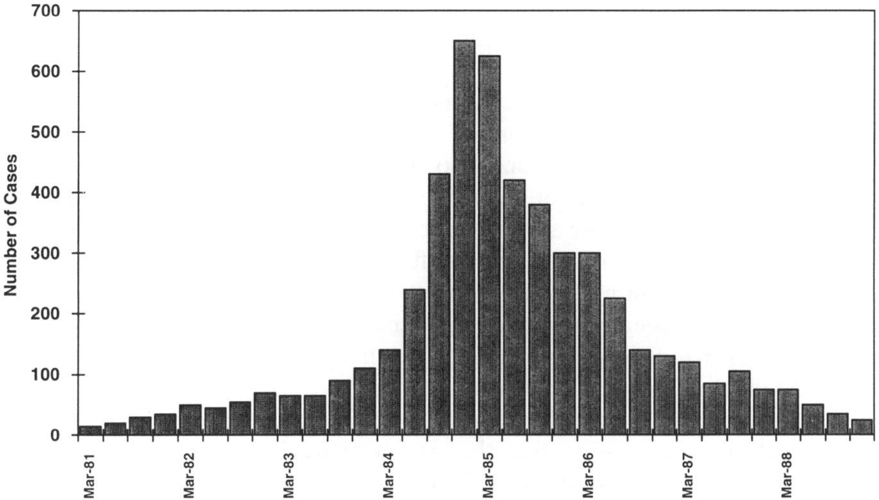

Figure 9.1 Cases of 'repetition strain injury' at Telecom by quarter, January 1, 1981 to December 31, 1988. Copyright © *The Medical Journal of Australia*, 1989, 150, 724; reprinted with permission.

In general there was no evidence of a linear dose–response relationship between keyboard work and incidence of RSI.

The epidemic in Telecom occurred in conjunction with epidemics in other Australian industry, particularly in offices. Rising trends dated from around 1979 but became marked by 1981. Data processors in the federal tax office and pharmaceutical benefits offices were particularly affected (Taylor and Pitcher, 1984). Unfortunately, none of the other epidemics appear to have been analyzed as closely as that in Telecom although it seems that the epidemic in the federal public service peaked nearly a year after that in Telecom.

I consider the reasons for both the rise and fall of the epidemic in Telecom to be equally obscure and uncertain. Regarding the rise of the epidemic there are various aspects to be considered.

First, the medical issues are still not resolved. The painful arms were originally attributed to tenosynovitis, tennis elbow, or carpal tunnel syndrome as recognized in manufacturing industry (Ferguson, 1971), but the symptoms and clinical findings did not match these classic conditions and the term 'repetition strain injury' (RSI) was introduced (see below). The early emphasis was on a peripheral lesion and one report, which was substantially criticized, claimed diagnostic muscle biopsy changes (Dennet and Fry, 1988). More recently interest has moved to neurogenic or central lesions. Helme *et al.* (1992) have reported evidence of an unusual neurogenic abnormality in a report yet to be confirmed. Cohen *et al.* (1992) have suggested a disorder of the dorsal horn pain mechanism and introduced the term 'refractory cervicobrachial pain' disorder. Again this has been criticized and needs confirmatory work. Even if any of the above postulated lesions were found to be consistent in RSI cases, it would still leave open the problem of the relationship between the impairment and the disability. As noted, this was highly variable with average time lost ranging from 21 to 38 days for Telecom staff with the same occupation in different parts of

Australia. Therefore while the clinical information must be considered, at present it does not provide a sufficient explanation for the patchy onset of the epidemic or its variable severity.

It is interesting that carpal tunnel syndrome was not a major concern, unlike in the American epidemic (see Chapter 6 of this volume).

Various psychiatric explanations also have been raised. The most notable, by Lucire, proposes an epidemic of conversion hysteria (Lucire, 1986). This postulates that people develop somatic symptoms by way of resolution of unpleasant past experiences and present interpersonal conflicts. Some evidence for this psychopathology has been found in psychiatric consultation with RSI cases. However, no controlled studies have been reported to show that nonaffected staff do not have these personal problems, nor is this personal psychodynamic explanation sufficient to explain the patchy spread of the epidemic.

The importance of job satisfaction was noted in some surveys of VDT operators in other industries suggesting that the system of work, including measurement of work rates, may be as important at the equipment (Ryan *et al.*, 1982; Taylor and Pitcher, 1984). In some work groups the new systems lead to deskilling of work which may affect job satisfaction. Graham studied two groups of telephonists in Adelaide (Graham, 1985). One group on international traffic had poor ergonomic equipment but a low incidence of RSI, whereas the group handling directory assistance had equipment that was good ergonomically (adjustable screens and chairs) but also had a high incidence of RSI. He found that the arrangements for work of the international operators allowed them to be human and social. They spoke to the client, the overseas operator, and sometimes the overseas connection, and gratitude was often expressed by the client. By contrast, directory assistance staff were deskilled from rapidly searching a suite of directories, were discouraged from engaging in pleasantries, time constraints were imposed, and there was a constant bank of calls waiting.

RSI was strongly associated with the introduction of VDT equipment, although Telecom subsequently had clusters of RSI in telephonists working on old 'cord and switch' equipment. The Japanese also experienced an epidemic in the 1960s of an RSI-like condition in telephonists using 'cord and switch' technology (Nakaseko *et al.*, 1982). This suggests that the VDT *per se* is not a unique or sufficient cause of RSI in telephonists.

Medical treatment initially emphasized splinting and not using the painful arm before returning to work, as well as prescribing various forms of analgesia. Lawyers in compensation cases emphasized the need for stability of the condition before finalizing a claim. All this led to prolonging the period of absence from work and the perception that it was extremely incapacitating.

In 1984 the NSW Health Department (Browne *et al.*, 1984) issued a statement using the term 'occupational repetition strain injury,' grading its severity and implying that it could progress to incapacitating degrees if not promptly detected and treated. This statement had the effects of legitimizing pain as a disease, and firmly linking the condition to rapid keystrokes in the mind of the workforce and many professionals. The statement also created a surge of education programs aimed to get keyboard workers to report any arm pain quickly so that incapacity might be avoided. Some unions and media amplified this message into the idea that any arm pain could lead to crippling incapacity. In addition, various ergonomic theories for the epidemic (keystroke rate, posture) were advanced and the importance of ergonomically designed workstations was emphasized. Ergonomic chairs, adjustable screens and tables, and training in keyboard technique were widely introduced and workers were educated in their importance to prevent the crippling effects of RSI.

The reasons for the decline in the epidemic are also not clear-cut. In Telecom the developing epidemic was discussed at federal and state health and safety committees and joint working parties were often formed to investigate the problem. Some of the VDT systems in telephony had reasonably good ergonomic work stations provided from the outset (e.g. adjustable screens and chairs) so supplementary training emphasized best use of this equipment. Wrist rests were made available, rest breaks were formalized, and in a few exchanges education about keying technique was given. However, there was no systematic evaluation of these interventions to determine their actual benefit.

Regulatory authorities claim that education and ergonomic equipment helped to lessen the epidemic (Emmett, 1992). The evidence for this is, at best, slight. Numerous interventions took place and it could be that all, some, or none have contributed. No controlled trails have been conducted so a placebo (Hawthorne) effect or coincidental temporal association cannot be excluded. For example, the Japanese considered that the introduction of lightweight headsets for telephonists was important in controlling their epidemic, but these were standard issue in Telecom prior to the epidemic which questions their importance in prevention and suggests a placebo affect for this ergonomic intervention. Also it is theoretically possible that the epidemic ended because of exhaustion of a pool of staff who were susceptible by virtue of their neuromuscular function (see Chapter 5 of this volume) and/or because of their workstyle (see Chapter 11 of this volume) or other unidentified factors. The major documents of Worksafe Australia were released after the decline began so it is doubtful that they were pivotal (Worksafe Australia, 1986, 1989). Additionally, the federal labour government was so concerned about the failure of Worksafe to manage the epidemic that it ordered the MacKay inquiry into its operations which led to the transfer of its then chief executive officer and extensive reorganization.

It should be noted that the Telecom RSI epidemic began to decline in January 1985. This was prior to a major compensation court case decision in May 1985 which did not support the plaintiff's claim (*Cooper* v. *Australian Tax Office*). Therefore while this court decision had substantial affects on public perception of RSI and its sufferers (see below), I do not believe that secondary gain (RSI = 'retrospective supplementary income') is a sufficient explanation for the onset of the epidemic, nor is it decline mainly explicable by loss of this sickness incentive (see Chapter 14 of this volume).

However, after the court decision, skepticism among the media, the public, and other keyboard workers increased regarding RSI and its sufferers. There have been several subsequent legal decisions which have nearly always not found for the plaintiff. In addition, medical opinion regarding treatment swung against immobilization to simple pain management and early graded return to work (RACP, 1988).

Later in the epidemic Telecom sought to keep affected staff coming to work for at least a part of the day even if to do very little. For some telephonists the use of a computer-aided voice recognition system[1] has been helpful as a rehabilitation device (Jack and Lenko, 1993). The decline of cases in Telecom was investigated by a joint union–management working party and found to be real. It was not due to underreporting of painful arms by staff for reasons of intimidation.

The above description of the epidemic is intended to give some feel of its dynamics and to indicate why simple explanations regarding the RSI epidemic should be treated cautiously. Systems of work which involve VDTs may be a necessary component but they and particularly their keyboards, are not a sufficient explanation for it.

A MEDICAL ANTHROPOLOGY MODEL

Anthropology offers insights into the social processes of groups of people and conflict situations that are considered relevant to the RSI epidemic and its uneven occurrence (Hocking, 1987, 1993).

Douglas (1975) has described how nearly all social groups can be described by two contrasting dimensions termed 'grid' and 'group.' 'Grid' is a hierarchical arrangement imposed on people which defines relationships and boundaries, e.g. in the military or hospital. 'Group' relates to the collectiveness of people, e.g. clubs, communes, or work groups. Groups tend to cohere more strongly in the face of an external threat, such as a perceived pollutant, and to define their boundaries more clearly. Groups are maintained by varying levels of arousal and additional levels of fear may produce various symptoms which require interpretation (see Report 4 in Hocking, 1987).

Noting this, I suggest that some groups of operators perceived pain and discomfort in their arm when working on new VDT systems possibly through mechanisms suggested by Westgaard and Blair (Chapters 5 and 6 of volume). Probably underlying the early cases was some apprehension about the health affects of the new VDT systems, which also deskilled the job, causing dissatisfaction and arousal (Graham, 1985). Due to multiple factors, including training courses, union and media publicity, and professional statements, the view became widespread that any pain and discomfort would lead to severe pain and long-lasting incapacity.

The situation may be compared to an iceberg (see Figure 9.2).

The iceberg represents a mass of ill-defined bodily sensations and subclinical disease, but only the tip is perceived as pain or clinically presented illness. However, the iceberg floats in a social sea. If this becomes 'denser,' the iceberg rises and the tip enlarges (and vice versa). Thus illness in a population or group of people is a relative matter. The size of the iceberg may increase (more arm pain after introduction of new systems) and/or the social environment may change (fear arousal with the group) and raise the iceberg (Hocking, 1993, 1987). This variously affects individuals as well as groups.

A further anthropological explanation relates to mechanisms of social change, conflict resolution, and coping with misfortunes. This properly involves an extensive discussion on witchcraft but is beyond the scope of this paper. Briefly the classic analysis is by Evans-Pritchard (1976), who emphasized how witchcraft provided not only an explanation of why a misfortune happened to an individual, but also could lead to a course of action to rectify the wrong. For example, a successful charge of witchcraft could lead to social change. Physical causes of misfortune and injury are recognized but not considered a sufficient explanation of 'Why me?' Douglas (1970) summarizes much literature as follows: 'The symbols of witchcraft are built on the theme of vulnerable internal goodness attacked by external power.'

Lewis (1976) has described 'possession' states in some cultures in which unusual symptoms manifest in socially subordinate people. For example, in Somalia women

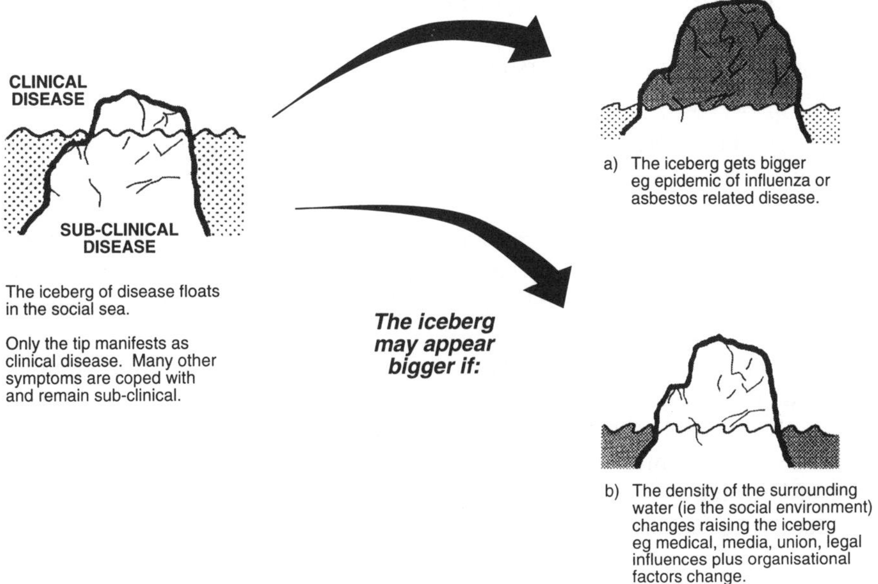

Figure 9.2 The iceberg of disease (Hocking, 1993).

may be possessed by a spirit that requires appeasement, such as by gifts. Lewis suggests that possession states are a milder and less radically challenging assault on authority than a charge of witchcraft and may be employed against persons whose authority is begrudgingly accepted by the powerless to bring about change. It is possible to interpret the RSI epidemic as also fulfilling this social function of conflict resolution, given the deskilling of work subsequent to the introduction of VDT systems and the concomitant symptoms of arm pain (see also Kriesler and Finholt, 1988).

These medical anthropological views are difficult to prove or disprove without extensive fieldwork. But such an argument may obscure their main virtue which is to enlarge our thinking about disease and to consider the social processes, internal and external to the workplace, giving rise to an illness. It should be emphasized that they relate to the behavior of normal people, as distinct from a psychiatrist's explanations based in psychopathology.

Another issue arising from medical anthropology is to question the relevance of the Australian epidemic for other countries. Given the interweaving of medical, political, and social factors, the condition is likely to be 'culture-bound' and therefore extrapolations overseas should be made with care; conversely, other countries may have their own disorders not apparent in Australian VDT workers. In Massachusetts a survey of 1,545 VDT operators found that while 32 per cent had noted arm symptoms, only 3 per cent had lost time due to arm pain and then only for a few days (Rossignol *et al.*, 1987). This contrasts with the 25 per cent of Telecom telephonists who lost time for an average of 24 days. Also the emphasis in America on carpal tunnel syndrome has been noted previously. Thus while it is true that arm pain does occur internationally, the Australian epidemic seems to have been fundamentally different and suggests caution when extrapolating to America. By contrast, in Scandinavia there has been a major problem of rashes on the face of VDT operators (Nilsen, 1982), a problem almost unknown in Australia.

Noting the limitations in understanding and extrapolating from the Telecom epidemic, the following is suggested in managing such epidemics elsewhere:

- A strategy should be aimed at biological and psychosocial factors within and external to the workplace. It requires consensus and cooperation from several stakeholders.
- Prompt, well-designed multidisciplinary research may be helpful. Failure to institute good research, particularly regarding clinical characterization of the condition, was probably the single biggest error by regulators and others in Australia. (See also Sandow *et al.*, 1987.)
- Basic ergonomics should be addressed, including training in use of the equipment provided. However, it is also important to consider broader issues about the system of work and other organizational issues (see Chapter 2 of this volume and Appendix 2) which may influence the psychosocial environment and contribute to unresolved conflict.
- The actions of regulators must be carefully weighed regarding inflaming or containing a situation (Hadler, 1992). Pejorative terms such as 'repetition strain injury' or 'occupational overuse syndrome' should be avoided in favor of terms such as 'painful arm' or 'office worker's arm pain' until diagnostic labels can be used with confidence.
- The media and unions can be sources of disinformation and need to be carefully informed or bypassed to ensure accurate communication with staff. In this regard usage of the iceberg concept (Figure 9.2) may be considered as an explanatory model which combines biological and psychosocial factors in a nonprejudicial way (see Chapter 13 of this volume).
- Professional education of doctors, lawyers, and occupational health workers is important. The release of authoritative statements, such as that by RACP (1988), can be influential in shaping attitudes.
- For individuals with RSI the Telecom experience points to the need for simple care of the painful arm while giving attention to psychological issues such as fear of VDT systems. The behaviorist approach of continuing attendance at work even though incapacitated appears to have been beneficial (Jack and Lenko, 1993). It is noted that the mere demonstration of a muscular or neural lesion does not necessarily equate to the degree of disability which may be due to learned pain behavior (Tyrer, 1986). Disability needs to by managed by vocational rehabilitation techniques in conjunction with appropriate medical treatments of the lesion (see Chapter 10 and 12 of this volume).

Lastly, it is suggested that there are other lessons to be learned from the RSI epidemic and medical anthropology (Hocking, 1993). It is proposed that the epidemic is indicative of a range of newly emerging work-related conditions (as distinct from the classic occupational diseases such as asbestosis). These will be subtle in manifestation and have complex origins which do not fit with the linear dose–response paradigm of occupational disease. For example, sick building syndrome was recently found to be disproportionately experienced by clerical VDT operators (Menzie *et al.*, 1993), and sick leave in general is due to a complex mix of biological and psychosocial factors. Since these conditions are likely to be partly linked to human resource management issues, Telecom has recently introduced a broad policy on work environment and distress. This policy (Appendix 1) covers matters such as organization of work, performance review, and so on, and is intended to optimize productivity while lessening major potentiating factors of new health issues.

In addition we have been developing models using nonlinear dynamical mathematics (Hocking and Thompson, 1992), to try to understand complex relationships in the workplace and how these may contribute to conditions such as RSI since simple linear models were found sadly lacking in the Telecom Australia RSI epidemic (Appendix 2).

FOOTNOTE: AUTHOR'S BIAS—A NOTE OF EXPLANATION

No one closely involved with the Australian RSI epidemic of the 1980s was left without prejudices and blind spots, such was the intensity of feeling that it engendered. Therefore the reader should know a little more about the writer.

I graduated in 1965 from Melbourne Medical School, a very orthodox, physical disease-orientated school. Subsequently I worked for several years in Asia and the Pacific, particularly in Papua New Guinea, where I had the fortune to meet several anthropologists. From them I began to appreciate the need to consider the social context in which biological phenomena such as disease occurs.

Therefore my approach to the RSI epidemic was one of a doctor schooled to look for a lesion (disease) but tempered with an awareness of social context influencing the pattern of illness (Hocking, 1987).

For the last 15 years I have been the Chief Medical Officer for Telecom Australia. My view therefore is further tempered by a senior executive of the company. This has the advantage for an anthropologist of living with the tribe and hence detecting cultural issues; on the other hand, the view is limited to this tribe and my role in it.

APPENDIX 1 AUSTRALIAN AND OVERSEAS TELECOMMUNICATIONS CORPORATION (AOTC) OCCUPATIONAL HEALTH AND SAFETY POLICY: WORK ENVIRONMENT AND DISTRESS POLICY AND GUIDELINES

It is AOTC's policy to create a work environment in which the work performance and potential of staff is optimized. Maximizing an individual's capacity to meet work requirements and providing a supportive work environment will be major factors in achieving this objective.

Discrepancies between the capacity of individuals and work requirements may lead to distress in the work environment. Nonwork factors may also lead to distress for individuals.

In order to maximize work performance, minimize distress, and enhance the well-being of staff, AOTC will, as far as is practicable:

Organize work, design jobs, and introduce new technology in a manner that recognizes the impact on and interaction of technology, changes to organizational structures, individual skills and personal well-being, and seeks to enhance work performance.

Relate to staff using a participatory style of management which supports individual skills and encourages staff participation, responsibility, and accountability for work performed.

Ensure that personnel practices adequately provide for addressing grievances including discrimination and harassment issues.

Ensure that feedback on work performance will be provided to and invited from individuals. This may be supported where necessary by changes to the work environment and/or by personal development such as career counselling, skills training, assertiveness courses, etc.

Promote general health, and provide a safe and healthy work environment so as to minimize stressors, e.g. physical, chemical, biological, etc.

Assist recovery from medical problems in accordance with AOTC's Rehabilitation Guidelines, facilitate referral for staff who require access to external professional counselling, and provide support where appropriate to staff whose distress is contributed to by nonwork factors.

Integrate the above approaches to managing the organizational environment into management practices, training, and development at all levels of the organization.

APPENDIX 2 CHAOS MODEL OF REPETITIVE WORK[2]

Nonlinear dynamical mathematics (chaos) has been applied to modelling repetitive work with a view to understanding parameters desirable to optimize production and to minimize potential ill effects. An introduction to chaos has been given elsewhere (Hocking and Thompson, 1992).

The job studied involved a worker (editor) making repeated data entry about clients' details onto a computer system. Each entry took about 2–3 minutes and in a day 150–200 entries were made. Editors work as a team but this preliminary model describes only an individual editor. Each day editors are assigned a workload by the team leader and unfinished work would be reassigned the next day. If needed, the team leader provides counselling about performance to editors. See Figure 9.3

The model assumes that an editor has a Gaussian efficiency profile (Figure 9.4). A Gaussian form is taken from $E(w)$ and the parameters a, b and c are adjusted to take account of team leaders' counselling and adjustments to any backlog.

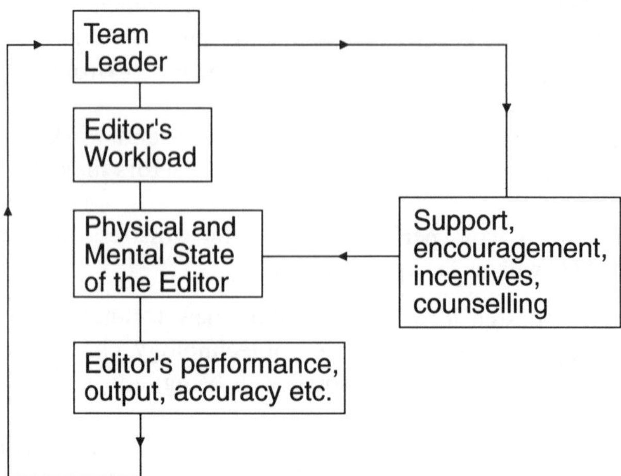

Figure 9.3 Qualitative model of an editor's work dynamics.

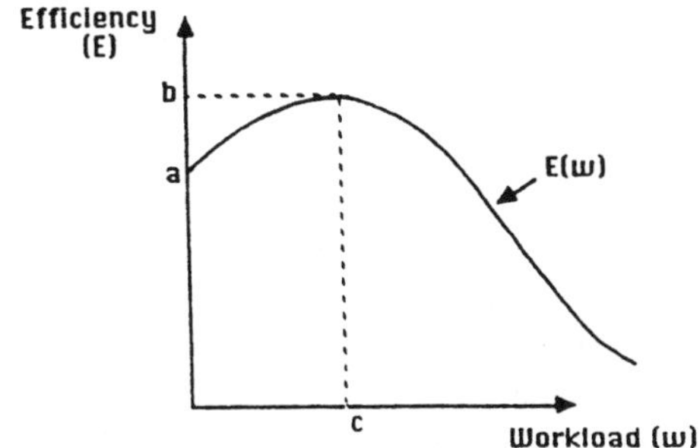

Figure 9.4 Efficiency curve for an editor.

a = the efficiency of an editor without workload

b = the peak efficiency

c = the workload that leads to peak efficiency.

The standard deviation, ^SSYMBOL 115\f"Symbol"^U canbe calculated from a, b and c.

The workload wn on 'day' n is taken to be a constant plus some fraction d of the previous day's backlog. The number of items processed by the editor on day n is then taken to be

$pn = wnE(wn)$

We define

wn = workload assigned to the editor on day n

pn = productivity of the editor on day n

bn = Max(0,wn-1-pn-1) is the backlog of work carried forward to day n.

If ^ SSYMBOL 97\f "Symbol"^U is the daily workload assignment we take

wn =^ SSYMBOL 97\f "Symbol" ^U + dbn

with

$d = (1 - r) \quad (0 < r < 1).$

The parameter r is a reduction factor by which a team leader can reduce the assigned workload by eliminating some of the backlog.

We assume that

$pn = wnE(wn)$

= wn exp^SSYMBOL 91 \f "Symbol" ^Uebn

– (c-wn)2/ ^SSYMBOL 115 \f "Symbol" ^U^ SSYMBOL 93 \

f "Symbol" ^U (9.1)

where

$$e = eo(1 + f) \qquad c = co(1 + f)$$

can be adjusted by a counselling factor *f*. The term *e* is a scaling factor for coping with backlog by an editor, and *c* has been defined previously.

Dynamics of the team leader–editor interaction can then be simulated by setting $wo = po = 0$, fixing parameter values (^SSYMBOL 97 \f "Symbol"^U, *d*, *r*, *eo*, *co*, *f* and ^SSYMBOL 115 \f "Symbol"^U) and iterating equation (9.1).

The simulation is robust in the sense that the same qualitative behavior (stability, instability, etc.) is obtained when relativities (e.g., ^SSYMBOL 97 \f "Symbol"^U > *c*) between parameters are maintained but absolute values are varied. The range of the simulation behavior is best seen from the demonstration software. See Figure 9.5.

The optimally efficient workload value of $wn = c$ (Figure 9.3) for a particular editor is an equilibrium solution for the model but it is an unstable equilibrium.

For workloads less than *c* the model editor typically relaxes into a 'two-cycle' (Figure 9.5a). No counselling or reduction of backlog assignment to the editor is required in this case (e.g., $d = 1$) and the dynamics is oscillatory but stable. Productivity in fact can be improved in some instances by reducing the assigned workload. Counselling tends to amplify the oscillations but the average productivity is increased (Figure 9.5b). However, there has been a change from a two-cycle to a three-cycle state, which indicates that chaos is close. When workloads are very much less than *c*, chaotic states with irregular oscillations are frequently obtained, which could presumably be linked to ill effects (Figure 9.5c). In cases of extremely small workloads, a very low productivity equilibrium is regained.

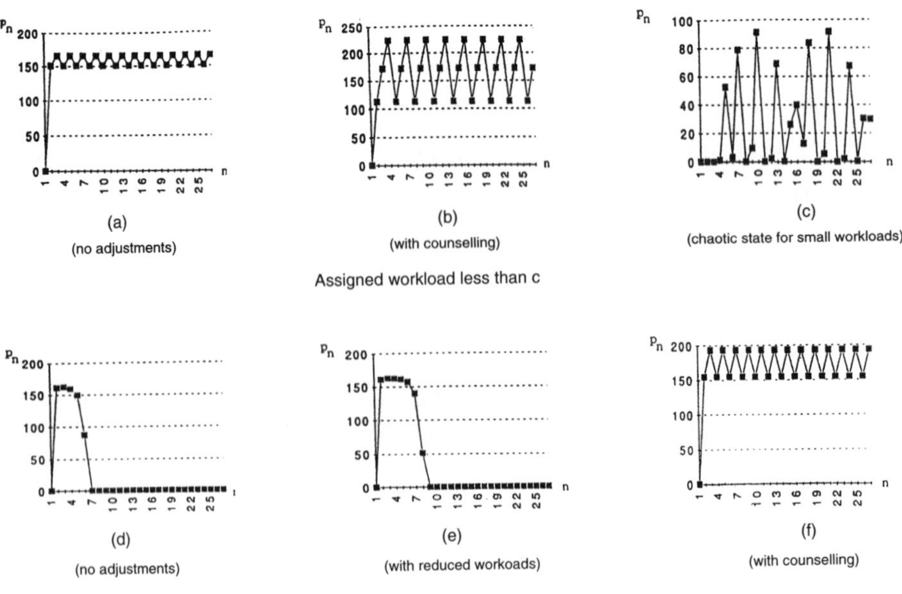

Figure 9.5 Computer simulation of productivity of an editor under various conditions.

For workloads in excess of c the dynamics is inherently unstable (Figure 9.5d, e, and f). Stability can, however, be restored in this case for workloads slightly above c by team leader counselling (Figure 9.5f), rather than by reducing the editor's backlog. For workloads moderately in excess of c stability can only be restored by eliminating some of the backlog from the assigned workload.

Finally we remark that the shape of $E(w)$ and an estimate for c could be obtained from suitable data and that this information could be of value to individual editors as well as to team leaders and management. Productivity could then be optimized on knowing the operators' capacity by assigning an appropriate workload and counselling when necessary. The optimal operating state is a two-cycle (Figure 9.5a) which is stable to minor changes, whereas a flat curve is unstable. Ill effects, which could include stress, are arbitrarily defined as occurring when the productivity curve deviates or oscillates outside acceptable boundaries (variance) (e.g. Figure 9.5c, d, and e).

The model has the potential of usefully matching workers' capacities to job requirements, but can be abused and will require care in any application. The model is being extended to include more complex interactions and more quantitative data.

NOTES

Thanks to B. Thompson for the computer modeling to produce Figure 9.5 and to Mr C. Langham for facilitating the study.

1 Voice recognition system available from Mission Critical Technologies, Concord, MA, USA.

2 By C. Thompson and B. Hocking. C. Thompson is Professor at the Department of Mathematics, Melbourne University, Victoria, Australia,

REFERENCES

BROWNE, C., NOLAN, B. and FAITHFULL, D. 1984 Occupational repetition strain injuries: Guidelines for diagnosis and management, *Medical Journal of Australia*, **140**, 329–32.

CAKIR, A., HART, D. and STEWART, T. 1979 *The VDT Manual*, Darmstadt: IFRA.

COHEN, M. *et al.* 1992 In search of the pathogenesis of refractory cervicobrachial pain syndrome: A deconstruction of the RSI phenonmenon, *Medical Journal of Australia*, **156**, 432–43, and see correspondence **156**, 670 and 815.

DENNET, X. and FRY, H. 1988 Overuse syndrome: A muscle biopsy study, *Lancet*, **1**, 905–8, and see correspondence **1**, 1465.

DOUGLAS, M. 1970 *Witchcraft Confessions and Accusations*, London: Tavistock.

DOUGLAS, M. 1975 *Natural Symbols*, Melbourne: Penguin.

DUNCAN, J. and FERGUSON, D. 1974 Keyboard operating posture and symptoms in operating, *Ergonomics*, **17**(5), 651–62.

EMMETT, E. 1992 New directions for occupational health and safety, Australia, *Journal of Occupational Health and Safety*, **8**(4), 293–308.

EVANS-PRITCHARD, E. 1976 *Witchcraft, Oracles and Magic among the Azande*, abridged, Melbourne: Oxford University Press.

FERGUSON, D. 1971 Repetition injuries in process workers, *Medical Journal of Australia*, August 21, 408–12.

GRAHAM, G. 1985 Job satisfaction and repetition strain injury (dissertation), Adelaide: Elton-Mayo School of Management, SA Institute of Technology.

HADLER, N. 1992 Arm pain in the workplace, *Journal of Occupational Medicine*, February, 113–19.

HELME, R. D., LEVASSEU, S. and GIBSON, S. 1992 RSI revisited; evidence for psychological and physiological differences from an age, sex and occupation matched control group, *Australia and New Zealand Journal of Medicine*, **22**, 23–9, and see correspondence 393–4.

HOCKING, B. 1985 Setting occupational health standards in Australia: The case of screen based equipment operators' eyesight tests, *Community Health Studies*, **9**(2), 139–44.

HOCKING, B. 1987 Anthropological aspects of occupational illness epidemics, *Journal of Occupational Medicine*, **29**, 526–30.

HOCKING, B. 1989 Epidemiological aspects of 'repetition strain injury' in Telecom Australia, *Medical Journal of Australia*, **147**, 218–22, and see correspondence **50**, 724.

HOCKING, B. 1993 The aftermath of RSI in Telecom Australia, *Journal of Occupational Health and Safety*, **9**(2), 131–5.

HOCKING, B. and THOMPSON, C. 1992 Chaos theory of occupational accidents, *Journal of Occupational Health and Safety*, **8**,(2), 99–108.

JACK, S. and LENKO, S. 1993 Rehabilitation of occupational overuse syndrome in keyboard operators using the voice recognition system, submitted to *Journal of Occupational Health and Safety*.

KRIESLER, S. and FINHOLT, T. 1988 The mystery of RSI, *American Psychologist*, December, 1004–15.

LEWIS, I. 1976 *Social Anthropology in Perspective*, Melbourne: Penguin, p. 89.

LUCIRE, Y. 1986 Neurosis in the workplace, *Medical Journal of Australia*, **145**, 323–7.

MENZIE, R., TAMBLYN, R., *et al.* 1993, The effect of varying levels of outdoor air supply on symptoms of sick building syndrome, *New England Journal of Medicine*, **328**, 821–7.

NAKASEKO, M., TOKUNAGA, R. and HOSUKAWA, M. 1982 History of occupational cervicobrachial disorder in Japan, *Journal of Human Ergolcogy*, **11**, 7–16.

NILSEN, A. 1982 Facial rash in visual display unit operators, *Contact Dermatitis*, **8**, 25–8.

RACP (ROYAL AUSTRALASIAN COLLEGE OF PHYSICIANS) 1988 *Repetitive strain injury*, Sydney: RACP.

ROSSIGNOL, A., MORSE, E., *et al.* 1987 Video display terminal use and reported health symptoms among Massachusetts clerical workers, *Journal of Occupational Medicine*, **29**, 118–22.

RYAN, A., HAGE, B and BAMPTON, M. 1982 Postural factors, work organization and musculoskeletal symptoms, in BUCKLE, P. (Ed.), *Musculoskeletal Disorders at Work*, London: Taylor & Francis.

SANDOW, M., YELLOWLESS, P., *et al.* 1987 Research into the regional pain syndrome, correspondence, *Medical Journal of Australia*, **146**, 389.

TAYLOR, R. and PITCHER, M. 1984 Medical and ergonomic aspects of an industrial dispute concerning occupational-related conditions in data process operators, *Community Health Studies*, **8**,(2), 172–80.

TYRER, S. 1986 Learned pain behavior, *British Medical Journal*, **292**, 1–2.

WORKSAFE AUSTRALIA 1986 *Code of Practice for the Prevention and Management of Occupational Overuse Syndrome*, Canberra: Australian Government Publishing Service.

WORKSAFE AUSTRALIA 1989 *Guidance Note for the Prevention of Occupational Overuse Syndrome in Keyboarding Employment*, Canberra: Australian Government Publishing Service.

CHAPTER TEN

A cognitive–behavioral perspective on pain in cumulative trauma disorders

FRANCIS J. KEEFE and JENNIFER R. EGERT

Persistent pain is a significant problem for patients having cumulative trauma disorders (CTDs) (Koch, 1986). Although CTDs may lead to significant impairments in physical and work performance, the main of concern of the patient is usually their pain. Many CTD patients have difficulty coping with what they view as the uncertain nature and future trajectory of their pain. Some patients may become so anxious and absorbed by the pain experience that they have difficulty functioning. Still other CTD patients develop significant behavioral problems such as avoidance of activities and dependence on medications that exacerbate their pain.

Recently, there has been growing recognition that persistent pain can be influenced by cognitive and behavioral factors (Keefe *et al.*, 1992). New methods for assessing and treating persistent pain have been developed by cognitive–behavioral pain researchers. These methods have been found to be helpful in managing both acute and chronic pain (Keefe *et al.*, 1992) and potentially could be quite useful in the management of CTD pain.

The purpose of this paper is to present a cognitive–behavioral perspective on pain in CTD. The first section outlines the basic elements of a cognitive–behavioral model of CTD pain. The second section describes assessment strategies that may be helpful in analyzing cognitive and behavioral factors affecting pain in CTD patients. The third section describes cognitive–behavioral interventions for helping patients manage CTD pain. The final section highlights important issues arising from the use of cognitive–behavioral interventions with CTD patients.

A COGNITIVE–BEHAVIORAL MODEL OF CTD PAIN

CTDs are usually evaluated and treated on the basis of biomedical model (Berger and Fromison, 1979; Dionne, 1984). The basic elements of this model are depicted in Figure 10.1. According to this model, cumulative trauma produces nociceptive input which is transmitted by small and large neural fibers to central nervous system pathways which then activate sensory areas of the brain responsible for pain sensation. This model maintains that pain can best be understood by analyzing its underlying tissue pathology and identifying the sources of cumulative trauma. Treatment

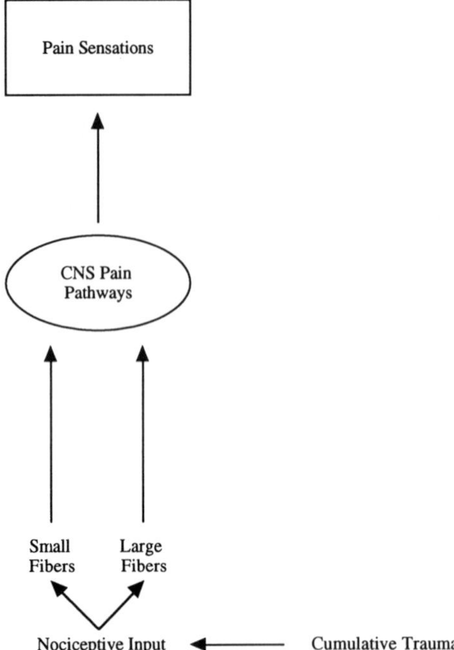

Figure 10.1 A biomedical model of CTD pain.

interventions based on the biomedical model are designed to decrease nociceptive input. This can be achieved either through medical management and/or by modifying the patient's physical environment to reduce or eliminate sources of physical trauma.

A hallmark of the biomedical model is that it views pain as a sensory experience. This model is simple: nociceptive input produces the sensation of pain, and reduction of this input will eliminate pain sensations. This view of pain as a sensory experience is pervasive, not only in biomedical settings, but also in society at large. Patients seeking biomedical treatment for CTDs often have an implicit sensory model of their pain. They expect the tissue pathology basis of their pain to be identified and effective treatment administered. Unfortunately, many patients having CTDs have repeatedly failed to respond to treatments based on such a biomedical model.

Recent developments in pain research and theory suggest that a cognitive–behavioral model may provide a useful alternative to the biomedical model in understanding CTD patients who suffer from persistent pain (Keefe *et al.*, 1992; Turk *et al.*, 1983). Figure 10.2 displays the basic elements of a cognitive–behavioral model of CTD pain. This model highlights the role that cognitive–behavioral responses to pain can play in modulating pain perception. Cumulative trauma produces nociceptive input which can be modulated at the spinal cord level via the gate control mechanisms described by Melzack and Wall (1965). The opening or closing of the gate determines whether central nervous system (CNS) pathways are activated and pain sensations are experienced or not. Pain sensations can trigger cognitive,

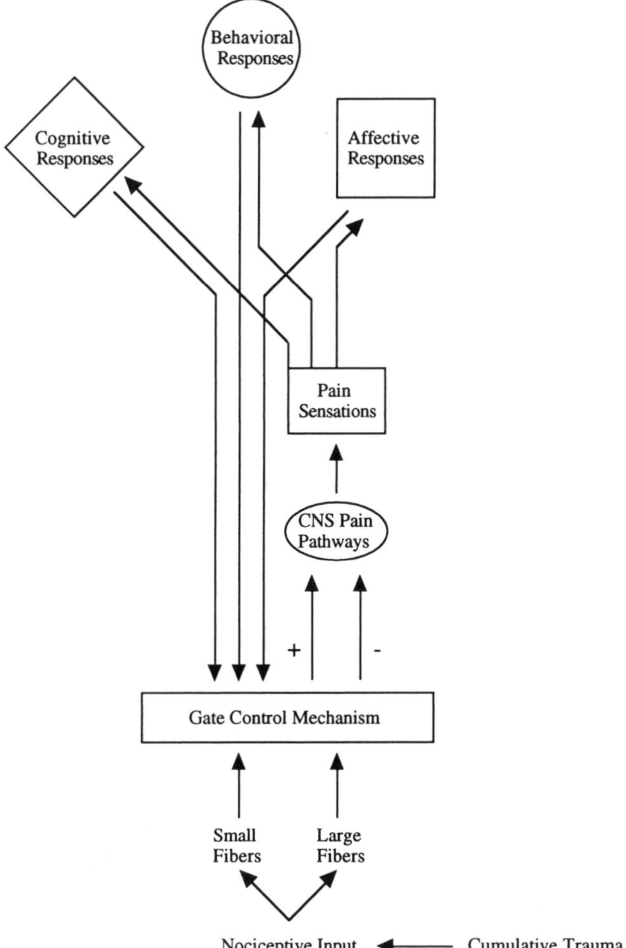

Figure 10.2 A cognitive–behavioral model of CTD pain.

affective, and behavioral responses which in turn exert a descending influence on the transmission of nociceptive input.

The cognitive–behavioral model has several important features that distinguish it from the biomedical model. First, it incorporates a systems theory perspective. Changes in one part of the system can influence and be influenced by changes in other parts of the system. This contrasts with the more linear view of pain sensations inherent in the biomedical model. Second, the cognitive–behavioral model directs attention to psychological variables that may be important in determining pain. Cognitive variables such as patient beliefs about pain, overly negative thinking, pain coping strategies, and perceived control over pain are thus seen as influencing pain sensations. The pain experience can also be affected by behavioral responses such as guarded pain avoidant posturing, an overly sedentary and dependent lifestyle, and dependence on habit-forming pain medications. Finally, the cognitive–behavioral model views affective factors such as anxiety or depression as important determinants of pain.

The cognitive–behavioral model not only provides a framework for understanding pain, it also serves to direct treatment interventions designed to reduce pain. Cognitive–behavioral therapy interventions teach CTD patients to control and decrease pain by altering cognitive, behavioral, and affective responses. Patients are typically trained with a variety of techniques including biofeedback, progressive relaxation training, activity pacing, cognitive restructuring, and cognitive pain coping skills (e.g. imagery and distraction). These techniques are described in detail later in this paper. For some CTD patients, cognitive–behavioral interventions may be just as important in reducing pain and disability as biomedical components of their treatment regimen.

Finally, the cognitive–behavioral model stresses the importance of early intervention to prevent CTD pain from becoming persistent. With the passage of time, there is more opportunity for cognitive, behavioral, and affective responses to affect CTD pain. Learned patterns of maladaptive responding can develop and become entrenched. Both behavioral theory and research suggests that training in techniques for the self-regulation of pain are more effective if they are applied earlier rather than later in the course of persistent pain (Ferster, 1965; Kanfer and Goldfoot, 1966).

COGNITIVE–BEHAVIORAL ASSESSMENT OF CTD PAIN

Cognitive–behavioral researchers have developed a variety of assessment measures that are applicable to CTD patients. In this section, we review a number of behavioral and cognitive assessment methods.

Behavioral Assessment

The three techniques most commonly used in the behavioral assessment of pain are behavioral observation, behavioral interviewing, and diary records.

Behavioral observation

Patients with CTD pain exhibit certain pain-related behaviors that can be directly observed and quantified. Observations of employees, for example, can be carried out in work settings to obtain information about body postures, movements, and ergonomic factors that may be contributing to the development and maintenance of CTD symptoms. The availability of inexpensive videotape cameras and recorders has made it much easier for clinicians and researchers to gather samples of pain-related behaviors from CTD patients.

Pascarelli and Kella (1993) videotaped 53 disabled computer keyboard operators at an experimental workstation. They identified certain styles, positions, and postures that could be potentially harmful because of biomechanical stresses placed on functioning anatomic structures. In particular, ligamentous hypermobility of the finger joints and inefficient keyboard styles appeared to relate to the severity of injury. One limitation of this study, however, is that it failed to compare injured and noninjured workers.

Feuerstein and Fitzgerald (1992) conducted a recent study comparing behavior patterns of sign-language interpreters who either had pain or were pain-free. They began their study by carrying out informal observations of sign-language interpreters at work to identify behavior patterns that might be related to pain. They noticed that interpreters with pain held themselves in postures that placed strain on the upper back and exhibited high frequency movements of the fingers, hands, wrists, and forearms with continuous shoulder exertions. To further test the validity of these observations, the authors videotaped interpreters during a simulated interpreting session. Videotaped behavior samples were recorded from two groups of interpreters: those working with pain ($n = 16$) and those working without pain ($n = 13$). Results indicated a number of significant differences in behavior between pain and pain-free interpreters. Interpreters with pain took fewer rest breaks per minute, and exhibited more hand–wrist deviations from neutral, and more excursions outside the work envelope (or area of optimal signing, 25 cm × 25 cm). Observer ratings also revealed that interpreters with pain exhibited a higher pace of finger/hand movement and exhibited more muscle tension.

The results of this study indicated that sign-language interpreters with CTD pain display a characteristic behavior pattern that differs from that of interpreters who do not have pain. This behavioral response to a difficult work task may increase subjects' risk for CTDs and is an important target for behavioral intervention.

Harber *et al.* (1992) used behavioral observation and ergonomic analysis to study the actions associated with grocery checking. Videotaped samples of behavior were collected from 50 individuals who worked as grocery checkers. One of the difficulties in analyzing these behavior samples is that the motions involved in grocery checking are not highly stereotyped. A large variety of items are checked of different weights and sizes each requiring different kinds of handling. In addition, some work periods are quite busy and demanding. To deal with these problems, two steps were taken. First, a series of standard 'indicator' objects (e.g. a bottle of milk, a quart of ice cream) were identified and behaviors occurring during the checking of these items were coded. Second, videotaped behavior samples were taken during a 15-minute slow period and a 15-minute fast period. Observers recorded the motions involved in checking (e.g. wrist flexion and extension, ulnar deviation, and lumbar flexion). The results were then combined to form a quantitative index of behaviors placing subjects at risk for CTD.

A second study by this research group (Harber *et al.*, 1993) examined the relation of behavior to pain and other CTD symptoms. The 50 individuals studied in the original report were interviewed to assess symptoms of CTD. The results indicated that there were relationships between several types of motion behaviors and symptoms. Wrist flexion and extension were particularly related to hand–wrist symptoms and carpal tunnel symptoms. Pronation and motions of the lumbar spine were found to relate to hand–wrist–lower-arm symptoms. The authors suggest that differences in the frequency of these motions were mainly a product of different workstations and that alternative workstations may minimize CTD risk. Another possibility is that workers engaging in these motions may be behaviorally responsive to work demands, such as in the Feuerstein and Fitzgerald (1992) study cited above. Regardless of interpretation, the observations were effective in identifying behaviors that deserve attention in treatment.

Taken together, the results of the studies reviewed in this section suggest that behavioral observation is a very useful technique for assessing behavioral factors influencing CTD pain.

Behavioral interviews

Behavioral interviews are frequently used in the behavioral assessment of persistent pain. Interview methods are particularly helpful in identifying behavioral and social factors that might be influencing pain.

Fordyce (1976) has discussed behavioral interviewing in detail. He has identified a number of important areas to be covered in the interview. These include:

1. Time pattern – identifying activities that precede pain, diurnal patterns of pain.
2. Environmental responses – determining how individuals in the patient's life (co-workers, family, friends) respond to pain-related behaviors with particular attention to the reinforcement by others of maladaptive behaviors.
3. Pain activators or diminishers – pinpointing the activities that increase or decrease pain.
4. Changes in activity because of pain – what changes in the patient's and spouse's life have occurred as a result of pain.

More recently structured behavioral interviews have been developed for use in chronic pain assessment. The Psychosocial Pain Inventory (PPI) (Heaton *et al.*, 1982) is one example. This interview gathers information from both the patient and spouse of 25 psychosocial aspects of pain. The PPI directly addresses work-related issues such as disability and income, employment history prior to pain, and changes in employment after pain onset. The behavioral interview can identify psychosocial factors that may have a strong relationship to pain complaints in CTD patients. Stutts and Kasdan (1993) interviewed 83 workers with upper-extremity pain who were applying for Workers' Compensation benefits. Their interview specifically asked subjects about the disability status of other family members. A control group of 318 asymptomatic working subjects were also interviewed about their work and the disability status of their family members. A highly significant difference ($p < 0.001$) in the occurrence of family disability was noted between the CTD patients and the control patients. A total of 52 per cent of the CTD patients had at least one family member who was disabled. Only 15 per cent of the control group of asymptomatic workers had a disabled family member. The authors conclude that a 'disabled' support system may serve to support and maintain disability in CTD patients. They also suggest that CTD-related disability may develop through a process of learning in which disabled family members model pain and illness behaviors and reinforce these behaviors when they are displayed by the patient.

Diary records

Diary records of activity and medication intake are frequently used in the behavioral assessment of chronic pain. Fordyce (1976) developed a diary that asked patients to make hourly entries of the time that they spent in three major activity categories: (1) sitting, (2) standing or walking, and (3) reclining. This diary format is widely used in pain assessment and is helpful in identifying problematic behavior patterns. A pattern often evident in the diary records of patients having CTDs is pain cycling (Gil *et al.*, 1988) in which the patient persists with a work activity until they reach the point of pain tolerance and then rest. As this pattern becomes habitual, tolerance for activity decreases and the amount of rest time decreases. Training patients to pace activities and take rest breaks on a time-contingent basis can break this cycle. Such activity pacing can also help patients to tolerate better activities that cause them pain. It also enables them to resume activities that they may be avoiding because of increased pain.

One advantage of diary records is that they can be tailored to address problems experienced by a particular patient. For example, a CTD patient who has increased pain during periods of stress and heavy work demands might be asked to keep diary records of workload, perceived stress, and pain. By examining these records, information can be gathered about the importance of workload and stress as determinants of pain. Research has shown that patients can keep reliable and valid records of a wide range of behaviors and environmental factors if they are provided with systematic training in record-keeping procedures (Affleck *et al.*, 1992; Follick *et al.*, 1984).

In the past five years, there have been important advances in the application of statistical techniques to the analysis of diary data. These analyses enable one to examine diary data gathered over extended time periods and quantify the relationships between variables such as activity and pain. They also permit one to establish temporal cause–effect relationships between behavior patterns and pain while controlling for confounding variables such as autocorrelation or day of the week. Affleck and his colleagues have demonstrated how these techniques can be applied to pain diary data gathered from arthritis patients (Affleck *et al.*, 1991). By applying similar methods to diary data collected from CTD patients, researchers may be able to provide important new information of the influence of behavioral responses on perceived pain.

Assessing Cognitive Variables

Persistent pain, a major symptom of CTD, can change an individual's thoughts, beliefs, and expectations (Keefe *et al.*, 1992). Individuals with chronic pain often have maladaptive beliefs about the diagnosis and treatment of pain and expect treatment efforts to fail (DeGood and Shutty, 1992). Such negative cognitions can not only increase the severity of pain (McGuire, 1992), but can also impair recovery by affecting compliance with a treatment regime (DeGood and Shutty, 1992). Overly negative cognitions can also lead to depression or anxiety which further impair workers' readiness to return to work and actual job performance.

Relatively few studies in the CTD literature have addressed cognitive factors influencing pain. This topic, however, has been receiving a great deal of attention in the chronic pain research literature. Researchers have developed a number of reliable and valid questionnaire instruments that are potentially quite useful for assessing pain-related cognitions in CTD patients.

The pain beliefs and perceptions inventory (PBAPI)

The PBAPI (Williams and Thorn, 1989) is a 16-item instrument designed to assess enduring beliefs that patients have about their pain. Factor analysis suggests that the PBAPI measures three basic dimensions of pain: (1) self-blame – the belief that they are to blame for their pain condition, (2) mystery – the belief that the pain cannot be explained and is a mystery to the patient and others, and (3) time – the belief that pain will persist in time.

In research with chronic pain patients, Williams and Thorn (1989) found that these three belief dimensions were not only related to pain but also to patients' compliance with treatment interventions. Patients who scored high on the time factor (who believed their pain would be chronic) and the mystery factor (who believed their pain was unexplainable) were found to comply poorly with physical therapy and cognitive–behavioral pain management. Those who scored high on the mystery factor also had higher levels of somatization and psychological distress.

Patients having CTD vary in their pain beliefs. While some patients appear to understand their pain, others have a poor grasp of what is causing their pain and are uncertain of the likely future course of their pain. Given that these variations in pain beliefs may impact treatment, there is a need to incorporate instruments such as the PBAPI into CTD assessment.

The coping strategies questionnaire (CSQ)

The CSQ (Rosenstiel and Keefe, 1983) is a 44-item scale that assesses (1) the degree to which patients use six cognitive and one behavioral pain coping strategies, and (2) the perceived effectiveness of these strategies in controlling and decreasing pain. The six cognitive strategies on the CSQ are: (1) diverting attention away from the pain, (2) reinterpreting pain sensations, (3) coping self-statements, (4) ignoring pain sensations, (5) praying or hoping, and (6) catastrophizing. The behavioral coping strategy measured by the CSQ is increasing activity.

The CSQ has been used in a number of studies of chronic pain patients (see Jensen *et al.*, 1991; Keefe *et al.*, 1992 for reviews of this literature). Typical of this research is a series of studies that we conducted on pain coping in patients with osteoarthritis of the knees (Keefe *et al.*, 1987a, b; Keefe *et al.*, 1990). In this research we identified a Pain Control and Rational Thinking factor on the CSQ through principal components analysis of patients' questionnaire responses (Keefe *et al.*, 1987a). Patients who scored high on this factor rated their ability to control pain as high and avoided overly negative thinking when coping with pain. This factor was a significant predictor of pain, physical disability, and psychological disability even after controlling for effects due to medical variables likely to affect knee pain. Patients who showed increases in scores on the Pain Control and Rational Thinking factor after undergoing cognitive–behavioral treatment, were also much more likely to have improvements in physical disability (Keefe *et al.*, 1990).

Spence (1989) has used the CSQ in a study of cognitive–behavioral treatment interventions for CTD patients with persistent upper-extremity pain. She found that patients undergoing cognitive–behavioral treatment showed a significant increase in the frequency of use of active coping strategies compared to a waiting-list control group. Patients were able to maintain their improvements in active coping over a six-month period. These results suggest that the CSQ is sensitive enough to detect treatment-related changes in CTD patients. Further research is needed to examine the relation of coping strategies to indices of pain, adjustment, and treatment response in CTD patients.

The cognitive errors questionnaire (CEQ)

The CEQ (Lefebvre, 1981) is a 24-item instrument designed to measure cognitive errors in patients with persistent pain. The CEQ has 24 short vignettes covering a broad range of life situations including work, family/home and recreational activities. At the end of each vignette is a brief statement which includes a cognitive distortion. Subjects rate on a five-point scale how similar the statement is to a thought that they would have in a similar situation. The CEQ measures four basic types of cognitive errors: (1) catastrophizing: interpreting or anticipating a catastrophic outcome from the event; (2) overgeneralization: assuming that the outcome of one event applies to the same or similar events in the future; (3) personalization: taking personal responsibility or attributing personal meaning to a negative event; and (4) selective abstraction: selectively attending to negative aspects of an experience. Two forms of the CEQ were developed, one focused on general life experiences and one specific to the problems of individuals with lower back pain (LBP). More recently, investigators have adapted the CEQ for use with other chronic pain populations, e.g. rheumatoid arthritis (Smith *et al.*, 1994).

Lefebvre (1980) used the CEQ to compare cognitive errors in LBP and depressed patients. He found that depressed individuals, either with or without LBP, made more cognitive errors than nondepressed individuals. Depressed LBP patients were particularly prone to make cognitive errors when responding to vignettes related to pain. The depressed LBP patients endorsed more cognitive errors on pain-related items than the pain-free depressed subjects. These results suggest that cognitive distortions are related to depression in patients with persistent pain. Assessing these distortions may be helpful in understanding pain report in patients who are depressed. Cognitive therapy interventions to reduce cognitive distortions and overly negative thinking also may be useful in managing pain.

COGNITIVE–BEHAVIORAL TREATMENT OF CTD PAIN

Behavioral and cognitive–behavioral interventions have only recently been applied to patients with persistent CTD pain. Although research on this topic is limited, three basic types of studies have been carried out: (1) those examining the efficacy of educational–behavioral interventions, (2) those examining the efficacy of cognitive–behavioral interventions alone, and (3) those in which cognitive–behavioral interventions have been combined with other treatments in a multidisciplinary program for CTD pain. This section describes and critically evaluates studies illustrating each of these three types of research.

Educational–Behavioral Interventions for CTD Pain

Educational programs for CTD are designed to provide patients with information about the causes of cumulative trauma in order to reduce further trauma pain and prevent future problems. Behavior change is a key target in many educational programs for CTD. Thus, a major goal of education is to reduce habitual behaviors such as the use of inappropriate or awkward hand movements during repetitive work tasks. Educational interventions typically use either a lecture–discussion format or provide didactic information through written or audiovisual materials. Many of these programs are implemented as part of prevention efforts, and thus are delivered before the development of CTD pain. They are thus designed to change habits which, left unchecked, may cause pain.

A good example of research on educational–behavioral interventions for preventing CTD pain is a study conducted by Dortch and Trombly (1990). Subjects in this study were 18 workers who performed electronic assembly jobs at a manufacturing plant. Before and after treatment, a behavioral observation was carried out at each subject's worksite to identify the frequency of movement behaviors that might be traumatizing or aggravating to the hand, wrist, and forearm. Subjects were randomly assigned to one of three treatment conditions. Subjects in the educational information group attended group sessions and were given handouts that provided information about the causes of CTD, the anatomical basis of this disorder, and methods for reducing mechanical stress on the wrist and hand. Patients in the education plus behavioral rehearsal condition received the same educational information, but also received an opportunity to rehearse skills for reducing cumulative trauma in the group setting. These subjects simulated their job performance, were given individualized instructions on how to avoid trauma, and then implemented behavior change efforts while being given performance feedback by the therapist. Subjects in the third condition received no educational or behavioral intervention and served as a control group.

Results of this study indicated that patients in both of the education conditions showed significant decreases in the frequency of traumatizing movements of the hand and wrist compared to subjects in the control condition. Although subjects in the education plus behavioral rehearsal intervention showed greater overall improvements than patients receiving education alone, this difference failed to reach statistical significance. This failure may have been due to the fact that very small sample sizes (n = 5–6 subjects per condition) limited the power of this study design to detect change.

The study by Dortch and Trombly has several limitations. These include the fact that none of the workers currently suffered from CTD pain, and the lack of long-term follow-up to evaluate the maintenance of behavior change. Nevertheless, this study is important since it demonstrates the potential efficacy of educational interventions either alone or in combination with behavioral rehearsal in reducing potentially traumatizing hand movements in industrial workers with repetitive jobs.

Cognitive–Behavioral Interventions Alone

Cognitive–behavioral interventions are based on the model of CTD pain presented earlier in this chapter. These interventions are designed to alter cognitive, behavioral, and affective responses to pain. In cognitive–behavioral treatment, CTD patients are taught coping skills for managing their pain. To enhance perceived control over pain, patients are taught a variety of skills and encouraged to apply the specific skills that they find most effective. Cognitive–behavioral interventions can be carried out either in group or individual therapy sessions.

Spence (1989) has carried out one of the few controlled studies evaluating the effects of cognitive–behavioral treatment for CTD pain. In this study, 45 subjects who had persistent work-related upper-limb pain were randomly assigned to one of three conditions: (1) group cognitive–behavioral therapy for pain management, in which patients attended nine 90-minute group sessions over nine weeks, (2) individual cognitive–behavioral therapy for pain management, in which patients attended the same number of individual therapy sessions, or (3) a waiting-list control condition, in which patients continued with their routine care. The cognitive–behavioral treatment was multimodal and addressed a number of pain-related problems. Table 10.1 lists the major components and treatment techniques used. As can be seen, training focused on behavioral issues such as time management, cognitive issues such as reducing the frequency of maladaptive thoughts, and affective issues such as anxiety reduction and control of depression.

To evaluate the outcome of treatment, patients completed daily pain diaries, and self-report measures of anxiety, depression, coping strategies, and disability before and after treatment and at the time of a six-month follow-up evaluation. Results indicated that the cognitive–behavioral interventions, whether delivered in an individual or group format, were equally effective. Patients in both cognitive–behavioral treatment conditions increased their use of active pain coping strategies and showed significant pre- to post-treatment improvements in pain, anxiety, depression, and disability. These improvements were generally very well maintained at the six-month follow-up evaluation. Little or no improvement was noted for patients participating in the waiting-list control condition.

Table 10.1 Major components of cognitive–behavioral intervention (based on Spence, 1989).

Components	Objectives
Cognitive restructuring	1. Challenge maladaptive pain beliefs 2. Accept role of psychological variables in pain experience 3. Reduce frequency of negative thoughts
Goal setting	1. Increase activity 2. Re-establish social contracts 3. Increasing reinforcing events and activities 4. Enhance time management skills
Relaxation training	1. Reduce overall muscle tension 2. Reduce tension during stressful events and repetitive work tasks 3. Interrupt pain–tension–pain cycle
Training in cognitive coping strategies	1. Divert attention from pain using imagery, distraction 2. Reinterpreting pain sensations – relabeling
Communication skills	1. Learning to make requests 2. Refusing unreasonable requests 3. Dealing with supervisors and co-workers
Sleep hygiene	1. Stimulus control methods to improve sleep 2. Relaxation to assist in decreasing tension

Spence (1991) conducted a two-year follow-up study to assess the long-term maintenance of improvements in the CTD patients treated in her original study. Results indicated that there was little relapse in outcome. Patients continued to report frequent use of active pain coping strategies and were able to maintain significant reductions in pain, depression, and disability.

Taken together, the results reported in the two studied by Spence are interesting. They suggest that cognitive–behavioral interventions may not only be effective in managing pain, but also in reducing pain-related psychological distress and physical disability. Limitations in this research are evident. The research, for example, failed to include an attention placebo condition against which to compare the effects of the cognitive–behavioral intervention. Interpretation of the long-term follow-up findings is also limited by the relatively small sample size ($n = 19$). Nevertheless, this research strongly suggests that cognitive–behavioral intervention can lead to significant and sustained improvements in patients suffering from work-related CTD pain.

Cognitive–Behavioral Intervention Combined with Multidisciplinary Treatment

In the past five years, multidisciplinary programs for CTD have begun to incorporate cognitive–behavioral pain management interventions into their treatment protocols. Patients undergoing treatment thus not only receive typical CTD treatment interventions such as physical conditioning, training in ergonomics, and work simulations, but also receive training in coping skills for managing pain. The rationale for multidisciplinary treatment is that CTDs are complex in etiology and when persistent pain and disability occur, multiple factors need to be addressed. Including a cognitive–behavioral component in multidisciplinary treatment is considered important because it can enhance patients' sense of mastery and control over pain.

A good example of how cognitive–behavioral interventions can be integrated into a multidisciplinary treatment program for CTD is provided by a recent report by Feuerstein and his colleagues (Feuerstein *et al.*, 1993). This report compared outcomes of patients who had undergone a combined cognitive–behavioral/multidisciplinary treatment regimen with a control group of patients who continued with their regular care. The patients were diagnosed as having nerve entrapment and tendinitis-related pain related to their work. All had persistent pain and were out of work for a minimum of three months.

The cognitive–behavioral intervention was carried out in daily group sessions conducted by a psychologist. Training techniques included (1) relaxation-based methods such as progressive relaxation and biofeedback, (2) training in cognitive coping strategies for managing emotional distress, (3) self-hypnosis for managing episodes of severe pain, (4) communication skills for improving patients' abilities to assert themselves with family, friends, and co-workers, and (5) training in problem-solving methods. The training also used extensive behavioral rehearsal to teach patients how they could apply each of these skills in actual work situations.

The rehabilitation program described by Feuerstein *et al.* (1993) was multidisciplinary. Thus, it integrated cognitive–behavioral treatment with: (1) physical conditioning – both aerobic and strength training; (2) work conditioning – which involved training in simulated work settings; and (3) vocational counseling – with a counselor with special expertise in CTD.

In analyzing their outcome data, the authors first compared the two groups prior to treatment. Their results indicated that, prior to the study, there were no significant differences in psychological status or perception of the work environment between the treatment and control groups. The authors examined return-to-work data collected 17 to 18 months after the patients entered the study. At that time, patients in the treatment group were found to be significantly more likely to return to work and remain working than patients in the usual care control condition. One of the most interesting findings at follow-up was that 80 per cent of the patients who had undergone multidisciplinary treatment were working full-time, while only 50 per cent of the control patients were working full-time. Based on clinical observations, the authors believe that the cognitive–behavioral interventions may have eased patients' transition to work by helping them relax, gain more control over pain and distress, and manage anger, frustration, and other emotional responses better.

Feuerstein *et al.* acknowledge that their study has several design problems. Patients were not randomly assigned to treatment and control conditions. In addition, because the cognitive–behavioral component was combined with other interventions, it was impossible to determine the unique contribution that this component made to outcome. The study also failed to include measures of change in pain, mood, and function.

Although this study does have drawbacks, it illustrates the potential of multidisciplinary, cognitive–behavioral treatment in returning CTD patients to work. Further research is needed to evaluate the role of cognitive–behavioral interventions in multidisciplinary rehabilitation programs for CTD.

SPECIAL ISSUES IN WORKING WITH CTD PATIENTS

A number of issues arise when cognitive–behavioral interventions are used to manage pain in CTD patients. Three of the most important issues are the relative importance of pain in managing CTD, applying pain coping skills in work situations, and issues related to maintenance of treatment gains.

Relative Importance of Pain in Managing CTD

The objective of most treatment programs for CTD is to improve function in order to facilitate return to work. The underlying assumption of these programs is that improvements in function will lead to reduced pain. One criticism that has been raised about using cognitive–behavioral interventions for managing CTD pain is that they view pain relief as the primary goal of treatment and thereby de-emphasize the goals of improved function and return to work. The basic concern is that patients may become so preoccupied with their pain that they avoid activities and exercises that, while increasing pain in the short run, are of crucial importance in improving functional status in the long run.

From the patient's perspective, relief of pain is almost always the primary goal of treatment. Pain is the symptom that motivates most CTD patients to seek treatment. Most patients judge the success of their treatment on the basis of how much it enables them to reduce or control pain. One reason that cognitive–behavioral intervention appeals to patients is that it acknowledges the central role that pain plays in determining the symptoms of CTD.

Patients learn in cognitive–behavioral treatment to reconceptualize their pain and the role that their own efforts to change behavior can play in determining pain.

Changing behavior through graded exercise or activation is seen as one of the most important ways of controlling and reducing pain. Thus, cognitive–behavioral therapists actively encourage CTD patients to exercise and help patients to learn methods to overcome obstacles to exercise such as a temporary increase in their pain.

In essence, the cognitive–behavioral perspective views pain reduction and improvement in function as compatible treatment goals. By acknowledging the importance of both of these goals, patients' motivation for and compliance with treatment is often enhanced.

Applying Coping Skills in Work Situations

Patients with CTD pain often experience pain during particular activities on the job. One criticism of cognitive–behavioral interventions such as relaxation training is that they teach patients to control pain in quiet, controlled settings, but cannot be applied in busy work settings where pain is likely to be a problem.

In cognitive–behavioral treatment, several methods are used to help patients to generalize pain coping skills to daily situations. One technique, covert rehearsal, involves having patients imagine themselves confronting problem situations and then applying coping skills. By reviewing patients' reactions to this type of rehearsal, problematic responses can be identified and specific recommendations provided on ways to cope with pain. A second technique, behavioral rehearsal, involves applying coping skills in simulated situations. Many programs for CTD have work simulation and conditioning programs that provide an excellent opportunity for rehearsing pain coping skills. Therapists can instruct patients on how they might apply a particular coping skill (e.g. a distraction or activity pacing technique) during a work task. The patient can then try to use the skill during the task while the therapist provides guidance and feedback on their performance. Behavioral rehearsal has been used in several studies of CTD patients (e.g. Dortch and Trombly, 1990; Feuerstein *et al.*, 1993).

A third technique to enhance generalization is the use of a practice hierarchy. Patients are usually able to identify specific home and work situations that are likely to increase their pain. These situations can be arranged in order from least to most difficult. Patients can then be given graded assignments from the hierarchy starting with those that are least difficult. By applying coping skills in these relatively easy situations first, patients can gain more confidence in their abilities to manage and decrease pain. Treatment can then progress to gradually more difficult situations.

In sum, cognitive–behavioral treatment recognizes the importance of generalization and incorporates methods designed to enhance transfer of learned skills to the work environment.

Maintenance Issues

One of the most important and neglected topics in the management of persistent pain is the degree to which therapeutic improvements can be maintained over time (Turk and Rudy, 1991). Maintenance is particularly an issue for cognitive–behavioral treatments for CTD pain because they rely on patients' abilities to continue to apply active coping efforts in work situations over extended time periods.

Several behavioral techniques have been developed to enhance the maintenance of pain coping skills. One method is to involve the patient's spouse in the treatment program (Fordyce, 1976). The spouse is often interested in assisting the patient in the learning of coping skills, but unsure what to do. Behavioral researchers have developed systematic training programs for spouses that not only provide spouses with information about the rationale for cognitive–behavioral treatment, but also provide specific training in techniques (e.g. prompting and reinforcement) to help the patient to maintain frequent coping skills practice (Moore and Chaney, 1985).

A second method for enhancing maintenance is to encourage the patient's supervisors to be more aware and supportive of the treatment program. The type of response that a returning worker gets from their supervisor may be important in determining the long-term outcome of interventions for CTD pain. In a study of LBP patients, Linton (1991) evaluated an educational program designed to teach supervisors techniques to facilitate patients to return to work. Supervisors were trained in communication skills and methods for reinforcing coping skills and work performance. The supervisors complied quite well with instructions to apply these skills in the workplace. Patients returning to work after an injury rated the supervisors who had received this skills training as much more supportive than supervisors who had not received the training.

To enhance maintenance, patients undergoing cognitive–behavioral treatment can also be trained in relapse prevention methods (Marlatt and Gordon, 1985). In relapse prevention training, patients are taught through covert rehearsal, review of prior relapses, and self-monitoring to recognize problem situations that are likely to lead to setbacks in coping with pain. They also behaviorally rehearse techniques for coping with setbacks and learn to apply these techniques early in order to prevent setbacks from developing into a full-blown relapse. Relapse prevention training has been found to be quite helpful in preventing relapse from disorders such as smoking (Hall *et al.*, 1984) and obesity (Perri *et al.*, 1984; Drapkin, 1990) and is a promising method for maintaining treatment gains in CTD patients with persistent pain.

CONCLUSIONS

The cognitive–behavioral perspective has much to offer those working with CTD patients. This perspective provides an important alternative to the traditional medical management of CTD. Unfortunately, cognitive–behavioral intervention is often reserved for patients who fail to respond to medical treatment. By integrating cognitive–behavioral approaches more fully into initial assessment and treatment efforts, health-care professionals may be better able to understand, treat, and prevent pain in CTD patients.

REFERENCES

AFFLECK, G., TENNEN, H. URROWS, S. and HIGGINS, P. 1992 Individual differences in the day-to-day experience of chronic pain: A prospective daily study of rheumatoid arthritis patients, *Health Psychology*, **10**, 419–26.

AFFLECK, G., TENNEN, H. URROWS, S. and HIGGINS, P. 1982 Neuroticism and the pain–mood relation in rheumatoid arthritis: Insights from a prospective daily study, *Journal of Consulting and Clinical Psychology*, **60**, 119–26.

BERGER, M. R. and FROMISON, A. L. 1979 Carpal tunnel syndrome, *American Journal of Nursing*, **79**, 264–6.

DEGOOD, D. E. and SHUTTY, M. S. 1992 Assessment of pain beliefs, coping, and self-efficacy, in TURK, D. C. and MELZACK, R. (Eds), *Handbook of Pain Assessment*, pp. 214–34, New York: Guilford Press.

DIONNE, E. D. 1984 Carpal tunnel syndrome, part I: The problem, *National Safety News*, **129**, 42–5.

DORTCH, H. L. and TROMBLY, C. A. 1990 The effects of education on hand use with industrial workers in repetitive jobs, *American Journal of Occupational Therapy*, **44**, 777–82.

DRAPKIN, R. G. 1990 Coping as a predictor of weight loss: The use of hypothetical high-risk situations, dissertation, University of Pittsburgh.

FERSTER, C. B. 1965 Classification of behavioral pathology, in KRASNER, L. and ULLMAN, L. P. (Eds), *Research in Behavior Modification: New Developments and Complications*, pp. 6–26, New York: Holt, Rinehart & Winston.

FEUERSTEIN, M., CALLAN-HARRIS, S., HICKEY, P., DYER, D., ARMBRUSTER, W. and CAROSELLA, A. M. 1993 Multidisciplinary rehabilitation of chronic work-related upper extremity disorders: Long-term effects, *Journal of Occupational Medicine*, **35**, 396–403.

FEUERSTEIN, M. and FITZGERALD, T. E. 1992 Multidisiplinary rehabilitation of chronic work related upper extremity disorders, *Journal of Occupational Medicine*, **35**, 257–264.

FOLLICK, M. K., AHERN, D. K. and LASER-WOLSTON, N. 1984 An electromechanical recording device for the measurement of 'uptime' or 'downtime' in chronic pain patients, *Archives of Physical Medical Rehabilitation*, **66**, 75–9.

FORDYCE, W. E. 1976 *Behavioral Methods for Chronic Pain and Illness*, St Louis, MO: Mosby.

GIL, K. M., ROSS, S. L. and KEEFE, F. J. 1988 Behavioral treatment of chronic pain: Four pain management protocols, in FRANCE, R. D. and KRISHNAN, K. R. (Eds), *Chronic Pain*, pp. 376–413, New York: American Psychiatric Press.

HALL, S. M., RUGG, D., TUNSTALL, C. and JONES, R. T. 1984 Preventing relapse to cigarette smoking by behavioral skill training, *Journal of Consulting and Clinical Psychology*, **52**, 372–82.

HARBER, P., BLOSWICK, D., BECK, J., PENA, L., BAKER, D. and LEE, J. 1992 The ergonomic challenge of repetitive motion with varying ergonomic stresses, *Journal of Occupational Medicine*, **34**, 518–28.

HARBER, P., BLOSWICK, D., BECK, J., PENA, L., BAKER, D. and LEE, J. 1993 Supermarket checker motions and cumulative trauma risk, *Journal of Occupational Medicine*, **35**, 805–11.

HEATON, R. K., GETTO, C. J., LEHMAN, R. A., FORDYCE, W. E., BRAVER, E. and GROBAN, S. E. 1982 A standardized evaluation of psychosocial factors in chronic pain, *Pain*, **12**(2), 165–74.

JENSEN, M. P., TURNER, J. A., ROMANO, J. M. and KAROLY, P. 1991, Coping with chronic pain: A critical review of the literature, *Pain*, **47**, 249–83.

KANFER, F. H. and GOLDFOOT, D. A. 1966 Self-control and tolerance of noxious stimulation, *Psychological Reports*, **18**, 79–85.

KEEFE, F. J., CALDWELL, D. S., QUEEN, K. T., GIL, K. M., MARTINEZ, S., CRISSON, J. E., OGDEN, W. and NUNLEY, J. 1987a Osteoarthritic knee pain: A behavioral analysis, *Pain*, **28**, 309–21.

KEEFE, F. J., CALDWELL, D. S., QUEEN, K. T., GIL, K. M., MARTINEZ, S., CRISSON, J. E., OGDEN, W. and NUNLEY, J. 1987b Pain coping strategies in osteoarthritis patients, *Journal of Consulting and Clinical Psychology*, **55**, 208–12.

KEEFE, F. J., CALDWELL, D. S., WILLIAMS, D. A., GIL, K. M., MITCHELL, D., ROBERTSON, C., MARTINEZ, S., NUNLEY, J., BECKHAM, J., CRISSON, J. E. and

HELMS, M. 1990, Pain coping skills training in the management of osteoarthritic knee pain: A comparative study, *Behavior Therapy*, **21**, 49–62.

KEEFE, F. J., DUNSMORE, J. and BURNETT, R. 1992 Behavioral and cognitive–behavioral approaches to chronic pain: Recent advances and future directions, *Journal of Consulting and Clinical Psychology*, **60**, 528–36.

KEEFE, F. J., SALLEY, A. N. JR and LEFEBVRE J. C. 1992 Coping with pain: Conceptual concerns and future directions, *Pain*, **51**(2), 131–9.

KOCH, H. 1986 *The Management of Chronic Pain in Office-based Ambulatory Care: National Ambulatory Medical Care Survey*, Washington, DC: US Department of Health and Human Services.

LEFEBVRE, M. F. 1980, Cognitive distortion in depressed psychiatric and low back pain patients, doctoral dissertation, University of Vermont; *Dissertation Abstracts International*, **41**, 693b (University Microfilms No. 80–17, 652).

LEFEBVRE, M. F. 1981 Cognitive distortions and cognitive errors in depressed psychiatric and low back pain patients, *Journal of Consulting and Clinical Psychology*, **49**, 517–25.

LINTON, S. J. 1991 A return to work after back injury is facilitated by an educational program for supervisors, unpublished manuscript, Orebro Medical Center, Orebro, Sweden.

MARLATT, G. A. and GORDON, J. R. 1985 *Relapse Prevention*, New York: Guilford Press.

MCGUIRE, D. B. 1992 Comprehensive and multidimensional assessment and measure of pain, *Journal of Pain and Symptom Management*, **7**(5), 312–19.

MELZACK, R. and WALL, P. 1965 Pain mechanisms: A new theory, *Science*, **50**, 971–9.

MOORE, J. E. and CHANEY, E. F. 1985 Outpatient group treatment of chronic pain: Effects of spouse involvement, *Journal of Consulting and Clinical Psychology*, **53**, 326–44.

PASCARELLI, E. F. and KELLA, J. J. 1993 Soft tissue injuries related to use of the computer keyboard, *Journal of Occupational Medicine*, **35**, 522–32.

PERRI, M. G., SHAPIRO, R. M., LUDWIG, W. W., TWENTYMAN, C. T. and MCADOO, W. G. 1984 Maintenance strategies for the treatment of obesity: An evaluation of relapse prevention training and post treatment contact by mail and telephone, *Journal of Consulting and Clinical Psychology*, **52**, 404–13.

ROSENSTIEL, A. K. and KEEFE, F. J. 1983, The use of coping strategies in chronic low back pain patients: Relationship to patient characteristics and current adjustment, *Pain*, **17**, 33–44.

SMITH, T. W., CHRISTENSEN, A. J., PECK, J. R. and LORD, J. R. 1994 Cognitive distortion, helplessness, and depressed mood in rheumatoid arthritis: A four year longitudinal analysis, *Health Psychology*.

SPENCE, S. H. 1989 Cognitive behavior therapy in the treatment of chronic, occupational pain of the upper limbs: A two year follow-up, *Behaviour, Research, and Therapy*, **27**, 435–46.

SPENCE, S. H. 1991 Cognitive behavior therapy in the treatment of chronic, occupational pain of the upper limbs: A two year follow-up, *Behaviour, Research, and Therapy*, **29**, 503–9.

STUTTS, J. T. and KASDAN, M. L. 1993 Disability: A new psychosocial perspective, *Journal of Occupational Medicine*, **35**, 825–7.

TURK, D. C., MEICHENBAUM, D. and GENEST, M. 1983 *Pain and Behavioral Medicine: A Cognitive–behavioral Perspective*, New York: Guilford Press.

TURK, D. C. and RUDY, T. E. 1991 Neglected topics in the treatment of chronic pain: relapse, noncompliance, and adherence enhancement, *Pain*, **44**, 528.

WILLIAMS, D. A. and THORN, B. E. 1989 An empirical assessment of pain beliefs, *Pain*, **36**, 351–8.

CHAPTER ELEVEN

Workstyle

Definition, Empirical Support, and Implications for Prevention, Evaluation, and Rehabilitation of Occupational Upper-Extremity Disorders

MICHAEL FEUERSTEIN

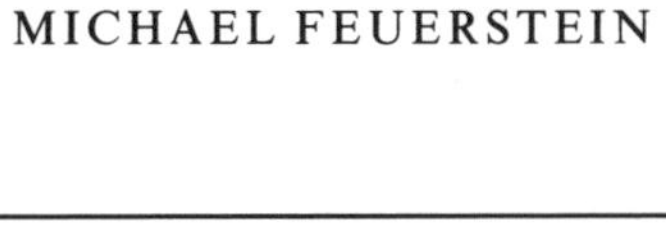

INTRODUCTION

There is much controversy as to the etiology of occupational musculoskeletal disorders of the upper extremities. Research suggests that a complex interaction among medical, ergonomic, organizational, and psychosocial factors contribute to the development, exacerbation, and maintenance of these broad ranges of symptoms and disorders (Armstrong *et al.*, 1993; Chaffin and Fine, 1993). Work-related upper-extremity symptoms may include pain, numbness, stiffness, and aching in the fingers, wrists, forearms, elbows, upper arms, neck, and shoulder regions (Putz-Anderson, 1988; Rempel *et al.*, 1992). These symptoms tend to fall into two classes of disorders: tendinitis-related and nerve entrapment-related (Putz-Anderson, 1988; Armstrong *et al.*, 1993). These symptoms and disorders appear to be affected by exposure to such biomechanical stressors as repetition, awkward postures, excessive force, inadequate work/rest cycles, vibration, and temperature extremes (Armstrong *et al.*, 1993; Ulin and Armstrong, 1992). The role of the more classic ergonomic stressors will not be addressed in this chapter other than to emphasize that the concepts presented must be considered in light of the complex interaction among medical, ergonomic, and psychosocial factors (Feuerstein, 1991). Also certain workstyles, coupled with work climate, work demand, and workstation factors may interact to increase exposure to ergonomic stressors, thus increasing the likelihood of symptom presentation or exacerbation and maintenance in an employee with preexisting symptoms. This chapter will focus on one psychosocial variable – *workstyle*, or how the individual worker approaches work.

The purpose of this chapter is to provide an operational definition of the construct of workstyle, illustrate the potential robustness of the construct by considering its presence in various types of hand-intensive work, and present preliminary evidence for the potential impact of workstyle primarily in the *exacerbation* of work-related upper-extremity symptoms. This chapter will also briefly describe research on interventions to modify workstyle and describe a hypothetical model linking workstyle to episodic, recurrent, and chronic symptoms, disorders, and disability associated with occupational upper-extremity disorders.

WORKSTYLE: OPERATIONAL DEFINITION

When one talks with supervisors regarding work-related upper-extremity symptoms/disorders in manufacturing and office environments alike, it is common to hear the question 'Why, when multiple employees work side by side performing similar tasks with equivalent workloads and apparently similar ergonomic exposures, do some develop upper-extremity symptoms and some do not?' When feasible, some supervisors even initiate measurement of cycle time, keying rate, posture, repetition rate, and force associated with specific tasks and at times such ergonomic stressors appear to be equivalent in the symptomatic and asymptomatic cases. It is feasible that the ergonomic assessment may not have been conducted properly or the measurement methodology was not sufficiently sensitive to identify differences. However, when this is not the case, what seems to differ between employee A, with symptoms, and B, without symptoms? There can be many factors that could potentially account for the presence of symptoms including predisposing metabolic differences, nonwork activities, pre-existing anatomic differences, or prior injuries or medical conditions (Chaffin and Fine, 1993). After ruling out these factors, what might help to explain the differences between symptomatic and asymptomatic workers?

Anecdotal evidence obtained through interviews and behavioral observations of workers performing work tasks along with discussion of their belief systems and approaches to stressors or challenges at work suggest that perhaps a differentiating factor between those who experience symptoms versus those who do not, may be in *how they perform their work, or their workstyle.* As our group observed this workstyle characteristic across a diverse set of work environments, we began to ask the following questions. Could the manner or intensity in which a given individual meets the demands of a work task give rise to increased levels of muscular exertion, excessive force, awkward postures, inadequate work/rest cycles, increased sympathetic nervous system arousal, and muscle tension? If so, could this response to work significantly contribute to the development, exacerbation, and/or maintenance of a complex set of upper-extremity symptoms/disorders? Could the persistence of a characteristic style of work subsequently contribute to prolonged functional decrements and work disability? Could there be a workstyle that predisposes a worker to upper-extremity symptoms/disorders as observed with the coronary-prone behavior pattern in relation to coronary artery disease (Jenkins, 1978)?[1]

As we continued to conduct assessments of workplaces for generic ergonomic risk factors, we also searched for evidence of the existence of these individual behavioral and cognitive patterns of workstyle. In addition, as workers with recurrent and chronic upper-extremity disorders were seen in our clinic, we also remained vigilant for the presence of these patterns. Indeed, as we continued to observe behavior during actual or simulated work tasks and questioned injured workers about their approach to work, a somewhat consistent pattern began to emerge. A subgroup of individuals presented to us with an intensity of effort that is generally not observed in patients with recurrent or chronic lower back pain. That is, many of the patients reported that they continued to work with pain for months because of their interest in keeping their job, the need to achieve at work, their perception of the important contribution of their work to the organization, or a strong work ethic. These individuals also tended to report difficulty pacing their work and a need to perform perfectly/optimally consistently day in and day out. They also displayed a certain heightened reactivity, increased level of intensity of effort, and increased need to improve their health *now* so that they could return to work immediately. While these observations are not all inclusive and only represent clinical anecdotal impressions, a pattern began to emerge that may help to explain a piece of the work-related upper-extremity disorder puzzle. This pattern is referred to as *workstyle*.

In order to measure objectively and validate a concept such as workstyle, it is essential to provide an operational or working definition. The proposed operational definition for workstyle is as follows:

1. Workstyle is an individual pattern of cognitions, behaviors, and physiological reactivity that co-occur while performing job tasks.
2. Workstyle may be associated with alterations in physiological state that, following repeated elicitation, can contribute to the development, exacerbation, and/or maintenance of recurrent or chronic musculoskeletal symptoms related to work.
3. Adverse workstyle (i.e. associated with increased occurrence of work-related upper-extremity symptoms) may be evoked by a high work demand (perceived or directly communicated by supervisor), self-generated by a high need for achievement and acceptance, increased fear of job loss or avoidance of a job-related negative consequence of inadequate or improper training, lack of awareness that a particular workstyle might be potentially high risk, and/or self-generated by time pressure.

Essentially, what this definition suggests is that a characteristic style or pattern of behaviors and cognitions exists in a given individual worker which is evoked in response to a set of work demands. This response to work demands can be characterized by heightened behavioral, cognitive, and physiological reactivity. The pattern may be triggered by excessive work demands that are either perceived by the worker, directly communicated by the supervisor, or self-generated by a high need to achieve. It may also be evoked by a fear of job loss or avoidance of some other negative job-related consequence (e.g. lack of co-worker or supervisor support).

It is hypothesized that this workstyle may predispose an individual worker to increased risk of developing work-related upper-extremity symptoms, particularly when coupled with exposure to other suspected ergonomic risk factors. This increased risk is not specific to an industry or type of work but rather the consequence of a complex interaction among work environment, individual response to work, and exposure to ergonomic risk factors. It is further proposed that workstyle itself can increase exposure to biomechanical stressors in the extremities by its association with concomitant increases in force, repetition, awkward posture and/or prolonged static loading of select muscles in the upper extremities, and inadequate work/rest cycles. It is important to emphasize that evidence suggests that exposure to ergonomic stressors has been associated with increased risk of upper-extremity symptoms/disorders without evoking the workstyle concept (Armstrong *et al.*, 1993). However, workstyle may increase the risk in an individual currently exposed to ergonomic stressors and/or serve to generate its own set of psychological and biomechanical stressors, thus predisposing the worker to upper-extremity symptoms/ disorders independent of workstation or work process-related biomechanical stressors. A similar process may exist in the exacerbation of symptoms/disorders and the prolongation of episodic or chronic pain and disability. This elaboration of the workstyle concept should serve only as a *working definition.* It most certainly will be refined as additional research related to the measurement and validation of the concept evolves.

EMPIRICAL RESEARCH

Findings from various epidemiological, laboratory, and outcome studies provide preliminary support for the role of workstyle, particularly in the exacerbation of upper-extremity symptoms. This section will provide an overview of this available research.

A few cautionary notes are important. The review does not consider a specific, well-defined disorder. Data will be presented that relate to various upper-extremity work-related musculoskeletal symptoms and, at times, disorders. As empirical research emerges, the concept may be more closely linked with certain symptoms (e.g. musculoskeletal pain) and not others (e.g. tingling, numbness, sensory loss), or certain disorders (e.g. tendinitis). However, at present, there is no apparent justification to assume this, and therefore this review will consider the full range of symptoms and disorders generally classified within the broad category of work-related upper-extremity disorders.

Epidemiological Surveys

Epidemiological research has suggested an association among a range of psychosocial factors, upper-extremity symptoms, and disorders. It is possible that these factors may evoke or contribute to the elicitation of a high-risk workstyle and are therefore reviewed below. In a study of medical secretaries in which 75 per cent worked more than two hours typing per day (computer keyboard or typewriter), 63 per cent reported neck pain while 62 per cent reported shoulder pain at some point during that same period (Linton and Kamwendo, 1989). These researchers noted a relationship between occurrence of pain and 'poor psychologic work environment.' Frequency of neck and shoulder pain was related to 'poor work content' but not to work demands or social support.

Research conducted by the National Institute of Occupational Safety and Health (NIOSH) in the context of two Health Hazard Evaluations provides further support for the role of psychosocial factors in work-related musculoskeletal symptoms and disorders of the upper-extremity, neck and shoulder regions (NIOSH, 1992, 1993). A Health Hazard Evaluation conducted in a large West Coast newspaper (NIOSH, 1993) indicated that 41 per cent met the case definition of at least one upper-extremity work-related musculoskeletal disorder. A self-administered questionnaire identified that the following factors were associated with the presence of work-related musculoskeletal symptoms: *hand–wrist* – more time spent typing on computer keyboards, greater number of hours on deadline, and less support from immediate supervisor; *shoulder* - less participation in job decision-making, greater number of years employed by specific employer, and greater job pressure; *neck* – greater number of hours on deadline, increased work variance (uneven workload during the day), more time on telephone and perception that management did not value the importance of ergonomics. There were 229 employees who subsequently participated in a case-control study. Variables that were identified with the more restrictive case definition of hand–wrist musculoskeletal disorder (positive symptoms *and* positive physical findings) were female gender and percentage of time typing on a computer keyboard. Hours spent on deadline and lack of supervisor support were not significant when considering the more restrictive definition. This investigation indicated that psychosocial factors were associated with *symptoms* in the hand–wrist, shoulder, and neck regions although the influence of such factors in hand–wrist *disorders* as measured by positive physical examination and symptoms were not supported.

In a study of the prevalence of work-related musculoskeletal disorders in telecommunications workers, 22 per cent met the case definition. Logistic regression analyses indicated that the following psychosocial variables were associated with upper-extremity musculoskeletal disorders: *neck* – lack of productivity standard, routine work lacking decision-making opportunities, fear of being replaced by computers, job requiring variety of tasks, high information-processing demands, and increased work pressure; *shoulder* – fear of being replaced by computers was the only variable identified; *elbow* – fear of being replaced by computers, routine work lacking decision-making opportunities, and surges in workload; *hand–wrist* – high information-processing demands; *upper-extremity overall* – fear of being replaced by computers, job requires a variety of tasks, and increasing work pressure. Odds ratios ranged from 1.1 to 3.5. In that same study, increased symptom severity (standardized composite score of frequency, severity, and duration) was associated with the following psychosocial factors: *neck* – increasing work pressure and uncertainty about job future; *shoulder* – increasing work pressure and overtime in past year (negative association); *elbow* – routine work lacking decision-making opportunities, uncertainty about job future, surges in workload, increasing work pressure, and lack of co-worker support; *hand–wrist* – high information-processing demands, uncertainty about job future, routine work lacking decision-making opportunities, increasing work pressure, and lack of supervisor support. While these factors were associated with increased symptom severity, the percentage variance that each accounted for was modest, ranging from 1 to 3 per cent. These findings suggest that lack of control, increased workload, and reduction in task diversity associated with VDT work may be contributing in part to increased reports of work-related upper-extremity symptoms/disorders (Bammer, 1987).

While we have addressed certain workplace psychosocial variables that may serve to trigger a high-risk workstyle and their association with presence and exacerbation of upper-extremity symptoms and disorders, what about the relationship among workstyle, work demands, perceived work environment, and symptoms? Feuerstein *et al.* (forthcoming) recently conducted a large-scale survey of 1,398 sign-language interpreters (58 per cent response rate), a group with a relatively high exposure to biomechanical stressors associated with upper-extremity symptoms (Feuerstein and Fitzgerald, 1992; Shealy, Feuerstein and Latko, 1991). The survey revealed that 20–32 per cent of the cases reported work-related symptoms. Figure 11.1 illustrates the percentage distribution by anatomic region.

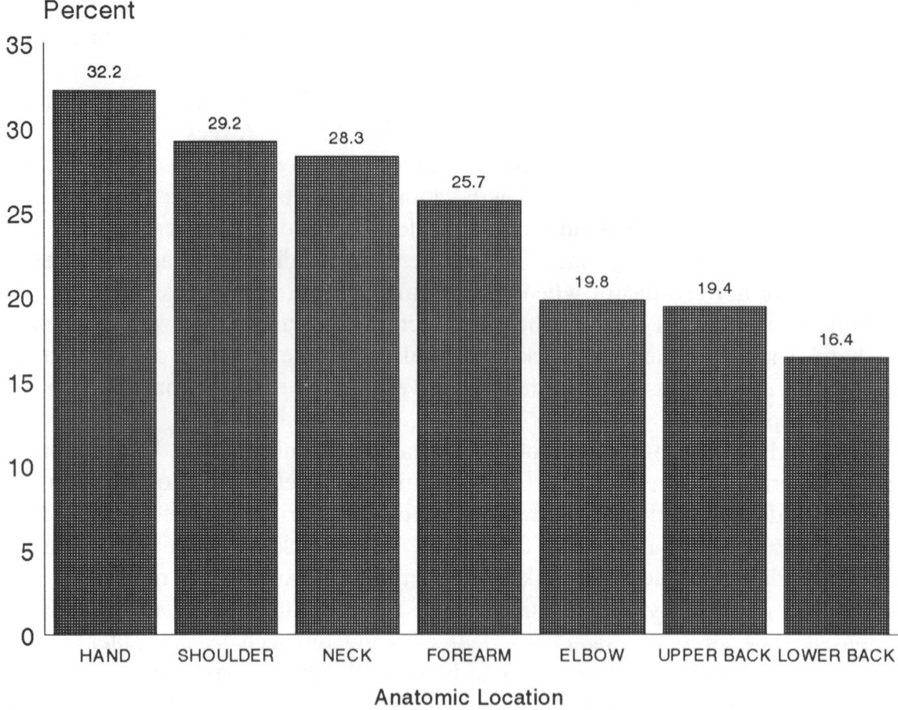

NOTE. Symptoms = Pain, aching, stiffness, burning, numbness, tingling
Based on NIOSH Symptom Survey.

Figure 11.1 Prevalence of work-related musculoskeletal symptoms in sign-language interpreters by anatomic region ($n = 1398$).

Of importance to the present discussion are the findings from the multivariate logistic regression analysis that considered years on the job, work demands, perceived work environment, and workstyle variables. Findings revealed that certification, years worked, physical conditions on the job, constant job pressure, fear of developing a pain problem at work, and tendency to continue to work with pain to insure high quality of work were associated with the presence of work-related hand–wrist symptoms. Professional sign-language interpreters who continued to expose themselves to repetitive, forceful movements and awkward postures despite pain to insure the quality of their work were more likely to be defined as cases. While the odds ratio for this variable was only 1.13, the finding does provide support for the need to consider how an individual performs work, as well as exposure to potential biomechanical stressors. It is important to note that other measures of workstyle included in the survey were not associated with case status for hand–wrist symptoms. In contrast, when considering factors associated with increased levels of pain and muscular tension at work as well as the impact of pain on function, a number of workstyle variables were associated with the exacerbation of pain, muscular tension, and disability. The workstyle-related variables and their relationship to pain, muscle tension, and the impact of upper-extremity symptoms on function are indicated in Tables 11.1, 11.2 and 11.3.

Table 11.1 Work demands, perceived work environment, and workstyle predictors of pain during work.

	Partial R^2	Model R^2	F	p
Upper limb (fingers, hands, wrists, forearms)				
Work in a painful way to ensure high quality	0.19	0.19	168.72	0.001
Fear of developing pain problem at work	0.08	0.28	82.13	0.001
Frequently moving as fast as you can	0.01	0.29	13.57	0.001
Years interpreting for pay	0.01	0.30	12.45	0.001
How often are unpleasant physical conditions at work	0.01	0.32	11.52	0.001
Frequently hitting hands together	0.01	0.32	6.21	0.05
How often are responsibilities clear at work	0.01	0.33	5.81	0.05
Interpreting affects consumer	0.01	0.33	5.76	0.05
Sole contact for interpreting service	0.01	0.34	5.19	0.05
Shoulder				
Work in a painful way to ensure high quality	0.16	0.16	135.50	0.001
Fear of developing pain problem at work	0.03	0.19	22.69	0.001
Sole contact for interpreting service	0.02	0.21	16.84	0.001
How often do you feel rushed	0.01	0.22	13.33	0.001
Hours of exposure per year	0.01	0.23	10.91	0.001
Perceived exertion	0.01	0.24	10.90	0.001
Back				
Work in a painful way to ensure high quality	0.10	0.10	79.97	0.001
Perceived exertion	0.04	0.14	30.43	0.001
How often do you feel rushed at work	0.02	0.16	17.89	0.001
Sole contact for interpreting service	0.01	0.17	11.02	0.001
Years interpreting for pay	0.01	0.18	6.65	0.01
Making forceful jerky movements	0.01	0.19	5.65	0.05
Preoccupied with accuracy and comprehension	0.01	0.20	6.35	0.05
Fear of developing pain problem at work	0.01	0.20	5.92	0.05
Deviate from neutral position	0.01	0.21	5.19	0.05
Hours of exposure per year	0.01	0.21	4.58	0.05
Anxiety	0.01	0.22	5.51	0.05
Neck				
Work in a painful way to ensure high quality	0.15	0.15	129.00	0.001
Fear of developing a pain problem at work	0.03	0.19	27.05	0.001
How often do you feel rushed at work	0.02	0.21	19.10	0.001
Perceived exertion	0.01	0.22	11.19	0.001
Sole contact for interpreting service	0.01	0.23	8.75	0.01
Hours of exposure per year	0.01	0.24	6.19	0.01

Note: $N = 824$

Another analysis conducted on the sign-language interpreter survey data related to identification of exposure, work demands, perceived work environment, and workstyle variables that differentiated cases with partial and full days of lost work due to upper-extremity symptoms from cases with no time lost from work. A discriminant function analysis was conducted on 277 lost-time cases and a randomly selected group of 277 cases with no lost time. The variables that discriminated lost-time from no-lost-time cases were high levels of fear of developing a pain problem at

Table 11.2 Work demands, perceived work environment, and workstyle predictors of muscle tension during work.

	Partial R^2	Model R^2	F	p
Upper limb (fingers, hands, wrists, forearms)				
Fear of developing pain problem at work	0.17	0.17	136.77	0.001
Work in a painful way to ensure high quality	0.08	0.25	74.79	0.001
Making forceful jerky movements	0.04	0.29	38.56	0.001
Perceived exertion	0.01	0.30	13.28	0.001
How often is there constant pressure	0.01	0.31	9.35	0.01
Deviate from neutral position at work	0.01	0.32	7.00	0.01
Shoulder				
Work in a painful way to ensure high quality	0.12	0.12	94.74	0.001
Perceived exertion	0.04	0.16	35.85	0.001
Fear of developing pain problem at work	0.01	0.17	11.97	0.001
Extend out of 'signing box'	0.01	0.18	9.35	0.01
Anxiety	0.01	0.19	7.98	0.01
How often do you feel rushed at work	0.01	0.20	4.90	0.05
How often are responsibilities clear at work	0.01	0.20	4.52	0.05
Deviate from neutral position	0.01	0.21	4.61	0.05
Neck				
Work in a painful way to ensure high quality	0.12	0.12	98.58	0.001
Perceived exertion	0.04	0.16	35.41	0.001
How often do you feel rushed at work	0.01	0.18	10.64	0.001
Fear of developing pain problem at work	0.01	0.19	8.69	0.01
Making forceful, jerky movements	0.01	0.19	6.22	0.05
Back				
Perceived exertion	0.08	0.08	62.73	0.001
Work in a painful way to ensure high quality	0.02	0.10	16.08	0.001
How often do you feel rushed at work	0.02	0.12	13.50	0.001
Anxiety	0.01	0.13	8.80	0.01
Years interpreting for pay	0.01	0.14	4.75	0.05
How often are unpleasant physical conditions at work	0.01	0.14	3.80	0.05

Note: $N = 824$

work, increased tendency to continue to work in a painful way to insure high quality, and less ability to use one's own initiative. These findings provide further support for the contribution of a combination of perceived work environment and a cognitive dimension of workstyle (i.e. concerns for high quality) to lost work time.

Interpreters who were more likely to continue to work in a painful way to insure high quality were more likely to miss time from work. This cognitive aspect of workstyle where an individual tends to drive oneself despite pain to insure quality, coupled with a fear of developing a pain problem at work and the perception of minimal control or initiative over the work, appears to contribute to establish a condition where work absence is more likely. The measures of the behavioral components of workstyle (e.g. work/rest breaks, moving hands as fast as one can, jerky forceful movements) were *not* associated with time off work. This may have been a consequence of the use of a self-report measure of workstyle in contrast to a behav-

Table 11.3 Prediction of the impact of upper-extremity symptoms on function.

	Partial R^2	Model R^2	F	p
Interference w/ function (total functional impact score)				
Fear of developing pain problem at work	0.21	0.21	174.16	0.001
Work in a painful way to ensure high quality	0.10	0.31	94.49	0.001
How often are you rushed at work	0.02	0.33	20.33	0.001
Years interpreting for pay	0.01	0.34	9.66	0.01
Perceived exertion	0.01	0.35	9.20	0.01
Control (hours worked/week and typical interpreting session)*	0.01	0.35	5.51	0.05
How often are unpleasant physical conditions at work	0.004	0.36	4.46	0.05
Frequently hitting hands together	0.004	0.36	3.92	0.05

Note: Based upon $N = 824$. Total functional impact score.
* Higher scores = greater perceived control.

ioral observation method or may suggest that cognitive components of workstyle contribute to time off work to a greater degree than the behavioral components. It is important to emphasize that these data are correlational and statements regarding the causal effect of workstyle on symptoms and disability cannot be made at this point. Determination of differences between behavioral and cognitive components of workstyle and their specific causal relationship to such outcomes as pain and function at work would be very useful in efforts to validate the workstyle construct.

Observational Research: Workplace, Laboratory, and Clinic

Research supporting the role of workstyle in the development, exacerbation, and/or maintenance of upper-extremity symptoms/disorders must demonstrate that the phenomena exists. Data based upon research that attempts to observe the behavioral, cognitive, and physiological dimensions of workstyle either in the natural work environment or during simulated work tasks can help to validate the occurrence of individual differences in workstyle. Studies that also link workstyle variables to either the presence or exacerbation of symptoms in the upper limbs using case-control methodology can provide support that the construct has some validity in relation to upper-extremity symptoms. While these studies are often retrospective or correlative in nature and do not indicate causality, such studies do represent a first step toward further documenting the existence of the phenomena and in determining its validity.

A prospective study of work technique and severity of upper-extremity disorders was conducted on 96 female electronics manufacturing workers (Kilbom and Persson, 1987). Disorders in neck, shoulder, and arm regions and frequency and severity of symptoms of pain, ache and fatigue were assessed. No subject had been on sick leave for any of the above disorders in the previous year. Subjects were followed at one and two years with a medical evaluation and assessment of work tasks. The purpose of the study was to determine the relationship among work technique, disorders, and symptoms. Work technique was measured using a standardized video protocol for the analysis of postures and movements of the upper arm, head, and shoulder – the VIRA method (Persson and Kilbom, 1983). The method was developed to measure short-cycle repetitive work. The authors observed a wide variation in work technique to an *identical* circuit-board assembly and soldering task (task was performed longer than a year prior to study). For example, work cycle time varied considerably across workers and ranged between 4.6 and 9.1 minutes. The total number of changes in posture varied between 170 and 452, as did the percentage of work cycle time in different postures (rest > 2 seconds: 4–42 per cent; 0–30°: 31–64 per cent; 30–60°: 2–43 per cent; >60°: 0–5 per cent). It is important to emphasize that these individual worker variations occurred in response to a standardized work task with a fixed work duration. This variability was observed in both subsamples studied. Of interest was the observation that work technique variables were significant predictors of progression toward a more severe disorder at any anatomic location both at one- and two-year follow-up intervals. These findings are summarized in Table 11.4.

In addition to posture and movement differences between symptomatic and asymptomatic workers, research on musculoskeletal response to standard work tasks (chocolate packing process) indicates that workers who experience pain, fatigue, and soreness in the neck and/or shoulders demonstrated higher static electromyographic (EMG) levels and fewer EMG gaps (periods with contraction levels consistently below 0.5 per cent maximum velocity contraction (MVC) than asymptomatic workers (Veiersted *et al.*, 1990). These investigators also observed that workers with a lower frequency of EMG gaps, also in response to a standard work task measured prior to symptom development, were more likely to experience symptoms in the neck and shoulder region (Veiersted *et al.*, 1993). Given the relatively modest effect of EMG gap frequency, its significance remains unclear. However, the tendency toward emitting fewer of these 'unconscious' EMG gaps (i.e. worker unaware of occurrence) to a standardized work task may represent a physiological concomitant of workstyle with potential etiological significance.

Table 11.4 Work technique and upper-extremity disorders in electronics workers: work technique variables predicting severity of disorder.

One-year follow-up

- Percentage of work cycle time with neck flexion
- Percentage of work cycle time with arm abduction >30°
- Percentage of work cycle time with arm abduction >60°
- Percentage of work cycle time with arm extension
- Number of shoulder elevations per hour

Two-year follow-up

- Number of shoulder elevations per hour
- Number of neck flexions per hour
- Percentage of work cycle time with neck flexion
- Percentage of work cycle time with shoulder extension
- Percentage of work cycle time with arm abduction 0–30°
- Average time with arm at rest (negative relationship)

From Kilbom and Persson, 1987.

In a cross-sectional laboratory analysis of workstyle, Feuerstein and Fitzgerald (1992) compared two groups of workers (working with pain, working without pain) on measures of repetitiveness of hand–wrist motion, work/rest cycle, postural stress, and smoothness of movement. The work groups were professional sign-language interpreters. The two groups were equivalent in age, gender distribution, years interpreting, and wrist and forearm endurance and flexibility. Subjects were exposed to a standardized work task and videotaped. Assessment of rest breaks, hand–wrist deviations per minute from neutral, mean work envelope excursions per minute, frequency of high-impact hand contacts and visual analog measures of pace of finger–hand movements, and smoothness of finger–hand movements was conducted. All measures were operationally defined and blind raters were trained. Interrater reliability was acceptable on all measures used. Correlation of workstyle measures with workers' ratings of pain, physical fatigue, and perceived decrease in upper-extremity flexibility were calculated. Findings indicated significant differences between the two groups on rest breaks, hand–wrist deviations, work envelope excursions, and pace of finger–hand movements. Increased pain was associated with increase in hand–wrist deviation frequency; fatigue was associated with fewer rest breaks and increase in hand–wrist deviations; and decrease in flexibility was associated with increased work envelope deviation and higher pace of finger–hand movements. These findings provide further support for the workstyle construct and its relationship to subjective symptoms of pain, fatigue, and decrease in perceived function.

Another source of evidence (indirect) for the existence of workstyle can be found in the research on psychomotor function in patients with carpal tunnel syndrome conducted by Radwin (1992). Although this research is directed at the development of innovative functional tests that may be useful in workplace surveillance, the observations of Radwin and associates are intriguing in relation to the workstyle concept. Radwin developed a rapid pinch-and-release psychomotor task which uses the muscles of the hand innervated by the median nerve. Using a strain gauge dynamometer with limited feedback, subjects were instructed to perform a rapid repeated pinch-and-release task. The strain gauge is repeatedly pinched to a predetermined force level – minimum upper force level (F_{upper}) – using the index finger and thumb and released as rapidly as possible to a second predetermined force level – maximum lower force level (F_{lower}). Variables measured were pinch rate or speed 'isometric force control' in terms of overshoot force (F_{over}) and time above the upper force level (T_{upper}) or the time in milliseconds force exceeded F_{upper} and T_{lower} or time below the lower force level threshold. A comparison of carpal tunnel syndrome (CTS) cases and controls indicated that the CTS cases generated fewer pinches per second than controls and demonstrated a pattern of overshoot to a greater degree than controls (28.3 per cent MVC in CTS versus 12.0 per cent in controls). Figure 11.2 illustrates the overshoot characteristic in a selected CTS and a control case (Radwin, 1992). While higher correlations were observed between nerve conduction findings and pinch speed, a significant correlation between median transcarpal latency and overshoot was also observed ($r = 0.412$, $p < 0.05$). In addition, T_{upper} was positively correlated with both median nerve motor and transcarpal latencies (Rodriguez *et al.*, 1993).

Both the Feuerstein and Fitzgerald (1992) and Radwin (1992) research are case-control studies and therefore it is impossible to determine whether the workstyle differences observed were present prior to the occurrence of the problem or rep-

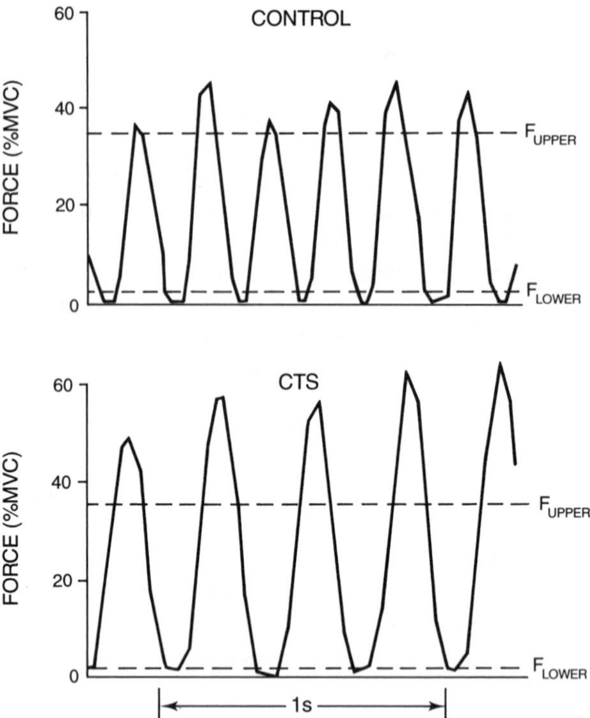

Figure 11.2 Illustration of force overshoot in selected control and case with carpal tunnel syndrome, duration one second (Radwin, 1992).

resent a secondary consequence of pain, nerve, or tendon pathology. However, the findings provide further evidence for the existence of some type of behavioral dysregulation and/or heightened reactivity that could potentially increase risk to high repetition, force, or awkward posture, thus increasing the likelihood of symptom exacerbation.

There are a cluster of recently published clinical and laboratory studies that have implications for the role of workstyle in office-related upper-extremity disorders and specifically keyboard-related problems. These studies have investigated disabled keyboard operators, as well as individual differences in key force variability in asymptomatic pianists and computer keyboard operators.

An interesting clinical series of 53 disabled keyboard operators presenting with pain in the forearms, elbows, wrists, shoulders, and hands was reported by Pascarelli and Kella (1993). Through the use of videotape observations, the authors identified several workstyles that may have contributed to the presenting problems. These investigators constructed a 'taxonomy of keyboard techniques' based upon videotape analysis. A summary of the taxonomy is listed in Table 11.5. It is interesting to note that 14 of the 53 cases (26 per cent) demonstrated a tendency to use the keyboard with considerable 'vigor and rapidity.' The force generated was associated with a loud clacking noise and these cases were referred to 'clackers.' Seventy-one per cent of this latter group had evidence of extension and flexion forearm pain, 36

Table 11.5 Taxonomy of keyboard technique $n = 53$.

Leaner ($n = 21$)
- Dorsiflexion of wrist
- Wrists resting on a desktop
- Fingers arched to reach proximal keys
- Wrist held in ulnar or radial deviation
- Alienated thumb or hyperextended fifth finger

Clacker ($n = 14$)
- Hit keyboard with vigor
- Rapidly pressing keys to end points

Pointer ($n = 3$)
- Use of index and middle fingers to strike keys and space bar
- Thumb used to strike space bar occasionally
- Primary movements were wrist flexion and extension in key strike combined with radial and ulnar movements and ulnar movements to locate keys

Lounger ($n = 2$)
- Horizontally oriented postures
- Lean to one side elevating one shoulder and flexing neck forward

Mouse Users ($n = 2$)

Not classified ($n = 11$)

From Pascarelli and Kella, 1993.

per cent had de Queváin's disease, and 21 per cent were diagnosed with carpal tunnel syndrome. The gender distribution was 33 per cent men and 23 per cent women. While they did not elaborate, the authors did suggest that these cases also had a higher incidence of epicondylitis. The systematic clinical observations of Pascarelli and Kella (1993) are intriguing. It is unfortunate that the authors did not present data on the validity and reliability of the methodology used to assess workstyle in order for others to replicate these findings. It would also be of interest to measure dimensions of workstyle in both symptomatic and asymptomatic word-processors in order to determine the specificity of the phenomena.

Investigations of piano keyboard technique provide additional support for the existence of individual differences in workstyle. It has also been suggested that repetitive, rapid, and precise movements over an extended period of time may predispose instrumental musicians to a range of upper-extremity symptoms or disorders and that such disorders may be associated with technique and ergonomic design of instruments (Fry, 1986; Larsson *et al.*, 1993). A recent study conducted by Wolf *et al.* (1993) in asymptomatic experienced pianists identified the presence of individual differences in keyboard technique that resulted in significant variations in force on finger joints and tendons. Using a biomechanical model of force based upon free-body equilibrium analysis (Harding *et al.*, 1989), Wolf *et al.* (1993) calculated force as a function of finger-segment size, finger geometry, angular position of the finger and keystroke force. Wolf *et al.* (1993) observed considerable variations in magnitude of keystroke force in response to a *standard* musical passage. Differences between the subject with the lowest and highest mean keystroke force varied by 178 per cent (2.00 N versus 5.56 N). While a strong inverse relationship between force and years of piano-playing experience was observed, a wide range of keystroke forces were associated with 'variations in interpretation' of identical segments of the music. The differences in interpretation of the 'work task' may represent an example of the role of the cognitive (interpretive) dimension of workstyle. For example, in this study differences in how a work task was interpreted was associated with wide variations in metacarpophalangeal (MP) joint force ranging from 6.94 N to 46.59 N in two subjects in response to an identical note (note 2). The intrinsic (INT) tendon force coefficient (sum of forces in the three intrinsic tendons of the hand) for note 2 between the same two subjects also varied significantly from 0.32 to 4.88 (13-fold difference). Thus, while only presented as an example, it is feasible that individual interpretations of work demands (e.g. extremely critical to job security or quality of work, therefore must be completed correctly and completed now versus less critical and therefore can be paced) can result in significant variations in the degree of force exerted. It is feasible that such cognitive interpretations of work demands in an office setting involving wordprocessing could result in increased force exerted on the computer keyboard, placing the upper limbs at greater risk for overexertion, fatigue, and pain. If such a response to a work demand is repeated over time, such a workstyle could contribute to recurrent or chronic upper-extremity symptoms, disorders, and subsequent disability.

A final group of studies related to the workstyle construct, particularly in relation to the office environment, was conducted on asymptomatic subjects designed to determine whether subjects exert more force than necessary to activate keys during a keyboarding or typing task (Armstrong *et al.*, 1991; Rempel and Gerson, 1991). Armstrong and colleagues developed a device to measure keyboard force related to three different desktop personal computer keyboards (Armstrong *et al.*, 1991). The device measures *keyboard* displacement using a linear voltage differential transformer driven by a rack and pinion system. The findings indicated that, on average, peak forces applied by subjects were 3.1 times greater than the force required for key activation. In addition, the study reported by Rempel and Gerson in 1991 indicated that an analysis of variance on keyboard × subject × row × finger revealed that the main effects for subject and keyboard explained the most variation in force. These findings highlight the presence of significant individual differences in the degree of force that a subject exerts on a keyboard to a standardized typing task. Whether individuals with upper-extremity symptoms/disorders demonstrate differential patterns of keyboard force and whether these force profiles are related to increased levels of pain, fatigue, numbness, or tingling represent important next steps in delineating the role of workstyle in office-related upper-extremity disorders. The author is presently conducting such an investigation.

PSYCHOBIOLOGICAL MECHANISM LINKING WORKSTYLE TO UPPER-EXTREMITY SYMPTOMS, DISORDERS, AND DISABILITY

The research reviewed provides preliminary evidence for the following:

1. While the magnitude of the effect is modest, workplace stressors such as job uncertainty, increased work pressure, lack of supervisor/co-worker support, surges in workload, and minimal decision-making opportunities are associated

with either the presence or exacerbation or work-related upper-extremity symptoms/disorders.

2. Clinical series, case-control, and prospective studies provide limited evidence that individual differences in how a worker performs a standard task exist and that these variations are associated with the presence and/or exacerbation of symptoms, disorders, and neurologic signs of disease.
3. Individual differences have been observed in such office work as keyboarding (keyforce) in asymptomatic subjects, suggesting the *potential* role of workstyle in the etiology, exacerbation, and/or maintenance of upper-extremity symptoms related to keyboarding tasks.

If workstyle plays a role in the development, exacerbation, and/or maintenance of work-related upper-extremity symptoms, disorders, and subsequent disability, how might this process occur? Figure 11.3 illustrates a possible pathway linking exposure to work-related psychosocial stressors and work demands with the evocation of a high-risk workstyle, and the experience of symptoms, disorders, and disability. The figure also highlights the potential role of biomechanical stressors that may co-occur with psychosocial stressors, work demands, and high-risk workstyle. The conceptual framework presented in Figure 11.3 proposes that workstyle may pre-exist as a characteristic approach to work demands and/or be triggered or exacerbated by the presence of workplace psychosocial stressors and/or increased work demands.

Many factors have been demonstrated to impact the response to a potential threat or stressor including predisposing temperament, social learning history, and social support (Feuerstein *et al.*, 1986; Levi, 1972; Lazarus, 1974). The proposed

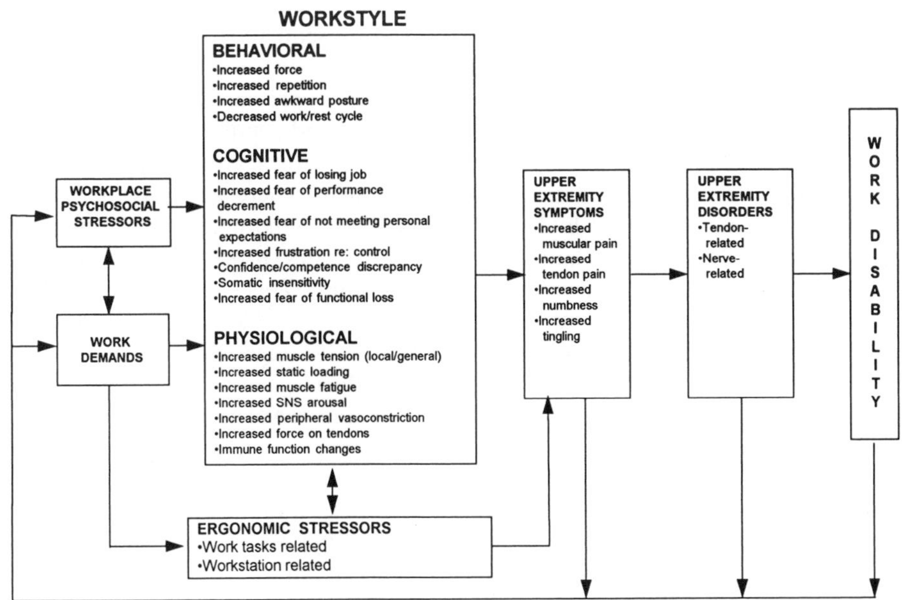

Figure 11.3 Workplace psychosocial stressors, work demands, workstyle, and upper-extremity symptoms, disorders, and disability.

model suggests that these factors can exert a modulating effect on cognitive filtering processes which in turn affect the level of perceived distress or threat. While workstyle may represent a learned or overlearned response to work in general and therefore is present at some static or baseline level, it is possible that the intensity of workstyle is influenced by the perceived level of threat. As workplace psychosocial stressors increase, the intensity of the workstyle response increases. Frequency and duration represent additional parameters of workstyle that may be modulated by the intensity of workplace psychosocial stressors and work demands.

Workstyle itself can be broken down into three components: behavioral, cognitive, and physiological. While the existence of each of these components needs to be validated and the degree of concordance among these components or dimensions is unclear at present, certain features or dimensions may be more pronounced in a given individual or in response to a specific job task and/or set of workplace psychosocial stressors. Nevertheless, the model assumes that workstyle is composed of *each* of these dimensions. The behavioral component represents the actual overt manifestations of movement, posture, and activity. These behaviors can set the stage for excessive biomechanical strain of muscles and tendons. The cognitive component of workstyle refers to the thoughts, feelings, appraisals of the situation, and the workers' evaluation of the success of any response in terms of reducing threat or enhancing personal sense of achievement regarding work. The final component, physiological, represents the biological changes that accompany the behavioral and cognitive reactions. These may include increases in muscle tension, force on tendons, changes in intracarpal tunnel pressure, increased catecholamine release, and stress-induced changes in immune function. It is when physiological changes are either recurrently evoked or are not permitted to recover or re-establish a homeostatic level that the stage is set for recurrent pain, numbness, tingling, inflammation, and decrement in function. As this continues, development of the tendon-related or nerve entrapment-related disorders can occur which, if unresolved, can lead to alterations in physical and psychological function and subsequent work disability.

Specifically, a number of psychosocial stressors may serve as precipitators of workstyle such as job uncertainty, increasing work pressure, lack of supervisor and/or co-worker support, surges in workload, and minimal decision-making opportunities. These factors may combine along with increased physical work demands to create a problematic work environment where an individual who is somewhat self-driven toward high performance/high achievement may not receive the latitude or flexibility to initiate the ideas or work processes that he or she believes are important to achieve optimal performance. This situation, coupled with minimal supervisor support and increasing surges in workload, can create a situation in which the high-risk workstyle is continuously triggered. In such a situation the individual may exert excessive levels of effort, generating significant biomechanical and physiological strain on muscles and tendons, thus increasing the likelihood of symptoms. As symptoms persist and the workstyle is continuously elicited along with its concomitant physiological correlates, very little opportunity is available for repair or recovery of tendons and muscles and the cycle of the behavior pattern and pain continues. Coupled with minimal support, such an individual may resort to their primary coping style which is to do more or continue to persist despite symptoms. This situation could set the stage for continuous exposure to increased or persistent biomechanical strain in the upper extremities, subsequently leading to potential nerve involvement and decrement in function.

A tendency to drive oneself despite symptoms is suggested by the research of Reid *et al.*, 1991. In an investigation of critical events and perceptions regarding the development of and subsequent evaluation and treatment for 'repetition strain injury' (RSI), Reid *et al.*, 1991 studied a group of 52 women either currently employed or work-disabled due to RSI (12/24 in a poultry processing plant, 15/28 in a telecommunications firm as keyboard operators). These investigators reported that 65 per cent of the interviewees depicted themselves as displaying hard-working habits as part of their pre-morbid lifestyle. Two quotations from these structured interviews depict this driving workstyle:

> 'If there was work to do, I did it. Some supervisors even came and told me to slow down because I was doing too much. I was doing another girl's share of the work. I am like that. I have to be on the go all the time.'

> 'I think I push myself too hard. I expect too much of myself. Preferable to telling people what I want done and how to do it, I will get in there and do it myself .... I think I am too conscientious and hardworking.'

While the Reid *et al.* research used a retrospective design, the findings provide additional indirect support for the hypothesis that a feature of this workstyle may be a heightened tendency to drive or push oneself. Such a tendency, particularly in response to increased work demands, may not allow time to attend to the range of premonitory signs of an impending upper-extremity problem. This tendency to drive oneself and become preoccupied with the demands of work may also serve to divert attention away from symptoms. Another possibility is that this behavior style may be associated with an attenuated perceptual sensitivity to symptoms. These potential psychophysiological processes need to be validated scientifically.

It is important to emphasize that workstyle is not intended to reflect a certain variant of psychopathology but rather a complex multidimensional response to work demands. In relation to this point, research investigating the presence of psychopathology among acute and chronic patients with work-related upper-limb pain, acute and chronic patients with accident injuries of the upper limbs, and noninjured keyboard operators (Spence, 1990) reported the *absence* of differences in depression, anxiety (state and trait), neuroticism, and psychoticism between the acute or chronic occupational upper-limb pain subjects compared to the accident-injured or noninjured controls. However, lower levels of extroversion were observed for the chronic accident-injured patients in contrast to the chronic occupational upper-limb group.

The model depicted in Figure 11.3 helps to identify entry points for evaluation and intervention. For example, efforts could be directed at reducing the prevalence and magnitude of workplace psychosocial stressors and work demands through organizational interventions. Systems-level interventions that restructure job tasks, implement total quality management (TQM) strategies to reduce fear in the workplace (Ryan and Oestreich, 1991), increase sense of control over certain features at work, and train employees in strategies to promote their own musculoskeletal safety and health through ergonomic and personal health initiatives may also exert an effect on workstyle and symptoms. Instruction of supervisors and employees in the identification and modification of high-risk components of workstyle coupled with line supervisor training to facilitate attitude and behavior change regarding musculoskeletal problems may also prove useful (Linton, 1991).

If workstyle and symptoms persist, more individualized interventions may be required including some combination of self-monitoring, cognitive intervention, videotape feedback, reinforcement, and behavioral rehearsal and psychophysiological interventions including biofeedback and/or relaxation techniques targeted at specific high-risk muscle groups or directed at facilitating a generalized reduction in musculoskeletal and autonomic levels or reactivity (Everly, 1989; Lehrer and Woolfolk, 1993; Schwartz, 1987). The specific interventions used should be based upon a comprehensive assessment of the presenting problem, including a determination of the existence of behavioral, cognitive, and psychophysiological components of a suspected high-risk workstyle. Such an approach is characteristic of cognitive–behavioral assessment and treatment (Hersen and Bellack, 1985).

In sum, the workstyle concept appears to have potential explanatory power in terms of improving our understanding of the role of psychosocial factors in upper-extremity symptoms/disorders while simultaneously assisting in targeting intervention efforts that provide a rational systematic approach to the complex interaction of ergonomic and psychosocial factors contributing to these disorders. However, only through well-controlled outcome research on the effects of various intervention strategies on workstyle and other variables of interest including symptoms, productivity, lost work time, and workers' compensation costs will the utility of various approaches to modifying workstyle be determined. Interventions will also need to address cost–benefit carefully. Efforts should be directed at developing approaches that exert minimal interference with ongoing work flow and are associated with the greatest impact on symptom prevention and management, lost work time, workers' compensation costs, productivity, and general quality of work life.

PREVENTION AND MANAGEMENT

Much research remains to be completed regarding the identification and validation of the workstyle construct across and within broad categories of work. However, given the preliminary data presented, it appears justified to embark cautiously on incorporating the concept in prevention and management efforts.

It is feasible for health and safety staff, consultants in ergonomics, or consultants with expertise in measurement of work method/work technique in a given industry to include a measurement protocol that not only evaluates exposure to ergonomic risk factors but also measures workstyle in workers with and without musculoskeletal symptoms/disorders. If this assessment identifies reliable differences between workers and workstyle appears to contribute to increased symptoms, efforts could be launched to assist the worker in modifying such a workstyle. Such an approach is not without its hazards, which those involved in such work must be aware of and make every effort to prevent. It is possible that while such an assessment and prevention/management effort is conducted to facilitate the health and safety of potentially higher-risk employees or employees experiencing symptoms, it could also be used as a means to blame a given worker for 'developing the problem.' That is, it is not inconceivable that a manager might respond to an employee with a potential high-risk workstyle in an accusatory manner and use the identification as an opportunity to reprimand or somehow limit opportunities for the employee. Such an approach can only exacerbate the problem. On the positive side, identification of an employee with a potential high-risk workstyle can be used as an educational tool in a constructive supportive manner to assist the employee in learning to recognize the style and the factors that influence it and to work on ways to modify it, potentially reducing exposure to excessive strain on the musculoskeletal system.

An additional cautionary note is that such an approach should never be used as a substitute for re-engineering the job to reduce ergonomic risk through redesign. At this point it is reasonable to assume that while modification of workstyle may be helpful in reducing exposure, if ergonomic hazards co-occur with a high-risk workstyle and are not addressed directly, workstyle modification will not be sufficient to reduce risk. This very important point should be kept in mind as efforts to modify workstyle are further developed.

This section will not provide a review of methods that have evolved to modify workstyle or work technique. While clinical reviews have suggested the potential of technique retraining (e.g. Bengtson and Schutt, 1992; Fry, 1986; Lambert, 1992; Larsson *et al.*, 1993; Pascarelli and Kella, 1993; Patkin, 1990), there are very few controlled outcome studies. Those that are available provide preliminary support for the utility of such interventions. Randomized outcome studies are needed that assess the outcome of well-defined protocols for specific types of workstyles and specific symptoms and disorders. In general, workstyle assessment methodologies, protocol development, and outcome research in this area has not evolved to this stage.

Our group developed a prevention and management program for upper-extremity symptoms/disorders for a specific work group (sign-language interpreters) which evolved from our preliminary analyses of the patterns of symptoms (Feuerstein and Jones, 1990), workstyle techniques (Feuerstein and Fitzgerald, 1992), biomechanics of sign-language interpreting (Shealy *et al.*, 1991), and the psychosocial factors that appeared to contribute to symptom exacerbation (Feuerstein and Jones, 1990). Of 42 sign-language interpreters who were medically screened, 20 (48 per cent) demonstrated signs or symptoms indicative of a range of medical diagnoses. The following diagnoses were observed in the 20 cases: tendinitis ($n = 10$), epicondylitis ($n = 2$), rheumatoid arthritis ($n = 1$), arthritis of the thumb ($n = 1$) and sprain/strain of shoulder or neck ($n = 3$).

The prevention and management program was conducted with 60 employed sign-language interpreters (both symptomatic and asymptomatic). The original program consisted of an 11-session group intervention provided to employees at the National Technical Institute for the Deaf of the Rochester Institute of Technology in Rochester, New York. Both prevention and management were goals. The interventions were multifaceted. Given the apparent important role of workstyle, coupled with the nature of the work of sign-language interpretation which generally does not involve the use of tools, machinery, or office equipment with the exception of a chair, a good deal of the intervention was focused on modification of the behavioral/ biomechanical, cognitive, and physiological concomitants of workstyle.

The intervention was conducted in two groups of 30 employees at the request of the employer. Sessions followed a set protocol with specific goals identified, rationale described, and skills taught. Participants asked questions during the sessions; however, given the nature and size of the groups, most of the discussion and questions and answers were addressed by the various work group managers during a regularly scheduled group meeting during the week following the session. Managers had a discussion outline available for each session and they all received training related to each of the areas presented throughout the 10-week intervention. Our group was continuously available to them. The Director of the Department of Interpreting Services and each of the managers were actively involved in all aspects of the initial research, and the prevention and management intervention phase. Indeed, the

Table 11.6 Upper-extremity cumulative trauma disorder prevention and management in sign-language interpreters.

Session 1 – Orientation: The UECTD – Interpreting connection
- Increase understanding of UECTDs and work disability in general.
- Increase awareness of factors that can affect pain, fatigue and disability in sign-language interpreters.
- Review and discuss COR's* findings from its investigation.
- Review UECTD Prevention and Management Program.

Session 2 – Overexertion: What is it? How can it be prevented or its impact reduced?
- Review Worksheet 1: Understanding Your UECTD/Interpreting Connection.
- Increase understanding of upper-extremity CTDs (e.g. carpal tunnel syndrome, epicondylitis, rotator cuff tendinitis).
- Increase understanding of the concept of overexertion in general, and specifically as it relates to sign-language interpreting.
- Identify individual 'hot spots' susceptible to overexertion.

Session 3 – Fitness training I
- Increase understanding of benefits of exercise and general methods of training related to problems of overexertion.
- Develop *individual* exercise program prescriptions.
- Discuss problems that may arise with a training program.

Session 4 – Fitness training II
- Review flexibility exercises from previous week.
- Review exercise routines to improve strength in upper extremities.
- Further refine personal fitness program.
- Discuss benefits/risks of exercise.
- Review fitness log/other monitoring forms.

Session 5 – Stress management I: From muscles to minds
- Increase awareness of sources and signs of stress at work.
- Provide a framework for thinking about stress and how its impact can be reduced – The Stress Chain.
- Increase awareness of single-channel thinking, the 'Shoulds of Interpreting' and methods to evaluate the utility of these modes of thinking.
- Discuss options for managing stress and review the importance of not attributing all symptoms to psychosocial stress.
- Distribute thought-refocusing diary.

Session 6 – Pain management
- Review symptoms of overexertion in sign-language interpreters as reported in questionnaire study.
- Review and discuss modern view of pain.
  - Multicomponent nature of pain.
  - Hurt versus harm.
- What steps can be used to prevent recurrent pain or manage/reduce persistent pain?

Sessions 7 and 8 – Biomechanics of interpreting I and II
- Review research findings on interpreting style and overexertion – The COR/NTID Study.
- Discuss implications of findings for interpreting style and steps to modify approaches to interpreting.

Table 11.6 (cont.).

- Discuss principles of movement and provide strategies to modify interpreting style to reduce risk.
- Review videotapes of interpreting styles.
- Follow up on efforts to modify workstyle.

Session 9 – Self-assessment/relapse prevention

- Review self-assessment of progress to date.
- Focus on concepts and strategies that have been helpful along with appraisal of those that have not been particularly useful.
- Review ways to facilitate change.
- Review strategies to maintain change/relapse prevention.

Session 10 – Stress management II

- Teach a relaxation approach to be used as an active coping skill prior to, during, and following interpreting sessions.
- Provide orientation to skin conductance biofeedback to facilitate training in relaxation response.
- Review overall strategy to assist in self-management of UECTDs.

Session 11 – Traversing the health-care system

- Review various UECTDs.
- Review evaluation and treatment options.
- Review algorithm for medical management.
  - 'Your Hunch – How to Proceed'
- Review roles of various health-care providers involved in prevention and management.

* Center for Occupational Rehabilitation

involvement, skills and genuine interest in the problem by management at all levels appeared to play a significant role in the program's success.

The intervention components are summarized in Tables 11.6 and 11.7.[2] Important features of the intervention were the focus on providing an understanding of the interactive role of predisposing medical factors, ergonomic and psychological stressors, fitness and its potential role in reducing fatigue and overexertion, and the need to identify and modify workstyle factors–behavioral, cognitive, and physiological. A series of upper-extremity and whole-body exercises were taught, directed at assisting the interpreter in improving flexibility, endurance, and strength and increasing awareness of bodily signs of fatigue and overuse. Preinterpreting stretching and warm-up exercises were also taught. Stress management strategies were introduced to begin to address cognitive concomitants of sign-language interpreting such as the strong need to interpret every word of the speaker perfectly or the tendency to respond to every need of the consumer. Progressive muscular relaxation techniques were introduced as well, to assist with the physiological consequences of job stress and high-risk workstyle. Training in increasing awareness and modification of potential high-risk workstyles was completed using videotape illustration

Table 11.7 Upper-extremity cumulative trauma disorder prevention and management in sign-language interpreters: supervisor involvement

- Provided input into program development.
- Received training regarding UECTD identification and management.
- Conducted session-by-session follow-up problem-solving groups for employees after each larger group session.
- Trained in identification of potential high-risk workstyles and conducted assessment.
- Attended problem-solving meetings with project manager during implementation and quarterly during a 1.5-year follow-up.
- Conducted continuous evaluation of program.

Note: Significant program support was provided by management at all levels. Continuous access to consultant staff was available during a 1.5-year follow-up period.

so that instruction in and alternate approaches for reducing biomechanical strain including movement technique was provided. This information was presented in a group format and reinforced by supervisors through periodic behavioral observation and feedback regarding workstyle.[3] A general overview of how to utilize the health-care system more effectively as it related to occupational upper-extremity disorders was also provided.

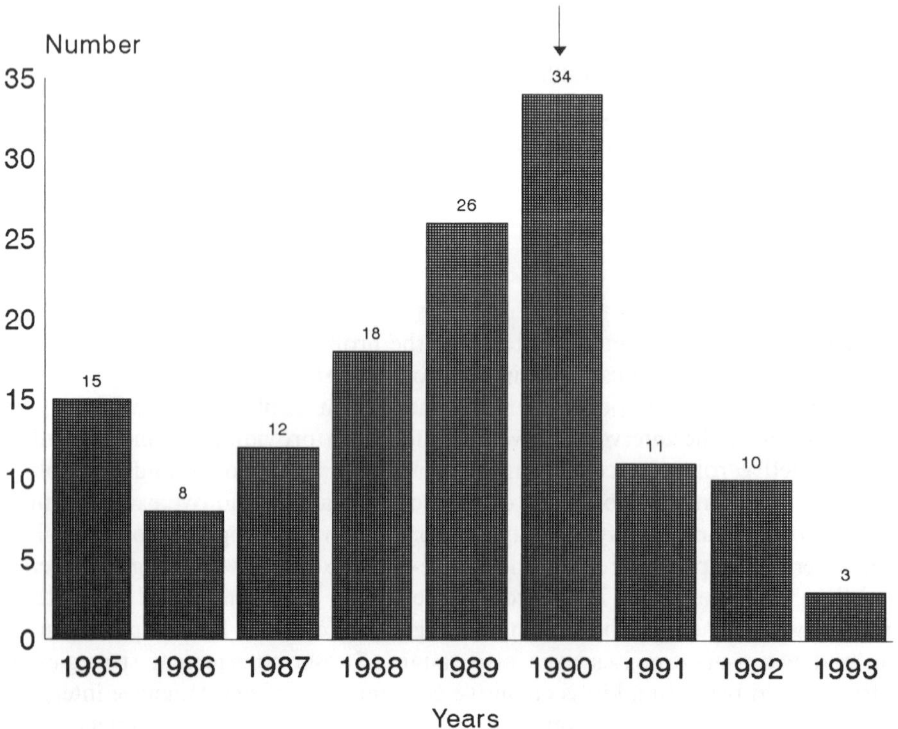

NOTE. Workgroup - Sign Language Interpreters

1990 Intervention Initiated

Figure 11.4 Upper-extremity CTD prevention and management program: accident reports.

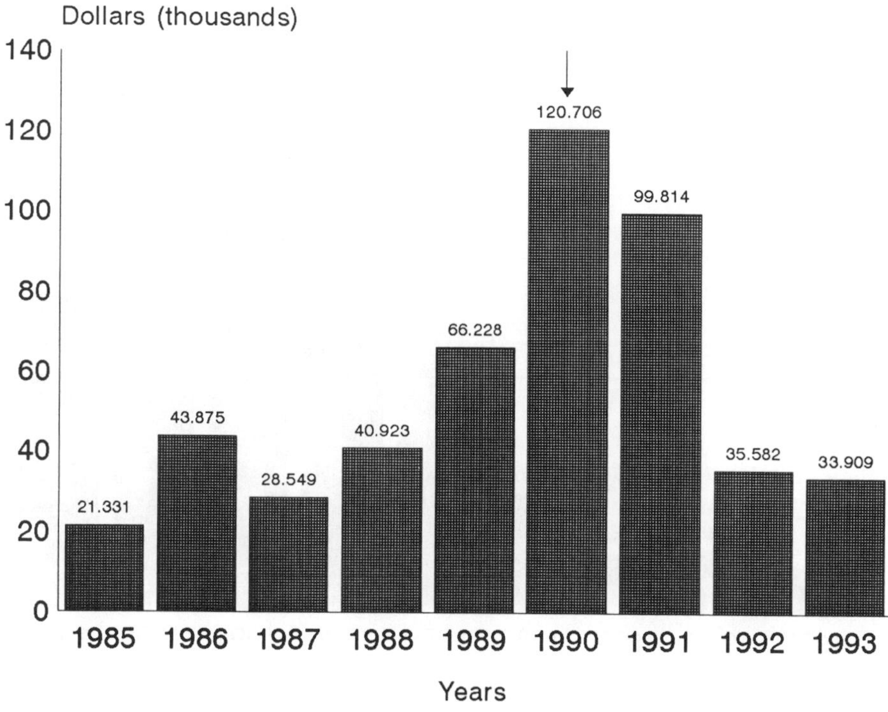

NOTE. Workgroup - Sign Language Interpreters

1990 Intervention Initiated

Figure 11.5 Upper-extremity CTD prevention and management program: Workers' Compensation indemnity costs.

Pre-post measures of symptoms (not reported in this chapter), as well as a full two years of follow-up data on 'accidents' reported to human resources, Workers' Compensation indemnity, and medical costs, suggest that the program was associated with short-term symptom improvement and long-term reductions in accident rates and Workers' Compensation costs (Feuerstein *et al.*, forthcoming). Figures 11.4, 11.5, and 11.6 present the accident report and workers' compensation indemnity and medical cost data prior to, during, and following the intervention.

This evaluation was conducted in the context of a consultation to assist with prevention and management of work disability associated with upper-limb pain. Consequently, the outcome evaluation was limited by the absence of a no-treatment or placebo control group. The absence of such controls precludes the ability to identify definitively the intervention as the primary factor contributing to the positive outcome. Also, there were no objective measures of pre-post changes in the behavioral, cognitive, and physiological concomitant of workstyle. Such measurement would help to identify the mechanism of change in relation to the workstyle construct. Also, given that the intervention was multicomponent by design, it is impossible to isolate specific effective treatment components. Despite these limitations, the results do suggest that a multicomponent intervention that identifies workstyle factors and intervenes to modify these factors along with a number of

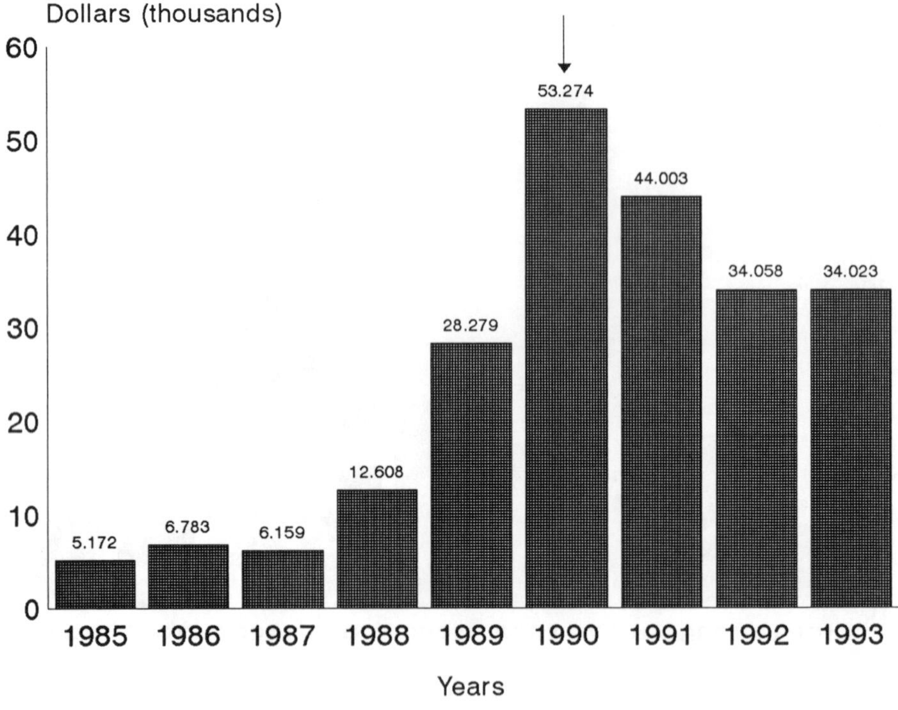

NOTE. Workgroup - Sign Language Interpreters

1990 Intervention Initiated

Figure 11.6 Upper-extremity CTD prevention and management program: workers' compensation medical costs.

other treatment components is associated with positive outcome in a group of employees who are exposed to biomechanical risk and experience a range of upper-extremity symptoms and disorders. Perhaps most importantly, the research provides preliminary support for the need to conduct controlled investigations on the effects of interventions specifically targeted at workstyle modification.

FUTURE RESEARCH

As further research accumulates regarding the existence of workstyle and its potential role in the exacerbation and maintenance of occupational upper-extremity symptoms/disorders, it could also emerge as an etiologic factor. The identification and validation of a potential risk factor for a set of symptoms, given disorder, or group of disorders requires that a number of levels of supportive evidence be established. These levels are presented in Table 11.8. It is also important to emphasize that the more evidence generated at each level, the stronger the potential role of the suspected risk factor. Only after repeated prospective studies have been conducted can one have sufficient evidence for the etiologic role of a given risk factor. However, it is also important to indicate that workstyle may play a role in the

Table 11.8 Criteria for evaluating the validity of a suspected risk factor.

1. *Strength* What is the value of the relative risk ratio?
2. *Consistency* Has the association been repeatedly observed in different places at different times by different observers (i.e. reliability)?
3. *Specificity* Is the association limited to a particular type of exposure and specific disease?
4. *Temporal relationship* How confident can one be that the suspected cause antedated to observed effect?
5. *Dose–response* Is there sufficient evidence of increasing risk with increased dose?
6. *Plausibility* Is the suggestion of causality biologically plausible?
7. *Coherence* Does the suggestion of causality conflict with other known data on the natural history and etiology of disease?
8. *Experimental confirmation* What is the effect of interventions?

From Feuerstein *et al.*, 1986.

exacerbation and/or maintenance of symptoms/disorders and disability and, given the magnitude of the problem of upper-extremity disorders, identification of exacerbating and maintaining factors can be quite useful for efforts at secondary and tertiary prevention. Developing approaches to assess and modify workstyle can potentially impact further symptom exacerbation and the subsequent development of work disability – major goals for effective management of these disorders.

While the concept of workstyle has potential in furthering our understanding of the role of biobehavioral factors in the development, exacerbation, and maintenance of a range of work-related upper-extremity disorders, much remains to be determined. Additional research is required in each of the eight criteria for determining the validity of a suspected risk factor.

In order to determine the strength of the effect of workstyle, a general consensus regarding a working definition needs to be established. Following this, specific assessment methodologies need to be developed and their reliability and validity determined. Once such an assessment approach is developed, further research on its specific contribution relative to other risk factors can be determined. In the interim, there are preliminary findings suggesting that certain features of the construct are related to occurrence of work-related upper-extremity symptoms and disorders (risk ratios between 1.0 and 3.0) as well as a relationship to symptom severity.

The need for a standardized measurement protocol is also critical to determining the consistency of the relationship. Also, clear case definitions and definitions of the symptom clusters and disorders are essential. Endpoints that are diffuse will only contribute to the lack of consistent or reliable findings linking workstyle to work-related upper-extremity disorders. In general, there are preliminary data that suggest that when work patterns or techniques are measured in response to a standardized task individual differences are observed and that these variations are associated with a range of symptoms particularly in the neck, shoulder, and wrist regions. Although the number of studies are small, these findings have been reported across different research groups.

In relation to specificity, *vis-à-vis* a specific type of exposure and specific disease, this question will need to wait for objective standardized measurement of the risk factor and more definitive definitions of the diseases. The problem related to this criteria is not specific to workstyle but to the occupational musculoskeletal disorders in general. These disorders appear to be multiply determined and clear-cut

Table 11.9 Future research questions.

- How can one develop simple psychometrically sound evaluation tools to identify high-risk workstyle at the workplace and in the clinic?
- Does the construct of high-risk workstyle generalize across types of hand-intensive work?
- Work factors trigger increases in high-risk workstyles?
- What are the specific behavioral and cognitive components of a high-risk workstyle?
- What are the specific psychophysiological correlates of high-risk workstyle?
- What is the specific association between workstyle and symptoms?
- What is the relative contribution of psychological style, work climate variables, ergonomic risk factors to workstyle?
- Can a high-risk workstyle be modified?
- What are the most effective intervention techniques for modifying high-risk workstyle?
- If modified, what are the short- and long-term effects on symptoms, productivity, worker satisfaction, OSHA recorded incidence, Workers' Compensation costs (medical and indemnity)?

endpoints for determining the relative contribution of specific risk factors is complex, thus making it difficult at this point to identify the *specific* role of workstyle.

The criteria of temporal relationship as mentioned in an earlier section of this chapter must await prospective longitudinal studies. Prospective studies typically follow a set of retrospective and cross-sectional analyses that support the suspected role of workstyle as well as a clear definition of the construct and sound measurement methodology.

In terms of dose–response, particularly in relation to symptom severity, in contrast to disease occurrence, there appears to be preliminary evidence indicating that the more the workstyle is exhibited (i.e. higher levels of self-generated force, fewer rest breaks, tendency to continue to work with pain to insure quality, etc.), the higher the level of symptom severity including positive nerve conduction findings. Whether this dose–response is a precursor or consequence is currently unclear.

The potential role of workstyle as a risk factor does appear to be biologically plausible. Increases in biomechanical and psychological strain potentially associated with the high-risk workstyle could contribute to muscular fatigue, pain, tendon strain, and increased sympathetic arousal which could contribute to increased intra-carpal tunnel pressure and entrapment of sensory and motor nerves of the hand as well as psychoneuro-immunologic changes which could contribute to episodic or persistent inflammatory processes. Given the role of the central nervous and autonomic nervous system on immune function and the effect of behavioral and psychosocial factors on the stress response and immune function, this link is plausible. Clearly, research on the biochemical correlates of workstyle variations and their relationship to symptoms represent a fruitful area for further research. Psychophysiological reactivity studies in those with and without symptoms as well as those with various levels of high-risk workstyle also seem warranted.

The question of whether the link between workstyle and upper-extremity symptoms/disorders is consistent with other known data on the natural history and etiology of these disorders will need to await further research on etiology. Anecdotal evidence suggests that individuals who develop persistent or recurrent pain problems in the upper-extremity have attempted to continue to work and persist despite pain, thus continuously exposing themselves to biomechanical stressors that can contribute to the development of a longer-term tendon or nerve-related problem. The etiologic role of many factors associated with these disorders is unclear at present and therefore very little can be addressed in relation to coherence.

The final criteria, experimental confirmation of the effect of interventions directed at modifying workstyle, suggest that such efforts have a potential positive effect. The uncontrolled group outcome study on the sign-language interpreters (Feuerstein *et al.*, forthcoming), anecdotal work by Pascarelli and Kella (1993), and outcome research with assembly workers (Parenmark *et al.*, 1988) suggest that focused efforts at modifying workstyle are associated with improvements in symptoms. At present, there are no randomized outcome studies investigating the effects of modifying workstyle on symptom development or symptom severity. Currently there is only anecdotal evidence that workstyle is modifiable.

Clearly, for workstyle to be considered an established, scientifically validated risk factor much remains to be accomplished. Some of the research issues were briefly eluded to above. A select list of specific research questions of interest are listed in Table 11.9.

SUMMARY

The construct of workstyle represents a viable concept that may help to explain how psychosocial factors in the workplace interact with work demands and biomechanical stressors to contribute to work-related upper-extremity symptoms/disorders/disability. The concept may help to serve as a bridging mechanism linking psychosocial stressors, work demands, generic ergonomic risk factors to behavioral, cognitive, and physiological responses with negative consequences regarding symptom development, exacerbation, and/or maintenance. This chapter defined the construct, reviewed literature supporting the existence of such a phenomena, illustrated the potential clinical utility of such a construct, and highlighted areas requiring further research. The construct holds potential for the development of innovative prevention, evaluation, and treatment approaches to assist in the alleviation of pain and suffering in individuals with these disorders as well as for reduction in the economic and productivity burden that these disorders represent to employers.

NOTES

I would like to acknowledge Susanne Callan-Harris, PT, MS, Anthony S. Papciak, PhD, Robert H. Jones, MD, Paul Hickey, MEd, William Armbruster, Jr., MS, and Ann Marie Carosella, PhD, colleagues who have worked at the Center for Occupational Rehabilitation at the University of Rochester Medical Center and during that time significantly contributed to the sign-language interpreter research effort. I would also like to thank James J. DeCaro, PhD, Dean at NTID/RIT for his consistent support of our work and Liza J. Marshall, Director of Interpreting Services at NTID and her talented, highly professional, and caring interpreting staff. Their willingness to contribute their insights into the biomechanical and psychosocial factors affecting upper-extremity problems at work as well as the time contributed as research subjects in our collaborative efforts to improve the health and safety of sign-language interpreters has contributed significantly to the work described in this chapter. I would also like to thank Marie Harring-Sweeney, PhD, epidemiologist at the National Institute for Occupational Safety and Health, for generously giving her time to discuss epidemiology and analyses, and Jennifer Boehles and Helen Hoffman for assistance with manuscript preparation.

The completion of this paper was supported in part by NIOSH Grant U6/CCU106156, the New England Center for Occupational Musculoskeletal Disorders and by the National Institute on Disability and Rehabilitation Research (Research and Demonstration grant number H133A00040, Michael Feuerstein, PhD, Principle Investigator).

1 While it should be recognized that much interest was generated around the construct of coronary-prone behavior as a risk factor for coronary artery disease, it only represents one factor in a complex multiply determined set of disorders – not dissimilar to occupational musculoskeletal disorders of the upper extremities.

2 A manual is available from the Department of Interpreting Services, National Training Institute for the Deaf, Rochester Institute of Technology, 1 Lomb Memorial Drive, Rochester, NY 14623, USA.

3 By necessity, given time constraints, this aspect of the program was limited to two one-hour sessions. Following this training, management and staff from NTID developed a videotape that provides an excellent review of four high-risk interpreting workstyles along with illustrations of alternative 'lower-risk' workstyles. This video, entitled *Biomechanics of Sign Language Interpreting*, is available from the Department of Interpreting Services at The National Technical Institute for the Deaf, Rochester Institute of Technology.

REFERENCES

Armstrong, T. J., Buckle, P., Fine, L. J., Hagberg, M., Jonsson, B., Kilborn, A., Kuorinka, I., Silverstein, B. A., Sjogaard, G. and Viikari-Juntura, E. 1993 A conceptual model of work related neck and upper-limb musculoskeletal disorders, *Scandinavian Journal of Work, Environment and Health*, **19**, 73–84.

Armstrong, T. J., Foulke, J. A., Martin, B. J. and Rempel, D. 1991 'An investigation of finger forces in alphanumeric keyboard work,' presentation at the meeting of the International Ergonomics Association, Paris, France.

Bammer, G. 1987 How technologic change can increase the risk of repetitive motion injuries, *Seminars in Occupational Medicine*, **2**, 25–30.

Bengtson, K. A. and Schutt, A. H. 1992 Upper extremity musculoskeletal problems in musicians: A follow up survey, *Medical Problems of Performing Artists*, **7**, 44–7.

Chaffin, D. B. and Fine, L. J. (Eds) 1993 *A National Strategy for Occupational Musculoskeletal Injuries – Implementation Issues and Research Needs: 1991 Conference Summary*, Department of Health and Human Services (NIOSH), Publication No. 93–101.

Everly, G. S. 1989 *A Clinical Guide to the Treatment of the Human Stress Response*, New York: Plenum.

Feuerstein, M. 1991 A multidisciplinary approach to the prevention, evaluation and management of work disability, *Journal of Occupational Rehabilitation*, **1**, 5–12.

Feuerstein, M., Carosella, A. M., Marshall, L. and DeCaro, J. forthcoming, 'Prevalence and pattern of occupational musculoskeletal symptoms of the upper extremities and spine in sign language interpreters.'

Feuerstein, M. and Fitzgerald, T. D. 1992 Biomechanical factors affecting upper extremity cumulative trauma disorders in sign language interpreters, *Journal of Occupational Medicine*, **34**, 257–64.

Feuerstein, M., Hickey, P., Callan-Harris, S., Jones, R., Marshall, L. and Thompson, W. forthcoming, 'Prevention and management of occupational musculoskeletal disorders of the upper extremity: Accident rates, symptoms and workers' compensation indemnity and medical costs.'

FEUERSTEIN, M. and JONES, R. 1990 *Comprehensive Multidisciplinary Approach to Evaluation. Rehabilitation and Prevention of Repetitive Motion Disorders in Sign Language Interpreters: Final Report*, Rochester, NY: University of Rochester School of Medicine and Dentistry.

FEUERSTEIN, M., LABBE, E. E. and KUCZMIERCZYK, A. R. 1986 *Health Psychology: A Psychobiological Perspective*, New York: Plenum Press.

FRY, H. J. H. 1986 Overuse syndrome in musicians: Prevention and management, *Lancet*, **ii**, 728–31.

HARDING, D. C., BRANDT, K. D. and HILLBERRY, B. M. 1989 Minimization of finger joint forces and tendon tensions in pianists, *Medical Problems of Performing Artists*, **4**, 103–8.

HERSEN, M. and BELLACK, A. S. (Eds) 1985 *Handbook of Clinical Behavior Therapy with Adults*, New York: Plenum.

JENKINS, C. D. 1978 Behavioral risk factors in coronary artery disease, *Annual Review of Medicine*, **29**, 543–62.

KILBOM, A. and PERSSON, J. 1987 Work techniques and its consequences for musculoskeletal disorders, *Ergonomics*, **30**, 273–9.

LAMBERT, C. M. 1992 Hand and upper limb problems of instrumental musicians, *British Journal of Rheumatology*, **31**, 265–71.

LARSSON, L. G., BAUM, J., MUDHOLKAR, G. S. and KOLLIA, G. D. 1993 Nature and impact of musculoskeletal problems in a population of musicians, *Medical Problems of Performing Artists*, **8**, 73–6.

LAZARUS, R. S. 1974 Psychological stress and coping in adaptation and illness, *International Journal of Psychiatry in Medicine*, **5**, 321–33.

LEHRER, P. M. and WOOLFOLK, R. L. 1993 *Principles and Practice of Stress Management*, New York: Guilford Press.

LEVI, L. 1972 Introduction: Psychosocial stimuli, psychophysiological reactions, and disease, in LEVI, L. (Ed.), *Stress and Distress in Response to Psychosocial Stimuli*, Oxford: Pergamon.

LINTON, S. J. 1991 A behavioral workshop for training immediate supervisors: The key to neck and back injuries?, *Perceptual and Motor Skills*, **73**, 1159–70.

LINTON, S. J. and KAMWENDO, K. 1989 Risk factors in the psychosocial work environment for neck and shoulder pain in secretaries, *Journal of Occupational Medicine*, **31**, 609–13.

NATIONAL INSTITUTE FOR OCCUPATIONAL SAFETY AND HEALTH 1992 *Health Hazard Evaluation Report: US West Communications*, US Department of Health and Human Services (HETA 90-0132277).

NATIONAL INSTITUTE FOR OCCUPATIONAL SAFETY AND HEALTH 1993 *Health Hazard Evaluation Report: Los Angeles Times*, US Department of Health and Human Services (HETA 90-0132277).

PARENMARK, G., ENGVALL, B. and MALMKVIST, A. K. 1988 Ergonomic on-the-job training of assembly workers, *Applied Ergonomics*, **19**, 143–6.

PASCARELLI, E. F. and KELLA, J. J. 1993 Soft-tissue injuries related to use of the computer keyboard: A clinical study of 53 severely injured persons, *Journal of Occupational Medicine*, **35**, 522–32.

PATKIN, M. 1990 Neck and arm pain in office workers: Causes and management, in SAUTER, S., DAINOFF, M. and SMITH, M. (Eds), *Promoting Health and Productivity in the Computerized Office*, London: Taylor & Francis.

PERSSON, J. and KILBOM, A. 1983 VIRA: en enkel videiofilmteknik för registrering och analys ava arbetsställningar och rörelser (English summary), *National Board of Occupational Safety and Health, Undersokningsrapport*, **10**, 23.

PUTZ-ANDERSON, V. 1988 *Cumulative Trauma Disorders: A Manual for Musculoskeletal Disease of the Upper Limbs*, Philadelphia, PA: Taylor & Francis.

RADWIN, R. G. 1992 'Automated psychomotor and sensory tests for functional deficits associated with carpal and tunnel syndrome,' presentation at the International Conference on Occupational Disorders of the Upper Extremities, University of Michigan, Ann Arbor, MI.

REID, J., EWAN, C. and LOWY, E. 1991 Pilgrimage of pain: The illness experiences of women with repetitive strain injury and the search for credibility, *Social Science and Medicine*, **32**, 601–12.

REMPEL, D. and GERSON, J. 1991 'Fingertip forces while using three different keyboards,' presentation at the 35th Annual Meeting of the Human Factors Society, San Francisco, CA.

REMPEL, D. M., HARRISON, R. J. and BARNHARDT, S. 1992 Work-related cumulative trauma disorders of the upper extremity, *Journal of the American Medical Association*, **267**, 838–42.

RODRIGUEZ, A. A., RADWIN, R. G. and JENG, O. J. 1993 Median nerve electrophysiologic parameters and psychomotor performance in carpal tunnel syndrome, *Electromyography and Clinical Neurophysiology*, **33**, 1–9.

RYAN, K. D. and OESTREICH, D. K. 1991 *Driving Fear Out of the Workplace*, San Francisco, CA: Jossey-Bass.

SCHWARTZ, M. S. 1987 *Biofeedback: A Practitioner's Guide*, New York: Guilford Press.

SHEALY, J., FEUERSTEIN, M. and LATKO, W. 1991 Biomechanical analysis of upper extremity risk in sign language interpreting, *Journal of Occupational Rehabilitation*, **1**, 215–23.

SPENCE, S. H. 1990 Psychopathology amongst acute and chronic patients with occupationally related upper limb pain versus accident injuries of the upper limbs, *Australian Psychologist*, **25**, 293–305.

ULIN, S. S. and ARMSTRONG, T. J. 1992 A strategy for evaluating occupational risk factors of musculoskeletal disorders, *Journal of Occupational Rehabilitation*, **2**, 35–50.

VEIERSTED, K. B., WESTGAARD, R. H. and ANDERSEN, P. 1990 Pattern of muscle activity during stereotypical work and its relation to muscle pain, *International Archives of Occupational and Environmental Health*, **62**, 31–41.

VEIERSTED, K. B., WESTGAARD, R. H. and ANDERSEN, P. 1993 Electromyographic evaluation of muscular work pattern as a predictor of trapezius myalgia, *Scandinavian Journal of Work, Environment and Health*, **19**, 284–90.

WOLF, F. G., KEANE, M. S., BRANDT, K. D. and HILLBERRY, B. M. 1993 An investigation of finger joint and tendon forces in experienced pianists, *Medical Problems of Performing Artists*, **8**, 84–95.

CHAPTER TWELVE

A psychosocial analysis of cumulative trauma disorders[1]

WILBERT E. FORDYCE

INTRODUCTION

This chapter addresses the problem of cumulative trauma disorders (CTDs) from a psychosocial perspective. It will be argued here that CTDs present problems relating to definition of illness. They cannot be understood if viewed solely as consequences of enduring neurophysiological effects from cumulatively stressing body structures or processes. It is held, further, that emergence and growth of the problem of CTDs relates significantly to psychosocial effects in society. A growing number of people have become ready to identify generalized suffering as a problem for which the health-care system has solutions. This increasing demand from society interacts with a health-care system too dedicated to biological reductionism: an insistence on 'finding' pathophysiologic or neurobiologic explanations for distress. The health-care system, eager to be of help, medicalizes suffering by applying ill-founded or poorly grounded diagnostic labels, to which treatments are then applied with, at best, mixed results.

Illness, the voicing of body complaints, and the seeking of health-care assistance involve a complex and dynamic interplay of somatic states or conditions, cognitive or mental processes, environmental influences, and political or social policy matters. This chapter will necessarily address these factors only briefly.

Two sets of data and conceptual analyses lie behind this chapter. One concerns nonspecific lower back pain (i.e. no fractures, no sciatica, no surgically correctable condition, no relevant systemic disease). The other draws on data and analyses from Australia concerning repetition strain injury (RSI), reported elsewhere in Chapter 9.

NONSPECIFIC LOWER BACK PAIN

Examination of the history of attribution of causes of lower back pain is instructive. Allan and Waddell reviewed the history of back pain, sciatica, and low back disability (Allan and Waddell, 1989; Waddell *et al.*, 1993). In summarizing their review, Waddell (Waddell *et al.*, 1993) comments:

> Back pain and sciatica have affected man throughout recorded history .... No evidence indicates that back problems have changed. The symptom of back pain appears to be no different, no more frequent, and no more severe than it has always been.
>
> What has changed is how back problems are understood and managed. Before the nineteenth century back pain was dismissed as 'fleeting pains' or rheumatics. Few became chronically disabled by simple backache. Two key ideas in the nineteenth century laid the foundations for our modern approach to back problems: (1) the pain came from the spine and (2) the pain was due to injury. The physical pathology of spinal irritation was never clearly defined ... and disappeared as a diagnosis, but the idea that the spine could be a source of pain was firmly established. The idea that a painful spine must somehow be irritable remains to this day.
>
> The other idea was 'railway spine.' The building of the railways was a key part. Early accidents led to a spate of serious injuries. Public concern led to legislation and the start of the modern compensation system. Only then did back pain begin to be blamed on trauma. It is not easy for us to realize that, all through history, chronic back pain had never been thought to be due to injury.

As the Allan and Waddell review points out, advances in general knowledge about pain and illness led to the emergence of plausible explanations for the common ailment of backache. The medical profession, long struggling to be of help but ill-equipped to do little more than provide comfort, came to be armed with a conceptual and quasi-empirical basis for their efforts to heal from newfound anatomic and physiologic knowledge. However plausible, those 'explanations' were not based on demonstrations of causative relationships between the neurophysiologic and anatomic factors alleged to underlie backache and its persistence into chronicity. Except for a very small percentage of cases meeting criteria for specific, as distinguished from nonspecific, lowerback pain, no functional linear relationships between body defect and pain, suffering, and disability were demonstrated. No solutions to the incidence and prevalence of disability from backache emerged. Decisive advances in knowledge about anatomic and neurophysiologic processes were not accompanied by corresponding reductions in the magnitude of the problem of lower back pain. Inspection of rates of incidence and prevalence of disability status attributed to lower back pain in a number of economically developed countries reveals quite an opposite picture (Frank, 1993; Frymoyer and Cats-Baril, 1991; Hager, 1993; Nachemson, 1992; Raspe, 1993). The incidence of back pain seems to be essentially stable. But assignment of disability status attributed to lower back pain has increased markedly and at an accelerating rate over the past several decades.

Studies of the meaning of symptoms to the suffering person and whether persons describing themselves as having backache seek care makes clear why there is not a close relationship between perceived backache and subsequent disability or functional impairment.

The one-year incidence of back symptoms ranges from 27 per cent to 60 per cent in working adults (Gyntelberg, 1974; Troup *et al.*, 1987), but only 2–5 per cent file back-injury claims or seek medical care (Spengler *et al.*, 1986; Waddell, 1987). When is a symptom not a symptom?

A review and summary of the problem of back pain in industry by Bigos and Battie (1991) suggests an explanation. They state:

> Most episodes of back pain do not seem to be caused by an injury in the typical sense of the word, but rather are a normal part of life and aging. Back pain is extremely common. Up to 85 per cent of the adult population recall having back pain by age 50,

and there is some indication that the remainder have forgotten such episodes. Approximately 50 per cent of people in the working age group admit to significant symptoms but only a small percentage (2–5 per cent) subsequently make the decision to file a back injury claim. Furthermore, only about one-fifth of patients with back problems can loosely associate the onset of their symptoms with an accident, injury or unusual activity.

The observations of Bigos and Battie, and the supporting studies that they cite, highlight the ambiguities inherent to lower back pain, and indicate clearly that something more is involved in the problem than nociceptive stimulation. Clearly, selective factors exert influence from the outset in work-related back-pain reports to determine whether a person decides that backache warrants seeking care.

Reviews of the effects of worksite-based programs on care seeking for back pain and on subsequent disability rates lend more support for questioning the state of the back as the determining factor in back pain reports. Findings of these studies indicate a greater impact on reduction of subsequent back-pain-related disability rates from policies and programs having little or no relationship to medical treatment (Hunt and Habeck, 1993). This will be commented on further below.

Health-care providers, as well as patients coming to the health-care system with complaints of backache, often do not understand the complex factors influencing such reports. Those misunderstandings impact diagnosis and treatment. They also impact the understanding of the relationship of pain to impairment and disability which provide the foundation from which insurance companies, compensation agencies, judicial systems, and employers make case decisions and set policy.

Adding to the difficulties in understanding the meaning of complaints of back pain, definitions of disability and criteria for its award have undergone changes that complicate the problem yet further. Disability benefits exist as a society's commitment to redressing the functional disadvantage of a person incurring a disabling condition. Subtle shifts have occurred. Definitions of what constitutes disability have broadened, making the problem of disability management yet more complicated. The medical profession is asked to judge or categorize people with respect to functional impairment when possible disability award is at stake. Those judgments provide the foundation for agency or legal mechanisms to determine whether the individual is entitled to disability benefits. Those judgments stand on shaky ground. The physician is led astray by insufficient understanding of the nature of pain and the factors that influence its report.

A CONCEPTUAL ANALYSIS OF PAIN

A brief examination of the conceptual basis for pain points out how complex emotional and metal or cognitive processes have come to be confounded with consequences of neurophysiologic or anatomic defect.

The concept of pain has been used in two rather different ways but with the differences often not appreciated. First, it has been seen as a sense. But reactions to nociceptive stimulation are concerned as much with impending or anticipated events as they are with current sensory input. That is a clear difference from the function of senses. Viewing pain as a sense or sensory system will not suffice.

The second use of 'pain' lumps the signal system with cognitive, emotional, and behavioral actions occurring subsequent to nociceptive stimulation, characterized as emotions, responses, or reactions. These reactions, corresponding to definitions of suffering and of pain behavior, do not occur exclusively as a response to painful or nociceptive stimuli. They may occur in relation to other events independent of nociception. The form and quality of these reactions, as well as the very perception of stimuli evoking them, are influenced by prior experience and anticipations of consequences deriving from that experience, as well as by ambient mood state. Pain behaviors also may be elicited by cues pointing to possible or probable consequences in the person's environment, thus relating pain behaviors to the contextual milieu in which the person is functioning.

There is a complex and dynamic interplay of information reaching the central nervous system from the mixing of inputs from sensory modalities with extant emotional state and mood. An aversive or nociceptive stimulus may lead to perception of pain. But currently active emotional states influence whether and how the aversive stimulus is perceived. Those emotional states also influence physiological processes (e.g. heart rate, blood pressure, muscle tension) which then feed back to color the perceptions of what is happening, the meanings assigned to it, and the actions taken in response. Perception of the nature and meaning of incoming sensory information, how one's body responds physiologically, and what actions are taken, as well as anticipations of what the future holds, are inextricably intertwined.

Thus, suffering and pain behaviors are variable in relation to the timing of nociceptive input and, within certain variable limits, with respect of their intensity.

SUFFERING AND THE MEANING OF SYMPTOMS

Pain behavior and its measurement is dealt with in more detail elsewhere in this volume (Chapter 10). Hearing a person complain or describe a 'pain,' or observing a person limping, rubbing a body part, or moving in guarded fashion, cannot be used as an indicator of the presence of nociceptive stimulation or of some neurophysiological defect ordinarily associated with pain and, potentially, with impairment. Alternative and equally viable explanations for their occurrence exist. Pain behaviors, including the verbal report of pain, should be seen as social communications and not simply as metrics of pain/nociception. Pain has tended to be viewed as if it were a discrete element within this interactive complex of forces when it is not. Factors influencing a person's decision to seek care should be examined further. Cameron *et al.* (1993) studied in a community-based population the decision to seek care or not for a range of symptoms, including pain. They noted from their findings that (p. 175) 'although pain may promote decisions to seek care, neither the level of pain nor perceived intensification over time seems to be a strong candidate for a determinant of care seeking.' That is not to say that intensity of experienced pain cannot determine care seeking but that, across a spectrum of persons and a range of severity of symptoms, other factors influence the decision. Many hurt but far fewer perceive it as a problem for which special help is needed.

The confounding of pain with suffering is basic to the issue. It is imperative to separate pain-as-a-signal from the reactions and emotions that people display when presenting to the world that they 'have pain.' Cassell (1991) pointed out that 'pain and suffering are distinct, and that there can be pain (or other dire symptoms) without suffering and suffering without such symptoms.' He characterizes suffering as an emotional state triggered by anticipation of threat to one's self or identity.

Budd developed yet further our understanding of the concept of suffering and the role that present mood state and the anticipated future have on body states (Budd, 1992). He characterized suffering as occurring 'when we assess ourselves in a situation and don't like where we are, where we have been, or where we are going *and* we can take no actions to close this gap.' Suffering may have been the ambient mood state at the time that a reported pain problem began or was first perceived and labelled. Alternatively, the mood may become one of suffering when anticipating what the future holds. When this occurs concomitantly with backache, that future may be clouded or aversive because of the anticipation of effects of perceived body damage on future functioning, whether correctly or not. For example, Waddell *et al.* (1993) have shown that anticipation of re-injury to the back is a more powerful predictor of return to work of those sidelined by backache than is medical diagnosis or treatment.

Anticipation of a negatively signed future may occur for reasons quite unrelated to pain. The previously cited (Cameron *et al.*, 1993) study presents further data to support this point. They report (p. 177): 'care seekers reported more life stresses in comparison with matched controls ... and reported a greater number of (non-illness) life stresses in relation to the entire sample of matched controls,' suggesting that negatively toned mood state makes care seeking more likely. They conclude that (p. 177) 'These findings, and the independent effect of life stressors on care seeking, are consistent with the hypothesis that care seeking will serve the critical function of reducing the load of emotional distress created both by symptoms and life stressors.'

Zola (1973) studied persons seeking aid for a symptom for the first time. He concluded from his findings (p. 645): 'they sought help because they could not stand it any longer. But what they could not stand was more likely to be a situation or a perceived implication of a symptom rather than any worsening of the symptom, *per se*.' Level of suffering may be intensified by ambient mood state to the point that the person becomes a care seeker.

The findings discussed here give a different perspective to the meaning of complaints of continuing pain in nonspecific lower back pain. Because of failure to differentiate suffering from 'pain,' both patient and physician are at risk and seemingly frequently do medicalize a suffering problem. This is often followed by award of disability status.

To summarize, it is contended here that the interaction of several forces has contributed to the dilemma of stable incidence but soaring disability rates for back pain. One is the emergence of plausible but not empirically validated neurophysiologic and anatomic rationales for chronic backache. A second is the ambiguous nature of pain complaints and their relationship to more generalized emotional distress. A third is a tendency for the health-care system and disability determination systems to view the problem rather exclusively from a medical model perspective. A fourth is a growing number of people who, when suffering for whatever reason, proceed as if the health-care system has a solution. A fifth is the gradual loosening of social/legal definitions of what constitutes disability, resulting in more readiness of utilize award of disability status as an element of medical 'management.'

REPETITION STRAIN INJURY

The Australian experience with RSI bears a striking resemblance to the historical course of nonspecific lower back pain. This history is discussed in more detail elsewhere (Chapter 9 of this volume; Bell, 1989; McPhee, 1986). Certain points will be made here to link the RSI experience to that of nonspecific lower back pain. Viewed together, experience is medical management of chronic nonspecific lower back pain and RSI suggests yet further that psychosocial factors play important roles in perception of disability and award of disability status.

The McPhee report on RSI (McPhee, 1986) draws the distinction between well-defined and poorly defined conditions. About the former, the report states:

> There is long-standing evidence in the scientific literature ... that work involving one or more of ... repetitious tasks, forceful movements and the maintenance of constrained postures for prolonged periods may be associated with a number of well-defined clinical conditions for which there are accepted means of diagnosis. The mechanisms of these ... are not always known. Rotator cuff syndrome, lateral and medical epicondylitis, carpal tunnel syndrome and tenosynovitis are examples.

About poorly defined conditions, the report (p. 4) states: 'There appears to be agreement that the majority of cases of RSI do not fall into (the well-defined) category.'

From the early 1970s to the mid-1980s, particularly 1983–1985, there was a rapid increase in Australia of cases diagnosed as RSI and for which disability status was awarded. Thereafter, the prevalence of the 'conditions,' and, more particularly, disability award for it, began a precipitous fall.

Ebbing of the epidemic of RSI coincided with the publication of a number of studies which highlighted the absence of systematic relationships between the alleged causative factors and occurrence of the condition. A number of these are described and discussed in detail in Chapter 9. Bell (1989), in synthesizing the data regarding RSI, noted (p. 280):

> The psychological basis of RSI is revealed by its rapid rise and fall ... RSI lacked a clear clinical definition or credible pathogenesis, its course was contradictory to experience with other illnesses, its signs were conspicuous by their absence and examination revealed no clinical abnormalities.

Bell went on to say (p. 281):

> A sudden appearance and rapid increase of a disorder that is not caused by a physical agent such as a poison or infection is likely to have psychological and social causes. The essential ingredient is the presentation with puzzling and novel complaints, which prompt medical practitioners to give complainants the benefit of the doubt. Perhaps the most devastating iatrogenic contribution of all was the many and varied attempts to treat RSI as a physical illness, which aided the community to accept the condition as an 'injury' ... new-found experts developed therapeutic empires with a vigorous entrepreneurial spirit that was undeterred by the ineffectiveness of their treatment methods. The measures that were introduced to manage the disorder were disastrously inappropriate and instead promoted its spread. The belief that the condition was an injury reinforced the hypochondriacal concern of the complainants and facilitated unjustified claims for compensation.

Review of the Australian experience is regard to RSI illustrates the hazards of a nonspecific condition interacting with a health-care system which analyzes patient problems within the framework of a medical model. There is considerable risk that medical 'diagnoses' become attached to personal suffering. It is a problem of medicalizing suffering. The resulting illness conviction by both patient and practitioner gains further strength by the application of unsuccessful but medically 'sanctified' treatment by physicians and others. Historically, increases in rates of disability assignment are modest *except* in nonspecific or ambiguous conditions in which linkage between symptoms or complaints and alleged neurophysiological or anatomic defect is tenuous or not demonstrated, as has been the case with nonspecific lower pack pain and RSI.

DISABILITY MANAGEMENT IN THE WORKPLACE

We can now return to another context to illustrate further the thesis presented here. In the past, industry has looked to medicine for help in resolving the problem of work-related back pain complaints and disability. Yet, despite advances in health-care technology, costs for back pain and incidence and costs of disability have continued to grow.

Viewed from the perspective of the health-care system and its medical model, amelioration of the disability management problem, as pertains to nonspecific lower back pain, has been assumed to reside mainly in establishing more effective diagnostic, treatment, and disability management programs within medicine. As has been shown, that strategy has not resulted in reductions in rate of award of disability for nonspecific lower back pain. Examination of studies pertaining to what transpires in the workplace prior to an injured worker's entry into the health-care delivery system suggests a rather different perspective on the problem.

Pertinent to this different perspective, a comment was made in the introductory remarks to the 16th Annual National Symposium on Workers' Compensation by William Hager, President of the National Council on Compensation Insurance (Hager, 1993). He said, 'Unless we get unneeded services and providers out of the workers' compensation system, the house will come down.' Frymoyer and Cats-Baril (1991) have raised the question: 'Have medical professionals of all types become part of the problem, rather than part of the solution?'

Rousmaniere (1990) has claimed that approximately 50 per cent of costs resulting from workplace injuries depends on how the company manages injuries after they occur. Habeck *et al.* (1991) reported confirming data when they found that firms performing disability management methods poorly, when compared with companies using effective disability management methods, had twice as many recordable injury events but four times as many workers' compensation claims.

Hunt and Habeck (1993) studied the relationship of three sets of employer policy and practice methods with disability outcome measures pertaining to all injuries or diseases, not just back pain. They studied 220 Michigan companies of 100 or more employees, distributed among seven industries. They examined policies focusing on safety intervention designed to prevent injuries from occurring, and disability management designed to minimize the disability consequences of a given injury, e.g. case monitoring and proactive return to work. They also studied health promotion: attempts to intervene with the individual worker to encourage more healthy life-styles in the expectation that this might reduce lost work time and the impact of applying ergonomic principles at the worksite. Results indicated that employer diligence on matters of work safety was strongly associated with fewer disability claims and shorter disability duration, as were policies providing for proactive return-to-work programs. They state (p. ii):

> the twin strategies of trying to prevent injuries in the first place, and working to ameliorate their disability effects through disability management techniques, are both shown to be productive in reducing workplace disability in those establishments that have implemented them rigorously.

The Hunt and Habeck study findings also indicated that neither ergonomic solutions nor efforts to enhance wellness in workers proved to be effective in influencing disability outcome. Indeed, ergonomic strategies to prevent injury and subsequent disability actually were followed by slightly higher disability rates.

The evidence seems clear that workers entering the health-care system with complaints of nonspecific back pain or RSI are being influenced by factors beyond the domain of pain/nociception and a medical model perspective. The currently prevailing strategies for work injury management operate from a health-care provider-based framework. It is a reactive approach. Habeck (1993) comments:

> As work disability increases, providers expand efforts to offer more and better rehabilitation services; however, due to the reactive nature of this model these efforts fail to address the underlying causes of the problem. As a result, many providers continue to function from a 'broken paradigm' that cam only offer limited solutions to work disability and may actually contribute to escalating costs of health-care and rehabilitation in disability benefit programs. The consequences of this broken paradigm are felt not only by payers and recipients of the system but are genuinely harmful to the viability of service providers.

That broken paradigm is one that fails adequately to differentiate pain from suffering and, having done so, treats suffering as if it were pain. An alternative to the reactive approach is to perceive the potential for interventions or disability prevention programs within the workplace setting to reduce health-care costs and the incidence of long-term disability. This is a proactive approach, one that seeks to prevent primary occurrence of injuries, e.g. work safety programs. But this approach also seeks to facilitate return to work both before referral to the health-care system and as an active part of medical management, should that referral occur. The relative successes of that approach indicate that conventional medical management by itself is of questionable relevance for chronic nonspecific lower back pain. The rapid and marked diminishing of incidence of RSI and disability award relating to it, as has been the Australian experience, points to a similar conclusion.

CONCLUSION

Analysis of the concepts of pain and suffering in the context of conditions having an ambiguous and questionable relationship to significant anatomic and neurophysiologic defects points to the importance of assessing psychosocial factors in disability determination. It is suggested here that the soaring rate of disability award for nonspecific lower back pain, as an example of CTD, has been influenced in significant degree by failure to distinguish 'pain' from suffering, thereby attributing the expressed complaints to body damage requiring remediation.

A second and related distorting influence has been the tendency to view the person undergoing 'cumulative trauma' as somewhat of an 'inert recipient.' Trauma, whether cumulative or singular, can have enduring effects on body structures and functions. The result can be clearly definable biomedical abnormality. However, trauma, cumulative or singular, happens to a dynamic organism; one equipped with automatic healing action and with the potential for moving ahead with full function. The presence of 'biomedical abnormality' does not in itself define whether, or to what extent, residual disability exists. To illustrate by a perhaps extreme analogy, cumulative trauma to a macadamized roadbed may result in pits and chuckholes for which remediation awaits highway road crews and the like. Cumulative trauma to a Michael Jordan may be followed by active engagement in remediating exercise or activity, or a resumption and maintenance of essentially unfettered performance without medical assistance somewhat irrespective of body effects attributed to trauma. The difference between a worker and an athlete cannot be regarded simply as the athlete being healthier or in better physical condition. That may be true but it is also the case that some workers differ from some athletes in their readiness to perceive themselves as ready and capable of proceeding with desired activity in the presence of trauma, singular or cumulative.

In a sense, then, the problem that we are faced with in judging residual effects of use or abuse of body parts, as is the implicit assumption underlying the concept of CTDs, is that of the interplay of body damage with the individual's readiness to undertake or maintain function. Clearly, neither can be ultimately defined independently of the other. A major difficulty now is that these problems tend to be viewed only in medical model terms. The medical model is useful but it is only a model. It captures only limited elements of the problems that suffering people bring to the health-care system. It also fails to come to grips adequately with the individual's self-starting and self-healing mechanisms. Nor does it take into account the influence of extant environmental or social feedback on individual performance readiness. The same model is at the core of award of disability status by legal and agency mechanisms and it fails there, too.

It is beyond the scope of this chapter to deal with strategies for dealing with chronic sufferers who heretofore have had their suffering medically sanctified. It is an important personal and social problem. It cannot be dealt with without first understanding the factors involved. The dramatic disabling effects of medicalizing suffering support the claim of Illich who, in commenting on similar diagnostically ambiguous conditions, said: 'medicine has become a disabling profession, turning citizens into patients to be saved by the experts' (Illich, 1977).

Diagnosis of CTDs should be required to assay psychosocial factors before proceeding. Depending upon the outcome of such assays, treatment should be required to demonstrate something broader than a medical model perspective on the patient's problem. The strategy for ameliorating the problem is to ensure that our health-care and disability determination systems recognize and consider psychosocial factors in illness definition and disability determination.

NOTES

1 Part of this chapter are adapted from W. Fordyce, 1995, pain in the workplace, a report of the IASP Task Force on Pain in the Workplace: Management of Disability from Low Back Pain.

REFERENCES

ALLAN, D. B. and WADDELL, G. W. 1989 An historical perspective on low back pain and disability, *Acta Orthopaedica Scandinavica*, Suppl. No. **234**(60), 1–23.

BELL, D. S. 1989 Repetitive strain injury: An iatrogenic epidemic of simulated injury, *Medical Journal of Australia*, **151**, 280–4.

BIGOS, S. and BATTIE, M. 1991 The impact of spinal disorders in industry, in FRYMOYER, J. (Ed.), *The Adult Spine: Principles and Practice*, pp. 147–53, New York: Raven Press.

BUDD, M. A. 1992 Human suffering: The road to illness or the gateway to learning, presentation at Lee Travis Institute for Biopsychosocial Research and the US Public Health Service, Boston, MA, pp. 1–17.

CAMERON, L., LEVENTHAL, E. and LEVENTHAL, H. 1993 Symptom representations and affect as determinants of care seeking in a community-dwelling, adult sample population, *Health Psychology*, **12**(3), 171–9.

CASSELL, E. J. 1991 *Recognizing Suffering*, Hastings Center Report, May–June, pp. 24–31.

FORDYCE, W. (Ed.) 1995 Backpain in the Workplace: Management of Disability in Nonspecific Conditions, Seattle, WA: IASP Press.

FRANK, A. 1993 Regular review: Low back pain, *British Medical Journal*, **306**, 901–9.

FRYMOYER, J. W. and CATS-BARIL, W. L. 1991 An overview of the incidence and costs of low back pain, *Orthopaedic Clinics N. America*, **22**, 263–71.

GYNTELBERG, F. 1974 One year incidence of low back pain among male residents of Copenhagen aged 40–59, *Danish Medical Bulletin*, **21**, 30–6.

HABECK, R. V. 1993 Achieving quality and value in service to the workplace, *Work Injury Management*, **2**(3), 2–8.

HABECK, R., LEAHY, M., HUNT, H., CHANG, F. and WELCH, E. 1991 Employer factors related to workers' compensation claims and disability management, *Rehabilatation Counseling Bulletin*, **34**(3), 210–26.

HAGER, W. D. 1993 *Workers' Compensation Back Claim Study*, Boca Raton, FL: National Council on Compensation Insurance, pp. 1–25.

HUNT, A. and HABECK, R. 1993 *The Michigan Disability Prevention Study*, Kalamazoo: W. E. Upjohn Institute for Employment Research.

ILLICH, I. 1977 Disabling professions, in ILLICH, I., ZOLA, I. and MCKNIGHT, J. (Eds), *Disabling Professions*, London: Marion Boyars, pp. 11–39.

MCPHEE, B. 1986 *Repetitive Strain Injury: A Report and Code of Practice*, National Occupational Health and Safety Commission, Australian Govt Printing Service, pp. 1–117.

NACHEMSON, A. L. 1992 Newest knowledge of low back pain: A critical look, *Clinical Orthopaedics*, **279**, 8–20.

RASPE, H. 1993 Back pain, in SILMAN, A. and HOCHBERG (Eds), *Epidemiology of Rheumatic Diseases*, Oxford: Oxford University Press.

ROUSMANIERE, P. 1990 Stop workers comp from shooting holes in corporate profits, *Corporate Cashflow*.

SPENGLER, D., BIGOS, S., MARTIN, N. A., ZEH, J., FISHER, L. and NACHEMSON, A. 1986 Back injuries in industry: A retrospective study, I: Overview and cost analysis, *Spine*, **11**, 241.

TASK FORCE 1985 *Repetition Strain Injury in the Australian Public Service*, Canberra: AGPS.

TROUP, J., FOREMAN, T. and BAXTER, C. 1987 The perception of back pain and the role of psychophysical tests of lifting capacity, 1987 Volvo Award in Clinical Sciences, *Spine*, **12**, 645–7.

WADDELL, G. 1987 A new clinical model for the treatment of low back pain, *Spine*, **12**, 632–44.

WADDELL, G., NEWTON, M., HENDERSON, I., SOMERVILLE, D. and MAIN, C. 1993 A fear-avoidance beliefs questionnaire (FABQ) and the role of fear-avoidance in chronic low back pain and disability, *Pain*, **52**, 157–68.

ZOLA, I. K. 1973 Pathways to the doctor: from a person to patient, *Soc. Sci. and Med.*, **7**, 677–89.

CHAPTER THIRTEEN

Social consequences of disclosing psychosocial concomitants of disease and injury

J. A. SKELTON

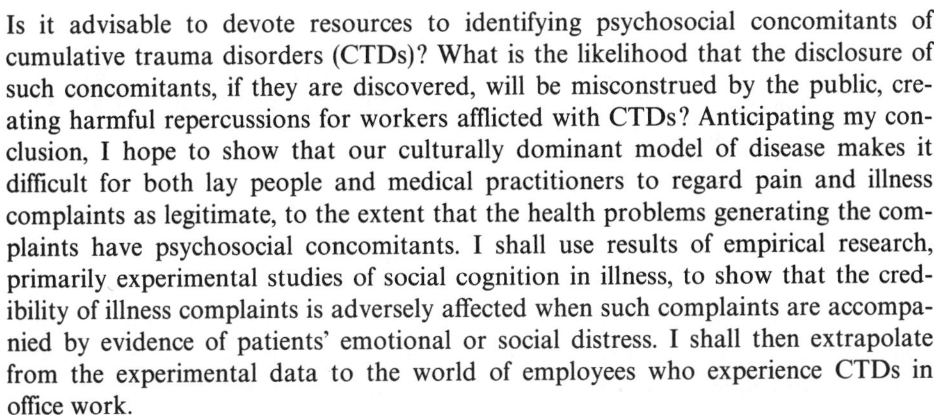

Is it advisable to devote resources to identifying psychosocial concomitants of cumulative trauma disorders (CTDs)? What is the likelihood that the disclosure of such concomitants, if they are discovered, will be misconstrued by the public, creating harmful repercussions for workers afflicted with CTDs? Anticipating my conclusion, I hope to show that our culturally dominant model of disease makes it difficult for both lay people and medical practitioners to regard pain and illness complaints as legitimate, to the extent that the health problems generating the complaints have psychosocial concomitants. I shall use results of empirical research, primarily experimental studies of social cognition in illness, to show that the credibility of illness complaints is adversely affected when such complaints are accompanied by evidence of patients' emotional or social distress. I shall then extrapolate from the experimental data to the world of employees who experience CTDs in office work.

In proposing that psychosocial distress undermines patients' credibility to observers, I am not claiming that work-related health problems represent the conversion of stress or worries into illness complaints.[1] Both lay people and medical professionals, however, are likely to believe that this is precisely what is going on when individuals' reports of pain and symptoms covary with information about the presence of psychosocial distress. The problem with identifying psychosocial concomitants of work-related musculoskeletal disorders, therefore, is that the truth may fail to make victims free; instead, it may cause them to be doubly victimized – first by their pain and then by psychogenic stereotypes. In other words, the problem is one of public perception or, more precisely, our mental model of what constitutes 'real' disease.

CREDIBILITY OF ILLNESS COMPLAINTS: AN OVERVIEW

Skepticism by Health Professionals

Empirical evidence concerning professional skepticism toward patients' illness complaints is not difficult to find. Wiener (1975) observed interactions between patients suffering from chronic lower back pain and nurses on an orthopedic ward. She concluded that professionals stereotype such patients by applying psychological labels, especially to those who prove to be 'difficult.' She also noticed that the mere presence of physical signs of pathology was not sufficient to dispel questions about the psychogenic etiology of patients' pain condition. Wiener's approach was observational and qualitative, whereas Burgess (1980) applied experimental methods and quantitative analyses to study the same problem. Burgess distributed to nurses case vignettes describing a stereotypic patient who presents for treatment of lower pack pain: an individual who has experienced pain for many months, who exhibits behavioral signs of psychological depression, and for whom no physical etiology has been determined. The nurse-subjects were asked to estimate how much pain the patient was suffering, using a 1–10 rating scale. Compared to a control patient whose back pain was described as short-lived, who exhibited no depressive signs, and for whom there were clear signs of physical pathology, the patient with the stereotypic profile was estimated to be suffering less.

Taylor *et al.* (1984) used a factorial experimental design to establish which characteristic comprising Burgess's stereotypic patient profiles – negative diagnostic signs, chronicity, or depression – undercut nurses' estimates of patient suffering. They verified Wiener's observation that positive diagnostic test results were not sufficient to allay health professionals' doubts about patients' self-reported pain, because hypothetical patients whose condition was described as chronic were estimated as suffering less than those whose condition was described as acute, even when both had positive diagnostic signs.

Peer Skepticism

Evidence is also accumulating that lay observers react with skepticism to illness claims. Subsequent to studies that sampled the views of health-care professionals toward patient suffering, I began a series of experiments on lay persons' responses to peers' illness complaints, and especially to psychosocial distress that co-occurs with illness; the earliest of these studies are reviewed in Skelton (1991). The starting assumption is that perceivers confronted with a peer's illness complaint or symptom report face the attributional question: why is this person claiming to be sick? By varying the context of the patient's illness claim, I have found two factors that consistently affect the lay perceiver's answer. The first is whether the patient's illness claim is corroborated by positive diagnostic signs. In two experiments, college students who read about a male peer who goes to the College Health Center complaining of a sore throat rated the patient as more credible if they were told that a diagnostic test had shown that the patient has a strep infection than if the test results were reported as negative (Skelton, 1991, Experiments 1 and 3). Such results reproduce the findings of Burgess (1980) and Taylor *et al.* (1984) and indicate that lay observers share at least some of the biomedical assumptions of health-care professionals.

The other factor that consistently affects perceivers' estimates of patient credibility is whether patients' symptom reports co-occur with reports of nonmedical problems. In each study conducted to date, some subjects are told only about the patient's medical problem (always a sore throat, a familiar health problem that is rarely life-threatening but for which medical help is sometimes sought). But other subjects are also told that the patient is experiencing personal problems, such as heavy schoolwork demands, a romantic breakup, a bout of insomnia, or even sickness in the patient's family. Subjects who receive this additional information rate the patient as more psychologically distressed and the illness complaint as less credible than subjects who know only about the sore throat (Skelton, 1991, Experiments 1 through 4). Denigration of patient credibility is independent of diagnostic evidence; even when the patient has a valid medical condition (indicated by positive diagnostic results), subjects regard the illness complaint as less credible when it is accompanied by information alluding to psychosocial distress in the patient's life. Patient descriptions have been presented in such varied formats as paragraph-length vignettes, Health Center files, written transcripts of interviews or conversations, and a video of a conversation between two students (Delaney and McNutt, 1992; Graham, 1994). I review one of those experiments here to provide a model of the paradigm and typical findings.

The patient was a male college student designated by the initials HC. He was interviewed by a Health Center nurse. In some interviews, HC reported only the symptoms, sore throat and nasal congestion. In others, he also reported a heavy midterm exam schedule, a three-day bout of insomnia, or both. Information about these personal problems was elicited through rather aggressive probing by the interviewing nurse, rather than being stated as simple matters of fact or being volunteered spontaneously by the patient. All interviews indicated that a diagnostic test had revealed a strep infection.

Subjects read one of four versions of the nurse–patient interview. Then they responded to a series of rating items. The mean of three items constituted the Credibility score: 'How believable is the student?,' 'How much is the student overreacting?' (reverse-scored), and 'To what degree does the patient have ulterior motives?' (also reversed). The items 'How much is the problem caused primarily by some biological factor?,' '... caused primarily by some psychological factor?,' and '... all in the student's mind?,' were averaged to produce a Psychological versus Physical Cause score, with high scores representing physical causation. Severity was measured by two items, 'How serious is the patient's problem?' and 'How unpleasant is ... the problem?' Finally, 'How much is the problem caused by the student's own behavior?' and 'How much is the student to blame for his problem?' comprised the Blame score. Values of Cronbach α for these scales ranged from 0.69 to 0.74. Subjects also completed a series of bipolar trait ratings, from which was derived a score representing the degree to which the patient was perceived as distressed.

Results for the four major measures are in Figure 13.1. Credibility ratings decreased markedly when HC's nonmedical problems were mentioned in the interview. The profile of Psychological versus Physical Cause scores was similar to that of Credibility scores; the correlation between the two measures was 0.62. Moreover, the size of Patient Problems' effect was very similar for both variables: $\eta^2 = 0.21$ for Credibility and 0.25 for Physical Cause.[2] Perceived Severity of HC's health problem was much less strongly affected by the presence of nonmedical sources of patient distress, $\eta^2 = 0.06$. Blame scores were likewise affected only weakly by Patient Problems, $\eta^2 = 0.05$, but blame rose when HC revealed both problems during the interview with the nurse, compared to interviews in which neither problem emerged, $r = 0.20$ for the 1-df comparison. The correlation between the Credibility score and ratings of patient distress was -0.35, similar in magnitude to relationships found in

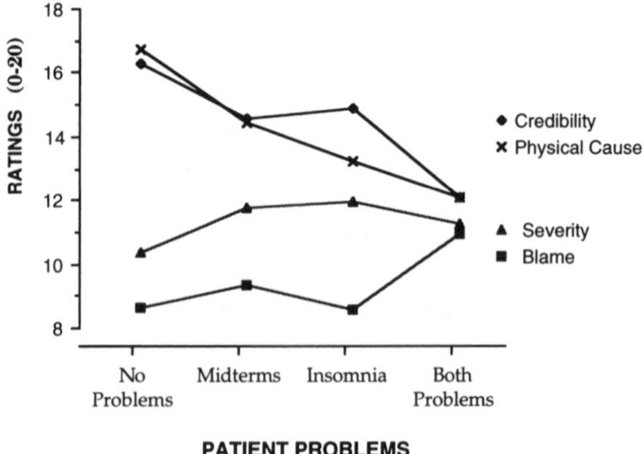

Figure 13.1 Effect of patient psychosocial problems on peers' ratings.

other experiments in the series; the more HC was regarded as distressed, the less credible was his complaint to observers.

Results of this and similar studies (Delaney and McNutt, 1992; Skelton, in press) converge on the conclusion that patients who experience psychosocial problems in conjunction with medical conditions risk their credibility when they reveal such problems. This is true not only for conditions having no known physical cause but also for those where there is demonstrably a physical cause. In the latter case, observers are likely to doubt the etiology of the medical condition (see the 'Physical Cause' line Figure 13.1, and cf. Wiener, 1975).

Why are Illness Complaints Discredited?

Why does the conjunction of medical with personal and social problems prompt such responses from observers? A number of theoretical accounts seem applicable. One has to do with our general reaction to distressed individuals. People neither like those who express negative affect nor wish to associate with them (Gurtzman *et al.*, 1990). One result may be a tendency not to credit the claims of 'negative' persons. For example, medical patients whom perceivers view as depressed elicit negative trait attributions from perceivers (Katz *et al.*, 1987).

Another possibility derives from Kelley's (1972) theory of causal schemata. This theory proposes that when people make causal attributions for a behavior they have observed – say, an individual's claim to be sick – they evaluate the presence of contributing factors and constraints. When an individual's behavior occurs despite forces that might have prevented it, people ordinarily infer that strong and unambiguous motives underlie the individual's chosen action. However, when an individual's behavior could have resulted from each a number of contributing factors, people find it more difficult to explain the behavior. A person claiming sickness may indeed be sick; but she or he might also be seeking sympathy, relief from obligations, or other social consequences of being defined as ill. If psychosocial distress information prompts observers to entertain such alternative explanations, then reductions in patient credibility may be simply a consequence of attributional *discounting.*

Appealing as the attribution theory explanation may be, it is sensible only if we can specify what counts as a 'contributing factor' in people's everyday attempts to understand the forces that prompt illness complaints. This, is turn, requires us to consider lay persons' *implicit disease models*, that is, the sociocultural schemata that define the meaning and the boundaries of health and illness (Skelton and Croyle, 1991). Fortunately, recent years have been witness to exponential increases in the attention paid by the social sciences to these models. Not surprisingly, the implicit disease models used by contemporary Western lay persons are strongly influenced by the biomedical model of health-care professionals. One characteristic of such models is that they distinguish physical from psychological causes of symptoms (Baumann *et al.*, 1989; Bishop, 1987) and biomedicine's essential materialism virtually requires that psychologically caused symptoms be defined as less *real* (Aronowitz, 1992; Gordon, 1988; Kirmayer, 1988). Thus, the patient who manifests both symptom complaints and psychosocial distress is making available to observers an alternative explanation for illness claims: the symptoms are psychologically caused. One intriguing implication is that such a patient will be perceived less as a medical than as a mental patient. And, once a resemblance to the category *mental patient* is made salient, negative perceptions characterizing lay persons' thinking about such patients (Purvis *et al.*, 1988) may come into play.

To summarize, acceptable illness complaints (from the standpoint contemporary, well-educated American lay persons) must not only satisfy the biomedical model's requirement that diseases are physically caused, but also must exclude nonmedical (especially so-called psychological) problems. Lay observers distinguish sharply between physical and mental causes of illness complaints, between symptoms that are prompted by 'stress' and those that are viewed as responses to physical causes. The research I have reviewed here indicates that the most credible complaints are those characterized by the absence of psychological complications.

IMPLICATIONS FOR THE STUDY OF OFFICE CTDs

My reasons for being pessimistic about the benefits of discovering psychosocial modifiers of CTDs should now be clear. Although we may take seriously the charge that appeared in our invitations to contribute to this volume – '*not* to argue the pre-eminence of a biomechanical or psychosocial source [nor] to debate how biomechanically "real" CTDs are in various circumstances' (Moon, 1993) – it may be difficult for onlookers to avoid doing so. Given a culturally dominant disease model that, even when amended by psychosomatic and biopsychosocial concepts, cannot transcend its own intrinsic dualism (Helman, 1988; Kirmayer, 1988), it may be too much to expect that disclosing psychosocial factors that predispose to CTDs can do anything *except* undermine the credibility of workers who experience these health problems.

Personological 'Drift'

At least two lines of evidence support a gloomy prognosis. First, psychosocially oriented research in the workplace has a history of drift toward personological levels of analysis. Kasl (1991), for example, has commented upon the tendency in occupational health research to psychologize workers by turning structural variables into personality traits. Tesh (1988) has compellingly reviewed the harm done to the cause of the Professional Air Traffic Controllers Organization (PATCO) when it attempted to use the concept of job-related stress to justify compensation demands to the Federal Aviation Administration in the early 1980s. PATCO employed 'stress' as a shorthand for job hazards to its members' health, but it was transmogrified by the FAA into an indicator that certain types of controllers are dispositionally prone to overreact to the job. In other words, 'stress' was interpreted in situational, job-related terms by PATCO, but the FAA preferred a personality-based interpretation. The FAA – abetted by President Reagan – won this war of definitions. The PATCO case nicely illustrates the old saw that 'when the psychologist[s] come in [to investigate psychosocial factors in the workplace], the case [for finding a physical cause of workers' illness complaints] is blown' (Singer, 1982, p. 132). Such a history does not inspire optimism.

But this is not a unique indictment of occupational health research. The drift toward personological explanations occurs time and again in the social and behavioral sciences and among everyday lay observers. Thus, the sheer ubiquity of dispositional explanation constitutes the second line that prompts a pessimistic appraisal of the social consequences of the search for the psychosocial concomitants of occupational health problems. Observers of human behavior have remarked repeatedly upon the seductive power of preferences for personological explanation (Heider, 1944; Icheiser, 1970; Jones and Nisbett, 1972; Nisbett and Ross, 1980; Ross and Nisbett, 1991). Social psychologists, perhaps the staunchest proponents of the view that situational variables constitute the prepotent influence upon people's behavior, are apparently just as susceptible to seduction as the lay person. For example, an eminent social psychologist (Snyder, 1987) has identified 'sensitivity to situational influences' as a personality trait! Roger Brown (1965) has shown how the concept of authoritarianism – originally devised to describe societal and family structures – devolved into a personality trait.

Examples are also available in psychological applications to health. Colleagues who a few years ago formulated theories of symptom-reporting behavior that emphasized situational factors such as the cueing of attention and the activation of perceptual schemata (Pennebaker, 1982) have more recently argued for the primacy of neuroticism as a determinant of symptom-reporting behavior (Watson and Pennebaker, 1989). The psychosomatic theorist, J. H. Weiss (1977), complained almost 20 years ago about the popular degeneration of psychosomatic concepts into personality characterizations. Personality-based explanations seem ineluctable; they may, in fact, be part and parcel of an individualistic world-view – as unavoidable as dualism.

From Work-related Factors to Individual Differences

It is a very short step from identifying work-related psychosocial factors that correlate with office-related CTDs to a dispositional interpretation of CTDs. Consider a recent study by National Institute for Occupational Safety and Health (NIOSH) investigators of directory assistance operators at US West Communications (Hales *et al.*, 1992). Regardless of whether workers' health status was defined solely by self-reported pain and symptoms – upper-extremity (UE) symptoms (p. 7) – or, more restrictively, by the concurrence of symptoms with positive physical signs – UE disorders (p. 11) – increasing work pressure and job insecurity were implicated as concomitant.[3] Overlooking the limitations upon causal inference that are inherent in the study design, we may read this finding as 'Jobs that involve increasing amounts of pressure upon workers or which do not have a secure future are more likely to prompt UE Disorders.'[4] But another reading of the same finding is: 'Workers who feel pressure and insecurity about their jobs are more likely to experience UE disorders.'

A DEMONSTRATION STUDY OF PUBLIC REACTIONS TO CTDs

My students and I conducted a preliminary investigation of personological renderings of the US West findings, adapting our methods from experimental studies of patient credibility. We devised an article that presents the US West findings in a format similar to that of a news magazine such as *Time* or *Newsweek*. In the style typical of those magazines, the story of office-related CTDs was told through the eyes of a directory assistance operator, Clara S., suffering from tendinitis. Both versions indicated that Clara has clinically verified signs of tendinitis. For this demonstration study, two article versions were prepared. One reported the finding that employees classified as cases spent 2.5 hours per day at the keyboard; in this version, there was *no* mention of psychosocial factors but only of work-related concomitants. The second version explicitly mentioned psychosocial concomitants of CTDs; the crucial paragraph was written so as to place a personological construction upon the findings:

> Musculoskeletal disorders such as Clara's become more likely when workers experience greater feelings of work pressure and job insecurity. For example, compared to workers at her company who do not have musculoskeletal problems, workers such as Clara are more fearful that their jobs will be eliminated by computers and feel greater work pressure, according to a NIOSH study.

The complete text of the article is reproduced in Table 13.1.

One hundred and thirty-two persons received one of the two versions, and they responded to a series of rating items about Clara, the worker described in the story. These items were similar to those used in previous studies. Four measures were derived from those items: (1) a three-item scale representing the *credibility* of Clara's health complaint (Cronbach $\alpha = 0.76$); (2) a two-item scale representing how much her health problem is *psychologically caused* (Cronbach $\alpha = 0.76$); (3) a single rating of how much Clara is to *blame* for her condition; and (4) a single item measuring how much respondents believe that Clara's condition is caused by *stress*.

As in previous experiments, the perceived credibility of the health complaint was related to the causes to which the health problem was attributed. The more Clara's tendinitis was attributed to psychological causes, the less credible was her complaint ($r = -0.70$) and the more she was blamed for the problem ($r = 0.45$). Similarly, the more her tendinitis was rated as stress-related, the more it was perceived as psychologically caused ($r = 0.43$) and the less credible was her complaint ($r = -0.33$).

Table 13.1 A 'news story' description of a CTD-in-the-workplace study.

NEW WORK HAZARD OF THE ELECTRONIC ERA?

Clara S. age 40, has worked for about six years as a directory assistance operator for a national telecommunications corporation. During a typical shift, she spends seven hours at a computer terminal. When a caller requests a telephone number, she types in the name of the person whose number was requested. Once the computer matches (or fails to match) the requested name with a telephone number, she notifies the caller. About once each month, she works overtime.

For the past year, Clara has noticed pain in some of the joints of her hands and wrists. The pain is not constant but it recurs every few weeks. On some occasions, the pain persists for more than a week before going away. She underwent a physical examination by a company-provided physician. The tests revealed that Clara has tendinitis in parts of both hands, and that the mobility of her left wrist is less than it should be.

As more workers in the US and other industrialized countries use computers as part of their work, health problems such as Clara's have become more common. The National Institute for Occupational Safety and Health (NIOSH) has been studying the prevalence of musculoskeletal disorder . . . (aches, pains, and movement difficulties associated with the muscles, bones, and connective tissue) in computer terminal operators. Rates vary from one industry to another, but 20% to 40% of such workers report symptoms in the hand/wrist areas, the elbows, the shoulders, or the neck. Clara's tendinitis is typical of about 15% of employees at her company.

Psychosocial factors not mentioned:

Musculoskeletal disorders such as Clara's become more likely when workers spend more time at the computer. For example, typical employees at a West Coast newspaper who have musculoskeletal problems spend 2.5 hours per day or more actually typing, according to a NIOSH study.

Psychosocial factors mentioned:

Musculoskeletal disorders such as Clara's become more likely when workers experience greater feelings of work pressure and job insecurity. For example, compared to workers at her company who do not have musculoskeletal problems, workers such as Clara are more fearful that their jobs will be eliminated by computers and feel greater work pressure, according to a NIOSH study.

The potential for injury claims resulting from work-related musculoskeletal disorders has naturally attracted the attention of the health insurance industry and government. It's expected that the underlying causes of these health problems will receive increased investigation as computer use becomes more widespread in American business.

For workers such as Clara, however, the issue is more personal. 'No one wants to live with pain and discomfort. It makes your work more difficult, and you can't do the things at home that you'd like. So I just hope they can come up with an answer for people like me.'

And what influenced subjects' attributions about the causes of Clara's tendinitis? Figure 13.2 shows that subjects were more likely to make a 'psychological' attribution if they had read the news story that mentioned psychosocial concomitant of CTDs ($r = 0.17$ for the main effect of story version, $p = 0.05$). In addition, male subjects were more likely than female subjects to make psychological attributions ($r = 0.21$, $p = 0.02$). This gender difference was particularly evident if the story did *not* mention psychosocial concomitants of CTDs ($r = 0.23$ for the simple effect of gender, $p = 0.01$); women and men were equally likely to make a psychological attribution when the story mentioned psychosocial concomitants, but men were more likely to do so even when the story focused on work-related factors in CTDs.

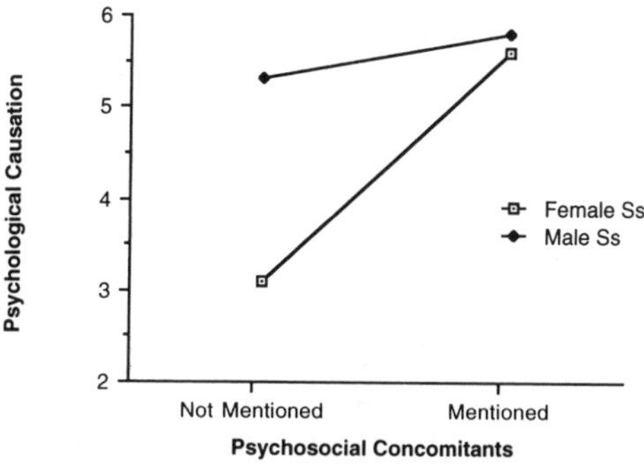

Figure 13.2 Effects of mentioning psychosocial concomitants and subject gender on attributions about Clara's tendinitis.

The effect upon Clara's credibility of mentioning psychosocial concomitants depended in an interesting way upon subjects' attributions about the cause of Clara's tendinitis. When we did not control for the extent to which subjects made psychological attributions, Clara's credibility was unaffected by the version of the story subjects received ($r = 0$ for the main effect), but women rated Clara as more credible than did men ($r = 0.28$, $p = 0.001$ for the gender main effect). When the data were analyzed with controls for the effect of subjects' psychological attributions, Clara's credibility was rated as greater by subjects who read the 'psychosocial concomitants' story ($r = 0.19$, $p = 0.032$ for the main effect of story version, controlling for psychological attributions). These results indicate that it was psychological attributions for Clara's tendinitis – and not the mere presence of information about psychosocial concomitants – that undermined her credibility to readers.

This interpretation is strengthened by the attenuation of gender differences in ratings of Clara's credibility, once the effect of psychological attributions was controlled ($r = 0.19$, $p = 0.037$ for the gender main effect). Considering that men were more likely to make psychological attributions in the first place, these results indicate the mediating effect of such attributions upon perceptions of patients' credibility.

This demonstration study has several limitations arising directly from our desire to gather some data quickly to evaluate the applicability of already-existing credibility research to the case of CTDs. First, the respondents were college students, administrators, and staff – people who differ in many ways from the general population. Second, although the news story that mentioned psychosocial concomitants of work-related tendinitis caused readers to make psychological attributions, what prompted these attributions is ambiguous. Information about psychosocial factors was deliberately confounded with a personological presentation of that information. So it remains to be shown that people spontaneously make personological interpretations. Moreover, it is possible that the statement 'workers experience greater *feelings* of work pressure and job insecurity' may have contributed to psychological attributions by creating the impression that work pressure and job insecurity are merely subjective perceptions, not objective conditions of the workplace. Third, the gender differences observed in the present study – never before obtained in our research on patient credibility – cannot be interpreted straightforwardly. Do they reflect stereotypes by men of women? By preponderantly *young* (18–22-years-old) males of middle-aged women? A social class bias interacting with gender biases? Thus, although we have made a provocative start in applying a theoretical model of patient credibility to real-world situations, it is only a start.

CASE DEFINITIONS AND THE CREDIBILITY OF CTDs

In foregoing discussion of CTDs, I have assumed that workers' reports of musculoskeletal pain and symptoms are confirmed positive diagnostic signs. This assumption was explicitly built into the stories used in the demonstration study. Despite being told that Clara's tendinitis was medically verified by physical signs, subjects who read the 'psychosocial concomitant' story nonetheless made psychological attributions for her problem, which in turn influenced their perceptions of her credibility.

In the real world of epidemiological data-gathering, however, things are rarely so neat. In two recent NIOSH reports on CTDs in the workplace (Bernard *et al.*, 1993; Hales *et al.*, 1992) some employees who reported musculoskeletal *symptoms* did not exhibit positive *signs*. The report authors accordingly defined 'cases' in two ways: (1) through employee symptom reports only, and (2) through physical examinations consequent upon positive symptom reports. In each study, the factors that predicted symptom-reporting were not isomorphic with those that distinguished cases from controls when 'problem' employees – those who report symptoms but fail to test positive for signs – were dropped from the case definition.[5] Neither report explicitly stated how many employees were 'problems,' and such selective reporting suggests that the investigators were aware of the negative implications of symptomatic but nonpositive employees.[6]

As mentioned earlier, our studies of patient credibility show that symptom reporting in the absence of positive diagnostic signs is heavily discredited by both health professionals and lay persons, independently of information about co-occurring psychosocial distress. CTD problem cases thus represent the worst possible situation, from the standpoint of negative attributions and patient credibility: if cases with verified physical signs invite psychological attributions by lay observers, problem cases are even more likely to elicit suspicion toward patients. I fear that, to the extent that CTDs are defined solely by symptom reports, they will tend to be regarded as having an elusive etiology, a euphemism for 'We don't know how seriously to take these symptom complaints.' Such reactions are, of course, a reflection of biomedical dualism and the tacit belief that diagnostic technology is immune to Type II (false negative) errors. But such beliefs appear to be strongly ingrained, and researchers should be prepared to take them into account when communicating to the public about the role of psychosocial factors in cumulative trauma disorders.

NOTES

1 This is not to deny that such conversion may actually occur in some cases. But its incidence may be greatly overestimated.

2 I use eta-squared (η^2), the correlation ratio, as an index of effect size when there is more than 1 df in the numerator of the F-ratio employed for hypothesis tests. For 1-df comparisons, r is the preferred measure of effect size (Rosenthal and Rosnow, 1991).

3 The authors report (p. 20) that fear of being replaced by computers was associated with UE disorders, whereas uncertainty about one's job future correlated with UE symptoms. I treat these as conceptually similar findings.

4 Observe that I am restricting attention to cases for whom there were positive physical findings. This makes it less appropriate for critics to argue that the workers' health problems are 'only psychological.'

5 Such employees are problems from the standpoint of a biomedical disease model that defines legitimate symptom reports as those for which signs of physical pathology can be identified (Leventhal, 1986; Skelton, 1991). I am not implying that these employees are fabricating or converting; indeed, it is possible that the diagnostic tests used in these studies lacked the sensitivity to detect physical signs that were, nonetheless, present. Because of this possibility, I have deliberately described such employees as 'failing to test positive,' not as 'having negative signs.'

6 Hales, *et al.* (1992, pp. 14–15) are rather more forthcoming about the decrease in cases that results from adding positive physical findings as a qualification. But they do not indicate the magnitude of relationship between UE symptoms and UE disorders in their study of US West employees.

REFERENCES

ARONOWITZ, R. A. 1992 From myalgic encephalitis to yuppie flu: A history of chronic fatigue syndromes, in ROSENBERG, C. E. and GOLDEN, J. (Eds), *Framing Disease: Studies in Cultural History*, pp. 155–81, New Brunswick, NJ: Rutgers University Press.

BAUMANN, L. J., CAMERON, L. D., ZIMMERMAN, R. S. and LEVENTHAL, H. 1989 Illness representations and matching labels with symptoms, *Health Psychology*, **8**(4), 449–70.

BERNARD, B., SAUTER, S., PETERSEN, M., FINE, L. and HALES, T. 1993 *Health Hazard Evaluation Report, Los Angeles Times* (HETA No. 90-013-2277), National Institute for Occupational Safety and Health, Centers for Disease Control.

BISHOP, G. D. 1987 Lay conceptions of physical symptoms, *Journal of Applied Social Psychology*, **17**, 127–46.

BROWN, R. 1965 *Social Psychology*, New York: Free Press.

BURGESS, M. M. 1980 'Nurses' pain ratings of patients with acute and chronic low back pain' unpublished master's thesis, University of Virginia.

DELANEY, K. N. and MCNUTT, K. S. 1992 *Health advice and illness perceptions: The impact of viewing live interactions*, Undergraduate report, Department of Psychology, Dickinson College.

GORDON, D. R. 1988 Tenacious assumptions in Western medicine, in LOCK, M. and GORDON, D. R. (Eds), *Biomedicine Examined*, pp. 19–56, New York: Kluwer Academic Publishers.

GRAHAM, C. 1994 *Perceptions of illness complaints in video depictions*, Undergraduate report, Department of Psychology, Dickinson College.

GURTZMAN, M. B., MARTIN, K. M. and HINTZMAN, N. B. 1990 Interpersonal reactions to displays of depression and anxiety, *Journal of Social and Clinical Psychology*, **9**(2), 256–67.

HALES, T., SAUTER, S., PETERSEN, M., PUTZ-ANDERSON, V., FINE, L. OCHS, T., SCHEIFER, L. and BERNARD, B. 1992 *Health Hazard Evaluation Report, US West Communications* (HETA No. 89-299-2230), National Institute for Occupational Safety and Health, Centers for Disease Control.

HEIDER, F. 1944 Social perception and phenomenal causality, *Psychological Review*, **51**, 258–374.

HELMAN, C. G. 1988 Psyche, soma, and society: The social construction of psychosomatic disorders, in Lock, M. and Gordon, D. R. (Eds), *Biomedicine Examined*, pp. 95–122, New York: Kluwer Academic Publishers.

Icheiser, G. 1970 *Appearances and Reality*, San Francisco, CA: Jossey-Bass.

Jones, E. E. and Nisbett, R. 1972 The actor and the observer: Divergent perceptions of the causes of behavior, in Jones, E., Kanouse, D., Kelley, H., Nisbett, R., Valins, S. and Weiner, B. (Eds), *Attribution: Perceiving the Causes of Behavior*, pp. 79–93, Morristown, NJ: General Learning Press.

Kasl, S. V. 1991 Assessing health risks in the work setting, in Schroeder, H. E. (Eds), *New Directions in Health Psychology Assessment*, pp. 95–125, New York: Hemisphere Publishing.

Katz, I., Hass, R. G., Parisi, N., Astone, J. and McEvaddy, D. 1987 Lay people's and health care personnel's perceptions of cancer, AIDS, cardiac, and diabetic patient, *Psychological Reports*, **60**, 615–29.

Kelley, H. H. 1972 Causal schemata in the attribution process, in Jones, E., Kanouse, D., Kelley, H. Nisbett, R., Valins, S. and Weiner, B. (Eds), *Attribution: Perceiving the Causes of Behavior*, pp. 151–74, Morristown, NJ: General Learning Press.

Kirmayer, L. J. 1988 Mind and body as metaphors: Hidden values in biomedicine, in Lock, M. and Gordon, D. R. (Eds), *Biomedicine Examined*, pp. 57–93, New York: Kluwer Academic Publishers.

Leventhal, H. 1986 Symptom reporting: A focus on process, in McHugh, S. and Vallis, T. M. (Eds), *Illness Behavior: A Multidisciplinary Model*, pp. 219–37, New York: Plenum Press.

Moon, S. 1993 personal communication.

Nisbett, R. E. and Ross, L. 1980 *Human Inference: Strategies and Shortcomings of Social Judgment*, Englewood Cliffs, NJ: Prentice-Hall.

Pennebaker, J. W. 1982 *The Psychology of Physical Symptoms*, New York: Springer Verlag.

Purvis, B., Brandt, R., Rouse, C. 1988 Students' attitudes toward hypothetical chronically and acutely mentally and physically ill individuals, *Psychological Reports*, **62**, 627–30.

Rosenthal, R. and Rosnow, R. L. 1991 *Essentials of Behavioral Research: Methods and Data Analysis*, 2nd Edn, New York: McGraw-Hill.

Ross, L. and Nisbett, R. E. 1991 *The Person and the Situation: Perspectives of Social Psychology*, New York: McGraw-Hill.

Singer, J. E. 1982 Yes, Virginia, there really is a mass psychogenic illness, in Colligan, M. J., Pennebaker, W. and Murphy, L. R. (Eds), *Mass Psychogenic Illness: A Social Psychological Analysis*, pp. 127–38, Hillsdale, NJ: Lawrence Erlbaum Associates.

Skelton, J. A. 1991 Laypersons' judgments of patient credibility and the study of illness representations in Skelton, J. A. and Croyle, R. T. (Eds), *Mental Representation in Health and Illness*, pp. 108–31, New York: Springer Verlag.

Skelton, J. A. Patient distress undermines the credibility of illness complaints, *Journal of Applied Social Psychology*, in press.

Skelton, J. A. and Croyle, R. T. 1991 *Mental Representation in Health and Illness*, New York: Springer Verlag.

Snyder, M. 1987 *Public Appearances, Private Realities: The Psychology of Self-monitoring*, New York: W. H. Freeman.

Taylor, A. G., Skelton, J. A. and Butcher, J. 1984 Duration of pain condition and physical pathology as determinants of nurses' judgments of patients in pain, *Nursing Research*, **33**, 4–9.

Tesh, S. M. 1988 *Hidden Arguments: Political Ideology and Disease Prevention Policy*, New Brunswick, NJ: Rutgers University Press.

Watson, D. and Pennebaker, J. W. 1989 Health complaints, stress, and distress: Exploring the central role of negative affectivity, *Psycholology Review*, **96**, 234–54.

WEISS, J. H. 1977 The current status of the concept of psychosomatic disorder, in LIPOWSKI, Z. P., LIPSETT, D. R. and WHYBROW, P. C. (Eds), *Psychosomatic Medicine: Current Trends and Clinical Applications*, pp. 162–71, New York: Oxford University Press.

WIENER, C. L. 1975 Pain assessment on an orthopedic ward, *Nursing Outlook*, **23**, 508–16.

CHAPTER FOURTEEN

A human capital perspective for cumulative trauma disorders

Moral Hazard Effects in Disability Compensation Programs

HAROLD H. GARDNER and RICHARD J. BUTLER

A HUMAN CAPITAL MODEL FOR HEALTH AND PRODUCTIVITY

Disability compensation programs, usually coupled with medical (health-care) services, in the private and public sector have been based on the implicit assumptions in a biomedical model: that successful diagnosis and treatment of disease with accompanying restoration of health and rehabilitation to work is the primary incentive for the worker, their treating physician, and disability-plan administrators. Following a claim of injury or illness, an employee and their manager are assumed to be economically passive participants in a medical/disability process that replaces lost earnings, pays for necessary medical care expenditure, including whatever is feasibly required for work rehabilitation, and restores the worker to a productive job. Similarly, the health-care provider is assumed to be professionally capable of objective categorization of the health condition followed by appropriate (medically necessary) treatment and timely return of the worker to the job. Lastly, the administrator is assumed capable of gathering and interpreting medical and disability information needed to assure the integrity of the process and to provide timely wage replacement to the worker and medical treatment fees to the provider.

If the injured and ill employee, their physicians, and health-plan administrators are passive, in the sense of not altering their behavior as economic incentives change, or even if they are not passive but the health status of the dysfunctional worker can be objectively observed, then this is likely to be an adequate model on which to base disability compensation, medical treatment, and corporate health and safety programs. However, it is generally known that there are dynamic economic incentives operative in all aspects of the medical and disability marketplace and health conditions are frequently difficult to define objectively.

Cicero is said to have commented of a friend, 'He remained the same when the same was no longer fitting.' The same can be said of disability programs that are based on the reductionist, condition-focused 'biomedical' model. In this paradigm, the socioeconomic environment plays no role and only the 'objective' treatment of the anatomical and physiological causes of the disability by a physician are important. While the biomedical model may have provided a workable conceptual framework for disability before the widespread expansion of insurance, it certainly does not provide an adequate theory of disability now. The proliferation of health-related costs (group health, group disability, workers' compensation), as generally subsidized by employers and governmental agencies, has caused a virtual explosion of inefficiencies in total employee health costs that threatens the economic survival of companies and the nation as a whole. The current debate regarding health-care reform, which has largely ignored the costly interactions between disability and health-care programs, is but one instance of reliance on the inadequate 'biomedical' paradigm. Similarly, most corporate health and safety services evolved from this same classical biomedical model of diagnosis and treatment of illnesses and injuries resulting from workplace exposures. While this clinically based model may have met needs previously, before the widespread expansion of a number of often overlapping insurance schemes, it clearly falls short of addressing today's business problems of escalating cost for employee health benefits and worker absence.

This chapter presents a different conceptual paradigm, one that acknowledges the presence that economic incentives may influence behaviors of the participants in the medical/disability process, followed by empirical evidence that all participants in the medical/disability process – workers, managers, and health-care providers – are sensitive to economic incentives present in the system: as workers' benefits increase, their reported severity and frequency of claims increases; as workers experience productivity failure, they are more likely to be placed in disability by management; and doctors in health-maintenance organizations (HMOs) have a greater tendency to classify claims as compensable in the workers' compensation system than do other physicians. This suggests that disability outcomes hinge crucially on factors other than those associated purely with objectively defined biomedical phenomena.

A Human Capital Health and Productivity Paradigm

We have adopted a new utilitarian model for our research of workplace safety and worker health behaviors developed by Gardner and Fiske (1994). The general features of the Gardner–Fiske Human Capital Health and Productivity Paradigm are shown in Figure 14.1 and are founded on the inherent economic value of 'the worker (employee) as human capital stock' to employers. By human capital stock, we mean the innate and acquired capabilities of human beings to pursue objectives relating to their perceived happiness. The stock of human capital will be affected by health and wellness, educational attainment, and productivity vectors, all of which contribute to satisfying and remunerative employment. Modeling health outcomes in terms of human capital stock is appealing in that maintaining and enhancing the stock becomes an act of investment in the various components affecting the level of the stock.

The human capital model establishes, through an employment contract, worker and management goal congruence around the twin productivity themes: a productive job for the worker and job productivity for the employer. Management and

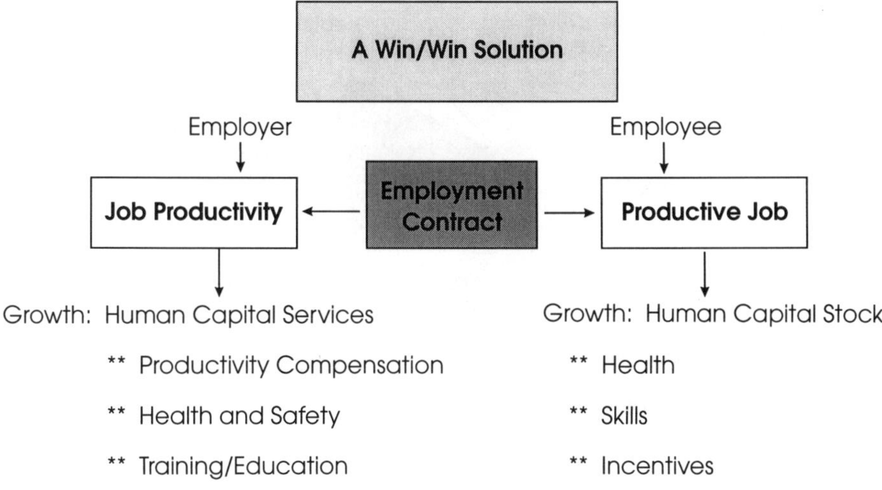

Figure 14.1 The Gardner–Fiske Human Capital Health and Productivity Paradigm.

workers are both motivated to protect health and generate productivity, rather than motivated to consume medical paid time off and health service benefits.

Employers value and reward worker productivity and invest in their human capital with performance compensation, training and education, and preventive health and safety programs. Traditional employee benefits, as embodied as alternative compensation programs, are funded with genuine health and productivity protection as the goal. Employees value a productive job with commensurate wages, and the opportunity to increase the worth of their human capital stock. Productive employment and skill development increases the value of a worker in the marketplace.

The employee benefits cost problem

Disability costs (medical paid time off) and medical care service programs (group health, workers' compensation medical and accidental medical) comprise an increasingly significant share of total labor costs as defined at a point in time for a large, private firm in the United States as shown in Figure 14.2. There is considerable relatedness among the major categories of alternative compensation costs as represented in medical paid time off, medical services, and administrative costs.

Medical expenditures comprise the largest fraction of employee health benefits, about 15 per cent. But the cost of medical absenteeism is 11 per cent and growing in proportion. Health program administration is also notable at 5 per cent and a relatively small amount (1 per cent) is spent on preventive health and safety programs. For some employers the cost of alternative compensation exceeds the compensation

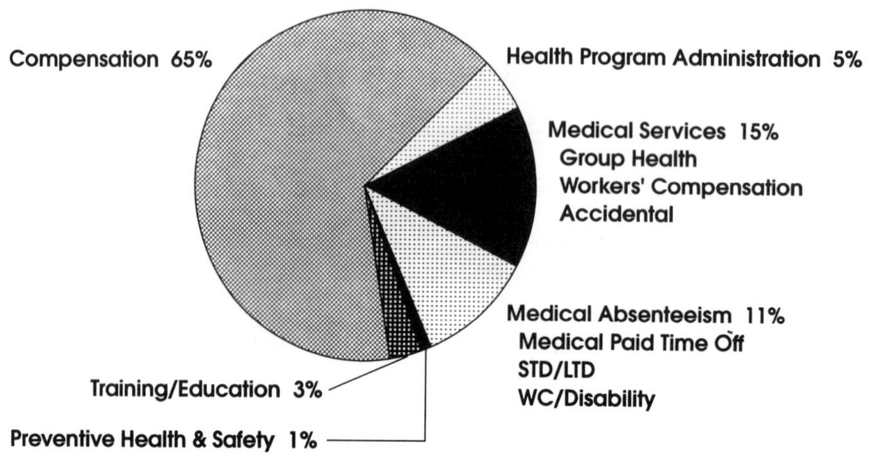

Figure 14.2 Human capital management: labor costs.

component of labor costs signifying the proliferation of employee health benefits costs.

Health-care expenditures in the economy as a whole are roughly $1 trillion, which suggests – to the extent that this company's experience is representative – that another trillion is estimated to be spent on other health costs. Effective cost containment of the health-care expenditures obviously must deal not only with direct medical outlays, but the substantial medical time-off and other health-related labor costs.

The biomedical paradigm that is the commonly used model for the observation and research of health and safety phenomena in the workplace and for the provision of occupational health and safety programs is limited in explaining the utilization and cost explosion. Partly this is due to its fixation on direct medical outlays which comprise less than 50 per cent of total health expenditures, and partly this is due to a failed understanding of the interaction among different programs as defined in integrated analysis.

Information asymmetry among the various participants in the many health programs accounts for a substantial percentage of the total health system inefficiency.

Human Capital Integrated Information Strategy

In order to manage, enhance, and protect worker human capital effectively, integrated information is required since person-based information may exist in isolation in several operating systems within the firm, as shown graphically in Figure 14.3. Gathering and analyzing health and productivity data from each is essential to risk identification and management.

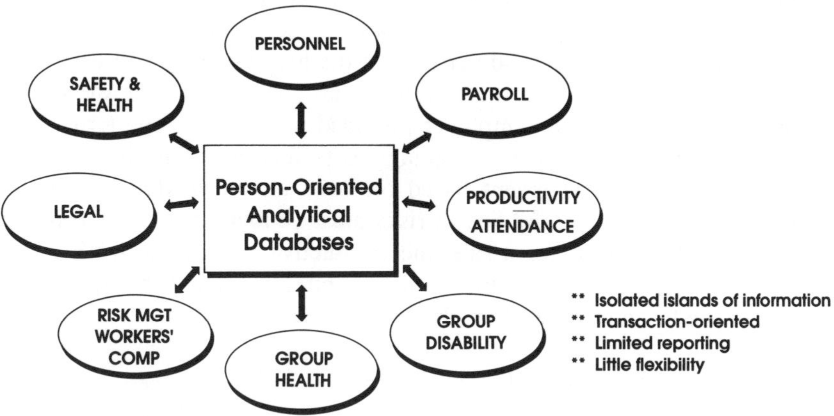

Figure 14.3 Human capital management: information integration/analysis.

We provide a few examples of integrated information outputs as previously reported by Gardner *et al.* (1994) to demonstrate the importance of integrated information.

Maldistribution of worker health costs: The Pareto phenomenon

As shown in Figure 14.4, there is significant maldistribution of health costs in the use of health-care resources, some of which is motivated by moral hazard problems. We begin by examining maldistribution of benefits usage overall, and then examine some specific moral hazard-related instances of benefit usage.

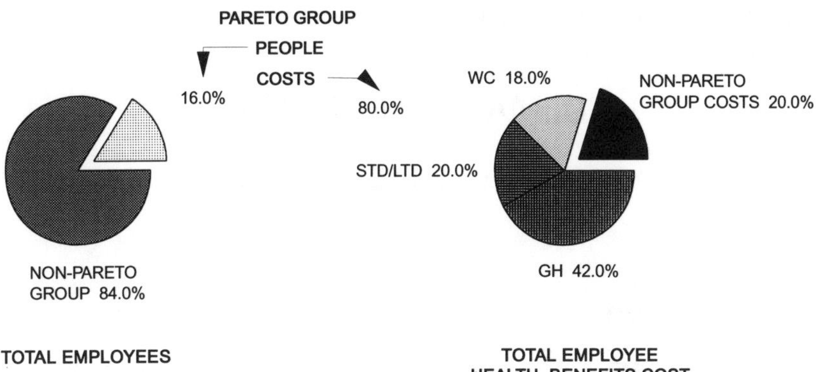

Figure 14.4 Pareto maldistribution.

As shown, a 16 per cent minority of employees incurred 80 per cent of the total health benefits cost. It is also of note that this Pareto group used all types of benefits (group health, STD/LTD, and workers' compensation). Obviously, identifying and successfully managing the health and costs of this group of workers is fundamental to cost management. The important issue of adverse selection comes into play when studying maldistribution. About 40 per cent of the firm's total health and disability costs go to disability claims for the Pareto group (20 per cent for workers' compensation and 20 per cent for employer-provided short- and long-term disability claims), with the remaining 40 per cent going just to their group health-care benefits. The value of strategic management based on good analytical data is apparent in these figures: worker's safety and health risks must be identified and job placement decisions made which allow for a safe and productive job for the worker and job productivity for the employer. This human capital management approach is a win–win situation for workers and employers.

Workers' compensation and group insurance demand migration

Our research shows that group health cost containment programs are associated with demand and cost migration from group health to workers' compensation. Figure 14.5 displays the relative group health and workers' compensation costs for a similar population of workers where the only notable difference was their selection of group health plan. The HMO-enrolled workers had 44 per cent higher workers' compensation costs. Financial incentives operate for both workers and medical providers to classify health conditions as work related. For the worker there is first dollar coverage and workers' compensation disability incentives and for the provider in a community-rated HMO there is incremental fee-for-service revenue if the demand is classified as work related. (We discuss this model further and present additional evidence on this migration below for another sample.) To be effective, safety and health programs must proactively identify human, as well as workplace risks and address them with prevention-oriented solutions. Safety and health program performance, as reflected in Occupational Safety and Health Administration (OSHA) reportable or workers' compensation claims, will often be adversely affected by demand migration. It is of note that the health conditions most associated with demand migration are of the cumulative trauma disorder (CTD) variety because of the difficulty with definitive and objective diagnosis. Because group health cost containment efforts increase workers' compensation system usage, safety and health programs will be faced with more worker injury/illness cases. It is strate-

DEMAND MIGRATION

HMO to Workers' Compensation

	N	WC Cost	
Non-HMO	18,984	$836	
HMO	4,084	$1,202	(44% Higher)

Figure 14.5 Demand migration.

gically important to focus safety and health interventions on prevention strategies and away from diagnostic and therapeutic measures. It is also important to assess safety and health program performance correctly. Such assessments will be critical to determining which risk-reduction interventions are working and which are not. Performance evaluations drive the need for, and the type of, interventions.

The disability compensation incentives

The relationship between disability compensation and medical service consumption behaviors has been studied and it was found that poor job performance is often associated with use of the disability system and medical services (which serve to justify the disability episode, see Table 14.4 on p. 247). One specific analysis showed that the availability of group disability compensation is associated with significantly higher group medical and workers' compensation costs for workers doing the same job. Those eligible for group disability benefits had total benefits costs 346 per cent greater than those with only the workers' compensation disability benefit (see Figure 14.6). Because disability usage is associated with job performance, it is critical that management be trained to manage employees at risk effectively. Critical to this management role is access to 'usable' information about an employee's health status and corporate policy.

Health and Disability Costs and CTDs

The focus of this volume, CTDs, is of major importance because of the increasing cost of this classification of health condition and the associated benefits utilization and cost. The CTD label itself is somewhat controversial, implying that motion itself may be traumatic when, in fact, motion within a fitness context is viewed as healthy. The Human Capital Health and Productivity Model serves as an alternative model for understanding and evaluating CTD in the workplace. The data analysis in the second main section of this chapter does not relate exclusively to 'CTD' claims, but to workers' compensation claims in general of which the majority fall into the CTD category. And, since lower back claims are the largest single category of claims in terms of cost, we argue that the dynamics described and the relationships demonstrated for workers' compensation claims generally apply fundamentally to a CTD category as well.

DISABILITY COMPENSATION INCENTIVES

	Worker with Group Disability	Worker without Group Disability	Variance
Group Medical	$658	$182	361%
Workers' Comp	$636	$232	274%
Group Disability	$139	$0	
TOTAL	$1,433	$414	346%

Figure 14.6 Disability compensation incentives.

To understand the risk of an employee population for CTD, it is essential to integrate claims data from group health, group disability, and workers' compensation with demographic and productivity information. Such integration can establish relationships between employee health benefit plans and programs and a host of other factors. The often perverse incentives of overlapping and frequently uncorrelated productivity, safety, health, and disability programs must be integratively analyzed and monitored so that a firm's overall strategic human capital goals can be achieved. This necessarily involves the following processes.

Managing health-related lost productivity, particularly in the form of medical paid time-off programs, is a major priority for the employer since health-related lost time, like total employee benefits use, is unequally distributed and disability compensation provides an incentive.

Figure 14.7 displays an integrated analysis of CTD claims for a population of workers who basically perform the same job. The percentage shown is of the total for each program. Note that for workers' compensation claims 57–67 per cent of total claims fall into the CTD classification. All of the health benefits given show a significant presence of CTD claims and costs.

The human capital model helps to clarify the most salient economic issues affecting worker CTD. The health component of human capital stock depreciates naturally over the life cycle through the natural physiological processes that give rise to the symptoms that we label as CTD. By considering incentives to invest in the stock of human capital, we obtain a more complete picture of CTD in its socioeconomic, as well as biomedical, setting.

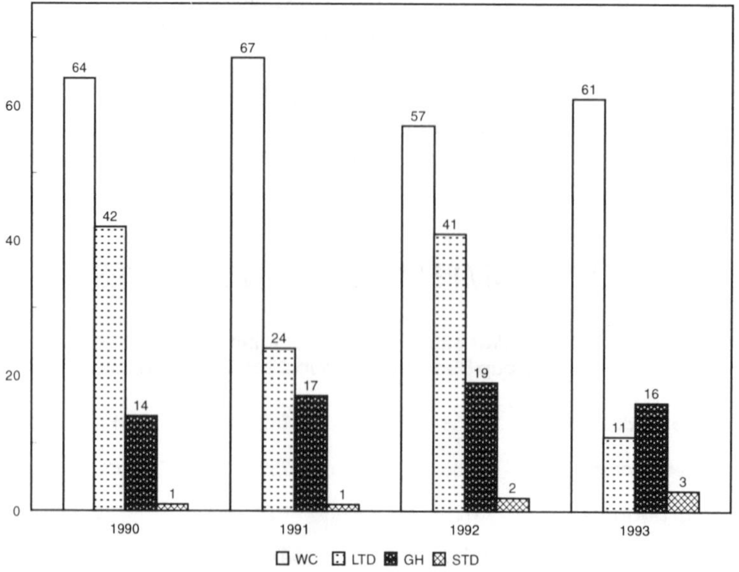

Figure 14.7 CTD claims benefits comparison.

In the human capital model, health events that depreciate the stock of human capital and precipitate entrance into the medical and disability process need to be viewed in the larger context of the workplace environment. If workers, managers, and health-care providers are engaging in self-interested behavior, then whether a health event becomes a disability will depend in part on the level of wages and benefits that workers receive, where workers are in their training, how satisfied they are with their working conditions, how work managers deal with productivity failure among the employees, and how health-care providers are reimbursed, etc. The disability system becomes not just a rehabilitation experience when health conditions, objectively defined, are serious enough, but it becomes an alternative to working itself – an alternative that depends on more than just the 'objective' nature of the health event itself. Hence the disability system affects human capital in ways other than the simple biomedical model indicates: to the extent that it lowers incentives to remain productive, or to misclassify management failure costs as 'disability' costs (an example we provide in the second main section), it actually lowers the stock of human capital.

Hence, the 'disability program' at work is more than a unidirectional assembly line that one enters when there is an 'objective need' and then leaves when the 'objective treatment' has been completed. Rather it is part of the workplace environment, with each aspect of the system (group health, workers' compensation, disability insurance, sick pay) interacting with all other programs. In all of this, the worker, workplace manager, and health-care provider are not unconstrained in terms of their choice of actions.

Firm owners trying to employ their scarce resources efficiently would, in fact, like to write enforceable contracts that make the whole health/disability process 'objective' in the sense of providing only the appropriate, well-defined level of medical care. However, such contracts are difficult to monitor. Indeed, the costs of monitoring every aspect of the disability participant's behavior generally exceed the benefits of monitoring, and worker, workplace manager, and health-care provided have considerable latitude in their behavior. There is asymmetry in the information between the owners of the firm and disability participants, an asymmetry that can be exploited to the participants' advantage because of high monitoring costs. When such informational asymmetries are used for personal gain there is said to be a 'moral hazard' problem.

For example, there is a possibility that workers may use company-provided health benefits more than they would if the firm were perfectly informed about their true state of health. This 'extra' usage of the system is known as 'moral hazard' in the economics literature since the cost of the extra usage (above that in a perfect-information world) is borne by all the other workers and the owners of the company indirectly through higher cost for health benefits (with offsetting reductions in wages and possibly company profitability).

EMPIRICAL ESTIMATES OF MORAL HAZARD

Moral Hazard in the Disability System

As we indicated in the previous section, 'moral hazard' is where the participants in the health-care process can change the firm's benefits insurance liability without the firm being able to monitor such behavior adequately. Moral hazard in a firm's employee health benefits cost can manifest itself in at least five different ways:

1. Employee health benefits cost may be misclassified (so that an employee may claim that a given condition arose from a job injury and seek workers' compensation benefits because their real condition of need does not qualify for short-term disability compensation; or a manager may wish to classify as 'disability' costs problems that are in fact 'management' costs associated with productivity failure of particular workers).
2. Individuals with varying tastes for health benefits utilization may look for firms or jobs with specific types of benefits (for example, a habitual or frequent user of health care may prefer a job with especially good group health benefits. This particular type of moral hazard differs from the others in that the decision margin is job choice rather than frequency or duration of health benefits within a particular type of job. In the insurance literature as well as in economics it is usually considered separately from other types of moral hazard and is known as 'adverse selection').
3. Health benefits, because they may operate as a 'risk-taking safety net,' may change the degree of on-the-job safety and hence alter job risks, with higher risks resulting in more accidents or an increased severity of injuries (so the health benefit actually induces a change in the frequency of injuries).
4. Individuals may choose to stay on claims longer than they otherwise would (in the absence of insurance).
5. Individuals may choose to file a claim that would go unreported in the absence of insurance (or at lower levels of disability pay).

Note that moral hazard types (1), (4), and (5) have been called claims-reporting moral hazard, while (3) has been called risk-bearing moral hazard (Butler and Worrall, 1991). We provide empirical estimates on three types of moral hazard, all especially relevant to CTD, that impact the effective strategic management of the human capital employed by the firm.

Moral Hazard Associated with Benefit Levels

If it is difficult to diagnose some work-debilitating injuries (as is the case with many cumulative trauma injuries such as lower back sprains and strains), then moral hazard may affect frequency of claims. Even if an incident is known to have happened with certainty, it may be difficult to monitor the extent of the injury so that moral hazard may affect the reported severity of an injury.

Estimates indicate that workers respond to the disability environment: claim frequency and severity increase as benefits increase, and as the waiting period falls. Claim frequency increases with higher benefits in studies using aggregate data (Butler, 1983; Butler and Worrall, 1983; Chelius, 1982; Krueger and Burton, 1990; Ruser, 1985; Worrall and Appel, 1982) as well as those using microeconomic data (Leigh, 1985; Krueger, 1990; Ruser, 1991). Claim severity has been found to be positively correlated with benefits in studies employing individual insurance claim data (Johnson *et al.*, 1995; Worrall and Butler, 1990; Butler and Worrall, 1985,

1993a); in studies employing insurance data for individual firms (Butler and Worrall, 1988); and studies using sample survey data (Johnson and Ondrich, 1990).[1]

In Table 14.1 we provide some additional data from aggregate (to the state/year) insurance claim data. We discuss this data set more fully in the next section. Of interest here is the coefficient of the expected benefit effect. This variable, LN(Benefit), has values of 0.222 and 0.439 respectively in the logarithmic regressions. We used the logarithmic regressions for ease of interpretation. For example, the 0.222 and 0.439 estimated coefficients indicate that a 10 per cent increase in weekly benefit payments (the indemnity payments made for lost wages) results in a 2.2 per cent increase in claim frequency and a 4.4 per cent increase in claim severity. By virtue of the way that these variables are constructed, the overall impact of an increase in benefits is to increase average claim costs per worker by about 6.6 per cent as indicated in the middle column. If there were no moral hazard effects, we would expect that an increase in benefits would have no impact on claim frequency. Although we cannot disaggregate claims by type of injury in this data, these moral hazard effects are believed to be particularly important for these claims whose 'work-relatedness' is most difficult to monitor, i.e. CTD claims.

Moral Hazard in Health Care

Not only are workers subject to benefit consumption because of the potential for moral hazard, but health-care providers are as well. We provide just one empirical example of this suggested in the first section of the paper: physicians in HMOs have incentives to misclassify claims as compensable in the workers' compensation system in order to maximize their income.

Physicians are generally paid on either a 'fee for service' basis, in which they are paid on a 'piece rate' basis in the sense that they get paid for each service rendered, or they get paid on a 'salaried' basis in which they work so many hours for a fixed payment. HMOs are per capita payment programs in which physicians contract to

Table 14.1 Workers' compensation utility: HMOs and moral hazard (standard errors–heteroskidascity consistent estimates).

	Indemnity			Medical share regressions
	LN Freq. Regr.	LN Sev. Regr.	LN AC Regr.	
Intercept	−0.428	4.605**	4.177**	0.090
	(1.14)	(1.79)	(1.80)	(1.01)
LN (Wage)	0.330**	0.270	0.600**	−0.359**
	(0.17)	(0.27)	(0.28)	(0.15)
LN (Benefit)	0.222**	0.439**	0.661***	0.303***
	(0.10)	(0.21)	(0.22)	(0.10)
HMO	0.001	0.020***	0.021***	0.010***
	(0.00)	(0.00)	(0.004)	(0.00)
LN (Value)	0.062	0.034	0.096	−0.035
added)	(0.05)	(0.12)	(0.12)	(0.07)
R^2	0.950	0.791	0.884	0.799

Note: State effects included in all of the regressions.
* = signif. at 10% level; ** = signif. at 5% level; *** = signif. at 1% level.

meet all the health-care needs of an individual (or family) for an annual fee. For the population in a given state, as the percentage of individuals covered by HMOs grew, we would not expect to see any differences in the number of workers' compensation claims field in the absence of moral hazard.

But HMO physicians are differentially influenced by the 'fee for service' payment practice of all workers' compensation programs. 'Fee for service' doctors get paid the same for treating a broken bone arising from an accident at home as they do for the same type of break occurring on the job. The fact that it is compensable in the workers' compensation system makes no difference to them. It does make a difference to the physicians in an HMO, however, since the treatment of an injury compensable by the firm's workers' compensation insurance represents a net increase in their income. They get paid on a 'fee for service' basis for workers' compensation injuries, on top of their per capita fees, and so are financially better off when as many as possible of their treatments are classified as work related.

This suggests that, holding other things constant, doctors in HMOs have an incentive to classify health conditions that might otherwise only be marginally work related or nonwork related as having 'arisen in the course of or out of their employment' (the requirement for compensability in the workers' compensation system). This is especially true for cumulative trauma conditions which may have a long latent period and be difficult to monitor as to whether they are work related or not. This suggests the following hypotheses concerning moral hazard behavior among HMO physicians:

1. As HMOs expand, the number of workers' compensation indemnity claims will rise (and reported severity may rise or fall) as HMO physicians encourage more of their patients to view their health conditions as work related.
2. As HMOs expand, medical costs as a share of total workers' compensation costs should increase.
3. As HMOs expand, those injuries that are most difficult to monitor as to their 'work relatedness' will rise as a share of all injuries. In particular, we would expect that the number of CTD injuries would be higher in HMOs.

While we do not have data on the latter hypothesis, we do on the first two hypotheses which we present in Table 14.2.

On average, across all 50 states, the proportion of the population covered by an HMO insurance agreement grew by 0.8 per cent annually. This is a relatively large rate of increase over the span of a single decade, going from 2.5 per cent of the population covered by HMOs in 1980 to about 10 per cent in 1988. To test whether this fourfold increase in HMO coverage affected workers' compensation claim frequency or severity, in Tables 14.1 and 14.2 we present a sample of roughly 28 states for which we generally have complete data during the 1980–1987 period on the claims reported to the National Council on Compensation Insurance (NCCI). We exclude some state/year observations for missing values (mostly on the NCCI claim data).[2]

NCCI is an actuarial advisory organization, supported by the insurance industry, which serves most of the states in helping them to formulate prices for their workers' compensation insurance. (Workers' compensation is a regulated line of insurance in most states, and rate increases in the insurance must be approved on a state-by-state basis.) In the process of formulating rates, the NCCI receives data on claims from all

Table 14.2 Variable means for HMO analysis (and standard deviations).

	Mean	Standard deviation
Dependendent variables		
Indemnity claims		
LN Freq. (indemnity claims/non ag. EES)	2.73	(0.34)
LN Sev. (indemnity payments/claims)	8.34	(0.36)
LN Ave. Cost (indemnity payments/non ag. EES)	11.08	(0.50)
Medical share		
LN Med (medical costs/total costs)	−0.86	(0.19)
Independent variables		
LN Wage	5.70	(0.14)
LN Benefits	5.11	(0.15)
HMO	3.87	(4.83)
Value added	9.01	(1.11)

Notes: HMO is the percentage of the population covered by licensed HMOs.
'Value added' is the value added by manufactures in each state for each year.
All monetary variables have been converted to real 1967 dollars.
LN is the natural logarithm.
Non ag. EES is nonagricultural employment.

the insuring agencies in the various states, and then applies standard actuarial techniques to price out workers' compensation insurance policies appropriately.

The NCCI has taken accident year data on a first-report basis (since a claim may take several years to close), and then converted it to a calendar year basis to match the other data available for the analysis. Data on HMO penetration rates (the proportion of the population covered by HMO services) is from annual surveys conducted by InterStudy, and collected in Kraus *et al.* (1992).

Although our main concern was the impact of HMOs on workers' compensation costs (claim frequency and severity), we wanted to control for other factors that might have also played a role in determining claims costs. As discussed above, from the employees' perspective, the opportunity cost of a workers' compensation claim will be determined by the difference between their wages and indemnity benefits. We expect that higher wages will tend to lower the number of claims, but higher benefits will increase the number of claims in the presence of moral hazard. Real value added by manufacturers is also included to control for industrial demand for employment (and hence proxy for job scarcity), and for the associated increase in new hires that comes with that expansion. Finally, dummy variables for each state in the sample are included as controls for administrative differences across states in program structure. All pecuniary variables have been converted into real dollars (with the price index normalized so that 1982–1984 period = 100).

The results indicate that benefits have a significant impact in increasing the frequency and severity of claims as indicated in the last section. Changes in the demand for labor (as measured by the value added variable) do not seem to have much of an impact on either claim frequency or claim severity once one controls for state effects (as we do here).

Most significantly, the HMO variable plays a very significant role in determining workers' compensation costs. It increases frequency (although the estimated impact is not statistically significant) and severity: the 7.5 increase in the percentage of HMO coverage during the 1980s translates into a 1 per cent increase in the frequency of claims, and about a 15 per cent increase in costs per claim. Since these are indemnity costs, there are probably no offsets in other programs. That is, to the extent that medical costs in workers' compensation go up, there may be a fall in the medical expenditures under group health coverage (although there will be a rise as well, as indicated by the examples in the first section of this chapter). However, these numbers are *not* for medical costs under workers' compensation, they are indemnity costs (weekly payments for lost work time) only. This HMO type of moral hazard appears, from this sample, to have a real effect upon the disability status of workers as our first hypothesis above suggests.

The final column in Table 14.1 tests our second hypothesis. As expected, as HMOs expanded, the share of medical costs in the workers' compensation system increased. The coefficient for the HMO variable indicates that from 1980 to 1988, the share of medical costs in workers' compensation increased 7.5 per cent due to the expansion of HMOs (where 7.5 per cent equals the estimated HMO coefficient multiplied by the change in the HMO variable from 1980 to 1988).

Moral Hazard in Management: Worker Productivity Failure and Disability

The economic model of moral hazard upon which this section is based is straightforward. The owners of capital hire managers and laborers to produce an output. A group of laborers is directed by a single manager, and the manager's compensation is determined by the wages and physical output of his or her unit. The total wage bill and physical product of each managed unit is monitored by the owners, although the performances of individuals within the unit are not generally known. That is, the owners have good information about total unit productivity and pay, but poor information about the productivity and pay of individuals within the unit. We also assume that they have poor information about workers' health and disability costs, either at the individual or unit level.[3] In other words, there is asymmetric information both about individuals' performance, and about nonwage fringe benefits.

This asymmetry leads to the following moral hazard problem: a unit manager, faced with maximizing unit 'profits' (the monetized value of physical output over wage costs), will – in the presence of productivity failure of some the unit's employees – tend to use the disability system as a means of getting rid of those less productive employees. Since health and disability costs are not charged to the unit (and individuals' performances are costly for owners to monitor), this amounts to a misclassification of employment costs. Instead of correctly labeling workers' failed productivity as 'management' costs, these are counted as 'health-care/disability' costs. While this misclassification raises the measured profits of the unit, it undoubtedly lowers total firm profits in the long run. The problem is that the asymmetry of information between owners and managers yields incentive for the managers (and laborers, who would rather be 'disabled' than 'fired') to misclassify some of the employment costs.

A key assumption here is that the health-care and disability costs of individuals or units are not monitored as closely as their wages and output. We make this assumption as an empirical matter, although it seems to us that profit-maximizing firms ought to be concerned with these costs at the unit level because of the moral hazard incentives that they potentially generate. But in the firm that we analyze, as in most firms of which we are aware, oversights for health-care and disability programs are separate from those of pay and performance. Our findings suggest that this separation tends to exacerbate the type of misclassification moral hazard that we measure here.

Empirical results

In order to minimize other aspects (that claim usage and discipline) of the disability system, we have focused on a sample of homogeneous workers in a single division from a single company. We examine the disability behavior of these workers at four different locations. Those locations, one in each census region, ensure that our disability response is not particular to any given area (and hence, to any particular administrative form of workers' compensation). We further restrict our sample to those employed after the date that our information on disability claims begins (to minimize initial condition problems). This tends to make our sample both relatively younger and less experienced. We follow this sample roughly from midyear in 1985 to midyear in 1992. These workers are employed in 'blue-collar' occupations, where the type of work performed in all locations is equivalent in the degree of inherent risk.

As indicated by the means in Table 14.3, there are over 25,000 worker years in our sample, four-fifths of which come from one location. Inspection of the means reveals that demographic characteristics vary considerably by region: locations 1, 2, and 4 have from 65–80 per cent nonwhite, while there is only 40 per cent nonwhite at location 3. Seventy per cent of those in location 4 are single, while almost half are married in location 3.

Table 14.3 Variable means for productivity failure analysis (and standard deviations).

	Location 1	Location 2	Location 3	Location 4
WC Claims	0.05	0.05	0.07	0.07
	(0.21)	(0.21)	(0.26)	(0.26)
Age	27.59	31.41	30.09	27.37
	(6.68)	(8.61)	(7.22)	(6.48)
Tenure	1.64	1.40	1.15	1.31
	(1.29)	(1.07)	(0.64)	(1.06)
Male	0.66	0.67	0.60	0.77
	(0.47)	(0.40)	(0.49)	(0.42)
White	0.35	0.18	0.58	0.32
	(0.48)	(0.38)	(0.49)	(0.47)
Married	0.39	0.41	0.45	0.29
	(0.49)	(0.49)	(0.50)	(0.45)
Disc-new	0.06	0.07	0.08	0.06
	(0.28)	(0.32)	(0.33)	(0.29)
Disc-old	0.10	0.06	0.04	0.04
	(0.44)	(0.31)	(0.28)	(0.25)
WC-Med	127.32	195.67	227.69	439.57
	(1041.56)	(1806.08)	(1847.31)	(2391.51)
N	19815	3123	2589	1410

This workforce is principally male, young, and relatively inexperienced at these jobs for sample selection reasons discussed above. Our confidence in any behavioral regularities that we measure ought to be enhanced since each of these locations is analyzed separately, and the workers' compensation system and worker demographics vary widely from site to site although the type of work does not.

The key variables in the analysis are the discipline variables and the workers' compensation/disability variables. Disc-new is a dummy variable indicating whether any kind of discipline notice had been given to the worker in the six months previous to his claim (or from January to June for those who had no disability claims). Disc-old is a dummy variable indicating whether any kind of discipline notice had been given earlier than the last six months (that is, from six months prior to the disability claim to the beginning of their employment). If our moral-hazard hypothesis is correct, we believe that the most recent disciplines will matter most to a manager or worker contemplating use of the disability system. So we anticipate the coefficient of Disc-new will exceed that of Disc-old, but that both coefficients will be positive.

Note that the rate of annual productivity failure (as measured by job performance warnings, Disc-new) is about 7 per cent. Since each observation is for a given person in a specific year, these annual productivity failures accumulate so that over a three- or four-year period over 20 per cent of the workforce will experience some sort of discipline. A visual examination of these performance warnings indicates that most of them arise from a definable failure to perform essential job functions, inappropriate language with customers or fellow workers, or excessive work absences. The progressive discipline policy in place for this company takes into account existing health problems that might be the cause of the job productivity failure. That is, job warnings would not be issued if, for example, 'excessive' absences were the result of some well-defined health condition.

On average, about 7 per cent of the workforce receive discipline notices in the 'previous' six months as indicated by the means of the Disc-new variable (averaging across the various employment groups). The Disc-old variable adds about another 7 per cent for previous notices,[4] making the number having received prior notices 10–16 per cent.

Although we have assumed that unit health/disability costs are not monitored very closely, workers and their managers may want to provide a rationale for their use of the disability system if they believe that it may be monitored. By frequent or severe use of medical care an employee could legitimize a subsequent large disability claim. This suggests that current and previous uses of medical care would likely be correlated with more frequent claims. The problem is that the current use of medical care is virtually guaranteed for a current disability claim – whether it is related to worker productivity failure or not. So to control for potential 'medical care signaling' of this type we include WC-med, the last six months of medical-care expenses received in workers' compensation, in the regressions. This also controls for other types of serial correlation in the claims including the possibility that managers may not be adhering to the company's policy of not issuing warnings if 'excessive absences' are due to a work-related health condition. Given the moral-hazard incentives discussed above, our model suggest that workers who are experiencing job performance failure will tend to use the disability system more than those who are not, *ceteris paribus.* To test this hypothesis in Table 14.4 we have regressed claim frequency on a number of demographic variables in our sample as well as the

Table 14.4 Linear probability model: productivity failure and disability usage (absolute *t*-statistics).

	Location 1	Location 2	Location 3	Location 4
Constant	0.026	0.020	0.084	0.040
	(3.81)	(1.31)	(3.39)	(1.27)
Age	3.7 E−4	2.9 E−4	2.1 E−4	6.9 E−4
	(1.61)	(0.63)	(0.29)	(0.65)
Tenure	0.002	0.004	−0.002	−0.004
	(1.57)	(1.15)	(0.26)	(0.59)
Male	−0.008	−0.005	−0.044	0.002
	(2.59)	(0.63)	(4.47)	(0.12)
White	0.004	0.025	−0.006	0.003
	(1.47)	(2.59)	(0.56)	(0.25)
Married	0.001	−0.003	0.002	−0.010
	(0.44)	(0.38)	(0.16)	(0.66)
Disc-new	0.018	0.080	0.053	0.053
	(3.57)	(7.06)	(3.48)	(2.38)
Disc-old	0.011	0.006	0.050	−8 E−4
	(3.10)	(0.46)	(2.69)	(0.03)
WC-Med	7 E−5	3 E−5	3 E−5	4 E−5
	(51.98)	(15.13)	(12.94)	(16.74)
R^2	0.352	0.295	0.282	0.423
Regression −F	350.32	37.15	27.84	38.08

Notes: All regressions are significant at better than the 1% level as indicated by the F statistics given on the last row.
Some estimated coefficients are sufficiently small so they are expressed in scientific notation (i.e. 3.7 E−4 = 0.000 37).

productivity failure variables (Disc-new and Disc-old). For each location, we expect that experiencing a productivity failure will significantly increase the probability of ending up in the disability system. That is, we expect that the coefficients of the performance warning variables will be positive in the claims frequency regressions.

While in general, older (Age) and female (Male) workers are more likely to go on a disability claim as one might expect from an opportunity cost standpoint, only the prior workers' compensation medical costs (WC-Med) and discipline (Disc-old and Disc-new) variables are consistently significant in explaining claim frequency. As hypothesized, WC-Med increases likelihood that one will subsequently go out on a disability claim. A $100 increase at the mean level of medical expenditures yields a 3–10 per cent (absolute) increase in the probability of a subsequent claim. This is a significant response, suggesting that more exhaustive research directed exclusively toward understanding this phenomenon might be a fruitful avenue for future examination.

The impact of productivity failure (performance warnings) on usage of the disability system is relatively large. Consider first the 0.08 coefficient in the second column of data in Table 14.4. This means that if a worker has received a disciplinary notice within the last six months, the likelihood of entering into a workers' compensation disability claim increases by 8 per cent. Since on average only 5 per cent of the workers enter into disability in any given year at location 2 (the second column and first row of Table 14.4), this means that the chance of going into disability more than doubles in location 2 if a worker is experiencing some productivity failure. Indeed, among the four units analyzed here, the probability of entering a workers' compensation disability claim increases from 55 per cent (location 1) to about 90 per cent (locations 2 and 3, when considering the overall impact of disciplinary notices). Moreover the fact that the most recent disciplinary notices increase the likelihood of entering into a disability claim more than prior notices (Disc-new coefficients are larger than Disc-old) provides further support for our hypothesis.

Concluding Remarks

One of the original purposes of the workers' compensation system was to expedite the return of able-bodied workers back into the workforce. Hence the existence of experience rating, rehabilitation services, and second injury funds. All these are intended to enhance productivity in the sense of providing firms with incentives to return workers back to the workplace. But worker productivity depends on more than the firm. It is also a function of the incentives that the system creates for workers (managers and laborers) and medical-care providers as well. In this larger setting, its not difficult to imagine that the current system of disability may generate incentives that are perverse, on net, to worker productivity.

In particular, disability may be seen as a reasonable alternative to work in the face of unpleasant job performance warnings representing productivity failure. Some workers experiencing such productivity failure may find, in a world with imperfect information, that it is possible to substitute the disability system for work both as a means of legitimizing their failure and as a means of generating some income. Their managers will also support this movement into the disability system to the extent that it enhances the monitored productivity of their unit. The reason for this form of moral hazard is that when worker 'productivity' is only partially monitored by the owners, good information on individual worker output and the true state of their health/disability status is lacking. In this paper, we have tried to test for the presence of this sort of moral hazard by looking at how job performance warnings, as a proxy for a productivity failure, affect subsequent use of the disability system.

This study, in conjunction with the many others examining moral hazard incentives in our current workers' compensation/disability system, should underscore the importance of analyzing financial motivations that are sometimes perverse despite the well-intentioned desires of the designers. It seems to us that moral-hazard problems are pervasive in the workers' compensation/disability system, and need to be further quantified for any rational analysis of workplace disability policy in a world of emerging health-care reform. Furthermore, this line of research indicates the importance of self-interested behavior of all the participants. Delivery systems based on paradigms that ignore this self-interested behavior (such as the biomedical model) are bound to be intrinsically less efficient in achieving their goals than those that account for incentive responses. The human capital model presented here is one such alternative paradigm.

NOTES

We would like to thank Torrey Powers of Options & Choices, Inc. and Desiree Adair for their help with the research, and Bob Hartwick of the National Council on Compensation Insurance for providing some of the data.

1 However, one desegregated analysis, a study done by Moore and Viscusi (1989), finds – contrary to the aggregate analysis by Butler (1983) – that a lower rate of fatal risk is associated with higher workers' compensation benefits. Their study of fatal injuries may be picking up changes in real risk behavior, and not measuring nominal or 'claims reporting' moral hazard. This is suggested in a simulation by Knieser and Leeth (1989), and in empirical research by Ruser (1990) and Butler and Worrall (1991).

2 The following states are included in analysis (by postal codes): AK, AL, AR, AZ, CT, FL, HI, IA, IN, KS, KY, LA, MD, ME, MI, MO, MS, MT, NC, NE, NM, OK, OR, RI, SC, TN, UT, VA, and VT. The following states were excluded because of missing benefit calculations: CO, IL, ID, GA, MA, NH, NY, SD, TX, and WI. The remainder of the sample was excluded because of missing claim data.

3 Interviews with various managers indicate that at the time of this study, managers were unaware of how much disability and health-care expenditures were generated by their units.

4 If all of the employees stayed with this firm then one might expect the mean of Disc-old to exceed the mean of Disc-new, because of an accumulation of notices in prior years. The reason that it does not is both because this is a sample of relatively new workers (as indicated above) and because there is a fair amount of turnover in the workforce.

REFERENCES

BUTLER, R. 1983 Wage and injury rate response to shifting levels of workers' compensation, in WORRALL, J. D. (Ed.), *Safety and the Work Force: Incentives and Disincentives in Workers' Compensation*, Ithaca, NY: ILR Press.

BUTLER, R. and WORRALL, J. 1983 Workers' compensation: Benefit and injury claim rates in the seventies, *Review of Economics and Statistics*, **65**, 580–9.

BUTLER, R. and WORRALL, J. 1985 Work injury compensation and the duration of nonwork spells, *Economic Journal*, **95**, 714–24.

BUTLER, R. and WORRALL, J. 1988 Labor market theory and the distribution of workers' compensation costs, in APPEL, D. and BORBA, P. S. (Eds), *Workers' Compensation Insurance Pricing*, Boston: Kluwer Academic Publishers.

BUTLER, R. and WORRALL, J. 1991 Claims reporting and risk bearing moral hazard in workers' compensation, *Journal of Risk and Insurance*, **53**, 191–204.

BUTLER, R. and WORRALL, J. 1993a Workers' compensation costs and heterogeneous claims, in DURBIN, D. and BORBA, P. S. (Eds), *Workers' Compensation Insurance: Claim Costs, Prices, and Regulation*, Boston: Kluwer Academic Publishers.

BUTLER, R. and WORRALL, J. 1993b Self insurance in workers' compensation, in DURBIN, D. and BORBA, P. S. (Eds), *Workers' Compensation Insurance: Claim Costs, Prices, and Regulation*, Boston: Kluwer Academic Publishers.

CHELIUS, J. 1982 The influence of workers' compensation on safety incentives, *Industrial and Labor Relations Review*, **35**, 235–42.

DUCATMAN, A. 1986 Workers' compensation cost-shifting: A unique concern of providers and purchasers of prepaid health care, *Journal of Occupational Medicine*, **28**(11).

GARDNER, H., BUTLER, R. and BRADSHAW, B. 1994 Employee health cost patterns by Pareto group: A case for human capital management, unpublished manuscript, Industrial Relations Center, University of Minnesota.

GARDNER, H. and FISKE, M. 1994 Human capital: A new paradigm for linking worker health & productivity, working paper, Cheyenne, WY: Gardner & Associates.

JOHNSON, W., BUTLER, R. and BALDWIN, M. 1995 First spells of work absences among Ontario workers, in THOMASON, T. and CHAYKOWSKI, R. (Eds), *Research in Canadian Workers' Compensation*, Ontario: Industrial Relations Centre, Queen's University Press.

JOHNSON, W. and ONDRICH, J. 1990 The duration of post-injury absences from work, *Review of Economics and Statistics*, November, 578–86.

KNIESNER, T. and LEETH, J. 1989 Separating the reporting effects from the injury rate effects of workers' compensation insurance: A hedonic simulation, *Industrial and Labor Relations Review*, **42**, 280–93.

KRAUS, N., PORTER, M. and BALL, P. 1992 *Managed Care: A Decade in Review 1980–1990*, Minneapolis, MN: Interstudy.

KRUEGER, A. 1990 Incentive effects of workers' compensation insurance, *Journal of Public Economics*, **41**, 73–99.

KRUEGER, A. and BURTON, JR., J. 1990 The employers' costs of workers' compensation insurance: Magnitudes and determinants, *Review of Economics and Statistics.*

LEIGH, J. 1985 Analysis of workers' compensation laws using data on individuals, *Industrial Relations*, **24**, 247–56.

MOORE, M. and VISCUSI, W. 1989 Promoting safety through workers' compensation: The efficacy and net wage costs of injury insurance, *Rand Journal of Economics*, **20**, 499–515; also in ch. 4 of MOORE, M. J. and VISCUSI, W. K. 1990 *Compensation Mechanisms for Job Risks: Wages, Workers' Compensation, and Product Liability*, Princeton, NJ: Princeton University Press.

RUSER, J. 1985, Workers' compensation insurance, experience rating, and occupational injuries, *Rand Journal of Economics*, **16**, 487–503.

RUSER, J. 1990 'The impact of workers' compensation insurance on occupational injuries and fatalities: Reporting effects and true safety effects', unpublished manuscript, Office of Economic Research, US Bureau of Labor Statistics.

RUSER, J. 1991 Workers' compensation and occupational injuries and illnesses, *Journal of Labor Economics*, **9**(4), 325–50.

WORRALL, J. and APPEL, D. 1982 The wage replacement rate and benefit utilization in workers' compensation insurance, *Journal of Risk and Insurance*, **49**, 361–71.

WORRALL, J. and BUTLER, R. 1990 Heterogeneity bias in the estimation of the determinants of workers' compensation loss distributions, in BORBA, P. S. and APPEL, D. (Eds), *Benefits, Costs, and Cycles in Workers' Compensation*, Boston, MA: Kluwer Academic Publishers.

CHAPTER FIFTEEN

The organizational response

Influence on Cumulative Trauma Disorders in the Workplace

GLENN PRANSKY, TERRY B. SNYDER and JAY HIMMELSTEIN

INTRODUCTION

Cumulative trauma disorders (CTDs) have become the fastest-growing cause of lost time in the US workforce. In industries where workers perform repetitive upper-extremity-intensive activities, these disorders represent the primary cause of work-related lost-time injuries (Roughton, 1993a). Outside of the manufacturing environment, similar trends have also become apparent in office and clerical settings (Brazier, 1993; Linton and Kamwendo, 1989). Specific ergonomic risk factors (excessive force, repetitions, awkward postures, vibration, and direct trauma) have been well described, and can be linked to a high incidence of CTDs in many work environments. However, nonergonomic factors can significantly influence the occurrence, reporting, and successful management of CTDs. In office and clerical environments, it has been suggested by some that these factors may account for most of the variance among different sites in rates of CTD (Hadler, 1992; Westgaard *et al.*, 1993). Through our review of the literature, and our consultation experience, we have identified three categories of nonergonomic factors that are significantly related to the CTD problem: *psychosocial* factors, *business* factors, and the *organizational response*.

NONERGONOMIC FACTORS AND CTDs

Psychosocial

Recent studies have identified the importance of psychosocial factors (e.g. locus of control, stress, job satisfaction, labor attitude, and others) in determining how workers perceive, report, and respond to musculoskeletal symptoms (Ursin *et al.*, 1988; Rundcrantz, *et al.*, 1991). Most investigators have focused on the psychologic state, attitudes, and perception of workers. Our experience shows that management's attitude is equally important in influencing the CTD problem, although this has not been thoroughly explored in the scientific literature.

Business

In our earlier workplace consultations, ergonomic problems were usually obvious to both workers and management. Not infrequently, we had been preceded by other consultants, who had given similar ergonomic recommendations as ours. Why had these recommendations not been followed? Why had high-risk job situations persisted? In other instances, companies enacted a wide variety of recommended ergonomic changes, only to see an increased rate of shoulder, arm, and hand complaints (Kadeforse *et al.*, 1992; Oxenburgh *et al.*, 1985). To understand these issues, we needed to step back from tasks, tools, and processes, to examine the business factors and practices that might be influencing CTDs. Although our clients may focus on problems occurring at the work bench, our experience has shown that we need to understand the business issues driving the work practices of the organization, in order to provide effective recommendations. Business issues and practices play a major role in influencing occurrence, reporting, and an organization's ability to respond to CTDs (Snyder *et al.*, 1991).

An examination of relevant business factors is based on data compiled from worker/management interviews, reviews of published literature such as annual reports, internal documents, and results of direct observation, an approach adapted from Haddon and Haddon (1987). We systematically review each functional area, focusing on how it affects the CTD problem. For example, questions that we raise to understand the role of these factors in CTDs may include the following:

Marketing sales What is the nature of the product? Is it a seasonal product? How accurate is the product mix forecast? Do these factors lead to excessive overtime and production pressure? How do they affect ability to plan and schedule production?

Operations/production Is this product highly customized? Can production be automated? How much inventory is carried to buffer the demand for labor? What alternative job duties are feasible?

Finance Is the company profitable? Can it afford to commit resources to decrease CTDs? What is the long-term financial goal of the company?

Human resource management Do worker compensation incentives (such as piece work) contribute to the CTD problem? Does excessive employee turnover prevent implementation of effective training programs? What effect does labor-management relations have on the CTD problem?

Health and safety Where does the safety director and the health clinic report in the organization? What CTD management programs exist?

Other business factors are examined, including the company's organizational structure, constraints of the local economy, and constraints of the particular industry. Business expertise is often needed to gather and analyze these data, since this is not part of the formal training of most occupational health or ergonomics consultants. This business analysis enables us to understand why obvious ergonomic problems are unresolved, and allows us to identify many hidden issues that often accelerate injury rates and contribute to poor management of injured workers, thus preventing resolution of CTD problems. With this understanding, we can make more effective, realistic, and credible recommendations in the 'language of the workplace.'

Organizational Response

However, companies with similar business factors often have very divergent levels of success in addressing the CTD problem, despite significant efforts to address ergonomic issues (Rigdon, 1992). Psychosocial factors alone do not appear to explain these differences fully, which are primarily related to the company's actions, and its ability to respond effectively (Terbourg, 1988). We define the organizational response as the actions taken within the company (including those of labor and management) to address CTD problems. This organizational response can be as important as ergonomic, psychosocial, and business factors in determining the success of the overall approach to CTDs. A positive organizational response might include setting clearly stated goals and priorities, committing financial resources to the CTD problem, forming problem-solving groups, empowering project leaders, restructuring the business organization, redesigning jobs and work practices, sending a positive message to workers, and effective injury and disability management. Negative organizational responses could include ignoring the problem, focusing on denial of work relatedness of CTDs, intimidating workers, or sending mixed messages about the employer's level of concern for employee health and welfare.

Definitions of 'success' with respect to CTDs in a particular company may vary. Management might define success in terms of short-term reduction in recorded injury rates, even though the level of worker complaints may continue to be high, or focus more on workers' compensation cost reductions, overall profitability, or Occupational Safety and Health Administration (OSHA) recordable injuries. A worker seeking to maximize earnings and benefits may support a high-risk situation such as an aggressive piece-work incentive program. That worker may label an organizational response that limits opportunity for high compensation as an 'unsuccessful' outcome, regardless of the impact on injury rates. Measurements of success are also hampered by limited data; workers' compensation data in typical manufacturing workplaces are biased towards underreporting, where symptom surveys may overrepresent the level and severity of work-related musculoskeletal symptoms. There is clearly a need for better outcome indicators that can be used across workplaces. As health and safety professionals, we define success as decreasing CTD injuries – not only those that are recorded and compensated, but also those that are perceived by the workforce. Based on our experience and this concept of a successful program, we have identified six characteristics of a successful organizational response, illustrated by case examples.

CHARACTERISTICS OF A SUCCESSFUL ORGANIZATIONAL RESPONSE

1. *Effective worker involvement* is an essential element of the successful corporate response. Early in the process, workers must receive a clear message from management that they are stakeholders in the ultimate outcome. Involvement of several levels of management, on a consistent basis, is necessary to reinforce the message that solutions are being genuinely sought, and that they will, in fact, be implemented. Training workers in basic group problem-solving skills is essential,

and appears to be more important than formal training in more complex ergonomic analysis techniques (Portis and Hill, 1989). Once a cohesive group of workers has completed this basic training, additional skills may naturally evolve, may be obtained through expert consultants (internal or external), or may be gained through additional training. However, maintaining a common-sense approach is most important for continued success.

Management and labor jointly create an opportunity for a team effort, beginning with allowing the time necessary for effective team-building. The organization, through a strong project leader, must empower the team with enough authority to investigate, design, implement, and monitor programs (Millar, 1993). Ongoing management involvement in the group problem-solving effort is essential in setting realistic goals in line with the long-term goals of the organization, and to insure that the team project is within the scope of the team members. Historically, trends in problem-solving group philosophy have varied along with group labels; these include total quality management (TQM) quality circles, management by objective (MBO) focus groups, and high-performance work teams (Roughton, 1993b; Kohn and Friend, 1993). Regardless of the group label, effective CTD problem-solving teams have certain common characteristics (Lawler and Mohrman, 1987).

Several tangible results are often achieved in those organizations that incorporate this level of earnest worker involvement. Because ergonomic principles are often intuitive to those performing the task, job design and ergonomic problem-solving become more efficient and cost-effective. As the level of worker ownership for recommended changes increases, implementation is greatly facilitated. Problem-solving becomes much more ongoing and iterative, with a higher level of on-line flexibility (Pipinich, 1993).

Industrial paper products – effective worker involvement

A division of a large producer of industrial paper products had persistently elevated rates of CTD injuries in production workers. For five years, the plant employed a full-time ergonomic safety engineer, who directed an appointed plant safety committee; its members were managers and selected supervisors, without any worker representation. Although this engineer had instituted several ergonomic changes, they seemed to have little effect on CTD rates. Several years later, high-performance work teams were instituted, led by experienced supervisors, skilled in facilitating problem-solving groups. These teams were charged with addressing quality, productivity, and ergonomic problems in their work areas. Each team elected a representative to the plant's new ergonomics group. Without formal ergonomic training, the high-performance work teams have generated and tested a variety of work practice and design changes throughout the plant. Although many of the changes did not survive an initial trial, these mistakes were expected, quickly recognized, and rectified. Other successful changes appear to be related to plant-wide decreases in musculoskeletal injuries and complaints, with significant cost savings, clearly justifying the investment in the problem-solving process.

2. *A strong project leader* is necessary. Successful project leaders may originate from various positions in the organization – safety manager, production engineer, office manager, occupational health nurse, supervisor, or the plant manager. This person must be empowered by both labor and management to maintain a lead-

ership position in guiding and selling the organizational response. Some basic industrial engineering knowledge may be required, but the project leader's ability to motivate labor and management is essential. In each case, the successful project leader is a good listener, and effective group leader and problem-solver. The project leader knows how to empower the team problem-solving effort, and effectively sells the resulting group ideas to labor and management (Roughton, 1993b). This leader can effectively use the language of the workplace in explaining costs and benefits to management (a high level of sophistication is not necessary, only clarity of presentation) and discussing constraints and short- and long-term benefits with workers.

Computer products supplier – successful project leader
A division of this company selected an experienced production line supervisor to chair the overall response to CTDs. Although he had no formal ergonomic or industrial engineering training, he had many years' experience as a production worker, and a strong ability to facilitate and direct group problem-solving. His workstyle was characterized by a positive attitude and commitment to meaningful worker involvement, focusing participants on generating tangible results. The problem-solving group that he chaired identified and remediated over 50 separate problems that contributed to CTDs, within 18 months of starting this process. Over a two-year period, the rates of reported CTD injuries decreased by 55 per cent, and workers reported fewer episodes of prolonged musculoskeletal complaints.

3. Organizational *flexibility* also characterizes successful responses; management and labor are willing to explore changes in the organizational structure, the empowerment of new individuals, and new business practices (Karasek, 1979). Borne out of an open-minded and solution-oriented approach, this flexibility may include changes in incentive programs, reorganizing work schedules to allow problem-solving team meetings, developing and empowering a labor-management safety committee, as well as a union's willingness to allow alternate job assignments (Silverstein, 1990). This same flexibility must also be a characteristic of the project leader. Flexibility is needed not only at the outset, but through an iterative process of feedback and change that characterizes successful responses.

Textile manufacturer-organizational flexibility
Historically, this company has been characterized by resistance to change. The plant facility is over 100 years old, and many production machines are at least 50 years old. Labor–management relations, business practices, and organizational structure have not changed considerably over the past 20 years at this location, or in the industry as a whole. Recently, a new plant manager's commitment to change and flexibility in addressing the CTD problem has motivated the plant management and labor organization to explore new, safer work practices. As a result, their successful approach to CTDs contains many new elements, including work reorganization, gradual elimination of piece work, temporary light-duty assignments, and initiation of problem-solving groups. Although CTD rates have dramatically escalated in other plants, the rates at this location have stayed low and stable over several years.

4. Action *must be consistent with the stated goals* of the organization. Before making commitments, management should carefully evaluate the organization's goals, to

insure that the actual approach represents a long-term solution for the CTD problem. Management may first need to refocus away from short-term goals of suppressing CTD reporting, in order to identify problems and thus achieve long-term success. An exclusive focus on short-term results and the latest management fad can lead to implementation of solutions that have negative long-term consequences in terms of CTDs, morale, and the credibility of any future group problem-solving efforts (Mahone, 1993). Long-term commitment is effectively communicated by top management participation in the process, which is targeted to reinforce the congruence between the team process and the overall goals of the company (Pipinich, 1993; Mykletun *et al.*, 1992). Management's responsive approach to the problem-solving team's suggestions is an important measure of this congruence for the team (Bers, 1992).

Goals should be clearly stated, including associated measures of success – decreased musculoskeletal complaints, decreased injuries, higher level of worker participation and satisfaction, decreased wastage, etc. The team leader and members should understand these goals, the metrics of success, and constraints of the company, its industry, and its product.

A utility company – problem-solving with no constraints
This utility focused their efforts on the problem-solving process rather than the goal of *appropriately* increased quality. As a result of establishing over 120 quality circles, they were the first US company to win the coveted Baldridge award for quality. However, management never communicated financial goals to the quality teams. The absence of these realistic constraints led to many impractical, costly, and inefficient solutions. For example, many projects targeted an improvement in the customer billing system, although customers did not perceive billing as a problem. The result was an extremely negative return on a substantial investment (Hayes, 1993).

5. All successful organizational responses appear to be based upon a certain level of *resource commitment*. Resources may include top management input, outside consultants, engineering and fabrication support, and purchase of new equipment. Management must carefully evaluate the range of resources available, and should present a clear, consistent message to the problem-solving group about the types and extent of resources that can be committed (Marash-Stanley, 1993). Making resource constraints known to the problem-solving group early in the process allows the group to focus on developing practical solutions that can be realistically implemented, rather than developing ideas that will never be realized. If constraints are communicated to the team too late in the problem-solving process, the entire credibility of the process could be in jeopardy, de-motivating the team effort and wasting resources (Loss control programs: the 10 most significant flaws, *Risk Management*, 1993).

Custom work station fabricator – working within constraints
A producer of customized metal workstations was faced with serious financial difficulties and layoffs in a shrinking market, as well as a monumental CTD problem. A plant ergonomics and CTD task force was instituted, which was empowered by management to examine all possible solutions to the problem. However, the financial situation precluded any substantial capital investment for several years. The team worked within these constraints to identify solutions, building upon the company's strengths – a loyal, highly trained work-

force, flexible organization, and innovative toolmakers. Over a three-year period, reported CTD injuries decreased by over 85 per cent, and direct workers' compensation costs decreased thirtyfold. This successful program included reorganization from piecework incentive jobs to team product-building concepts, alternate work assignments, job sharing, and worker training programs. Safer, alternative methods, of using existing equipment were devised, and the limited available capital was used for prioritized equipment modification.

6. In most manufacturing and intensive office work settings, *injury management* must be part of the response, as it is impossible to eliminate all risk of CTDs occurring or presenting in the workplace. In successful organizational responses, the injury management approach often evolves with labor and management input, so that medical opinions and recommendations are accepted with a high degree of trust. Coordination between internal and external services is important, with appropriate and frequently re-evaluated alternate duty. Early reporting is encouraged, and there is an established plan for addressing nondisabling musculoskeletal pain in the workplace (Solomon, 1993). Ergonomic changes designed to facilitate worker reintegration usually will enhance job safety for other, uninjured workers (Adams, 1993).

   Industrial storage equipment – managing CTDs
   A key element of the joint labor–management effort to address CTDs at Steelcase (Laabs, 1993) was the formation of an injury management program. To define a program that was acceptable to both management and labor required extensive negotiations, which at times seemed to be at impasse. Finally, a multifaceted program was created that was quite different from the expectations at the outset. Innovative elements of this program included early reporting and intervention, highly flexible alternate duty, and dispute arbitration as an alternative to the formal workers' compensation system. This program resulted in a substantial decrease in CTDs over a four-year period. Although generally regarded by labor and management as successful, some felt that the focus on injury management diverted resources from more important ergonomic issues.

ORGANIZATIONAL RESPONSE: A CASE EXAMPLE

The following case example demonstrates two divisions with very similar business and ergonomic factors, but divergent levels of success in addressing CTD injuries, primarily because of differences in their organizational response. Many of the typical characteristics of successful and unsuccessful responses are contrasted here.

Confectionery Company: Contrasting Divisions

Company history

This medium-sized, highly successful bakery company was consistently profitable, with a national demand for its high-quality products. This company started as a small family operation, but has had substantial financial growth over the last 10 years. As the number of employees and facilities has grown dramatically, the company felt the growing pains of adopting more formal reporting structures and controls.

Business analysis

A business analysis identified a broad product mix, expanding sales that were limited only by production capacity, rapid financial growth, and obvious opportunities for expansion into new markets. Production facilities varied, including old, rebuilt mill buildings and new, state-of-the-art custom facilities. Profits were consistently reinvested into capital equipment and facilities. The labor force was extremely stable and well compensated (especially in relation to the impoverished surrounding community), but had a fairly low level of training. Management and labor, loyal to the company in its original form, were uncomfortable and often resistant to the cultural changes required to run what had become a large organization. The health and safety structure varied from division to division; the corporate safety focus appeared to be on environmental impact to the surrounding community, rather than on injury prevention and management.

Contrast between two divisions

We were consulted because of elevated rates of CTDs in one division, compared with another nearby division. Our investigation began with a look at ergonomic factors, which explained only part of the differences among departments and divisions in worker musculoskeletal complaints and CTDs. The overall business issues were quite similar for both divisions. However, the organizational response differed in many respects.

A successful organizational response

In the division with low CTD injury rates, worker involvement was solicited throughout the entire design, pilot testing, and implementation of plant operations. A project leader was chosen who was open to new ideas and had strong team leadership and interpersonal skills, as well as the ability to communicate effectively with corporate-level management. Workers involved in designing new production lines had been given the time to obtain necessary skills and were also given the necessary capital commitment to select optimal equipment and develop a workable layout. This substantial investment in worker involvement effectively created the trust that management would incorporate worker input in the final implementation. This division used the corporate safety department to provide added reinforcement to the successful CTD management plan at their site. CTDs were usually accepted as work related if designated as such by workers or management; the organization's response focused on improving or altering work conditions to enable an expedient, safe return to work.

An unsuccessful organizational response

In contrast, in the division with high CTD rates, management encouraged worker involvement only when corporate headquarters requested divisional representation to a corporate problem-solving group. However, on a site level, workers were not given adequate time, training, or supportive resources to make a substantial contribution. These workers were never given clear expectations that their needs would be considered in the outcome, or that their input would be of any consequence in the final implementation of the production process. When workers were allowed to participate in a problem-solving effort, they were given a task well beyond their skills, with inadequate time and resources to engineer realistic solutions, and therefore became disillusioned with their inevitable failure.

The unsuccessful division's safety director had alienated both workers and management, and retreated from the more difficult ergonomic and work organizational issues to other regulatory compliance concerns, where he felt more comfortable. He neither sought input from workers, nor was he able to sell his ideas to labor or management. He was unable to see the possibility that worker involvement could be of value.

Although the employee newsletter was plastered with corporate goals that showed commitment to worker involvement and health and safety grograms, corporate-level management did little to empower this process at the unsuccessful division. The unsuccessful division had failed to attempt to define a list of prioritized actions, and had failed to communicate site-specific long-term goals. Although corporate-level resources were readily available, they were not requested by the unsuccessful division and therefore never appeared. This raised great resentment among long-time employees, who felt abandoned by the leadership that was once so accessible.

The injury management and psychosocial attitudes towards workers differed greatly from the successful division. There was often considerable distrust towards workers who were disabled because of CTDs; the primary focus was to determine whether a problem was work related. The entire injury management program targeted disabled workers, with very little coordination between the external provider and those on the job, especially those with early, mild symptoms, who might benefit most from appropriate intervention.

It is interesting to note that our consultation showed, as did others before us, that many of the ergonomic problems facing the unsuccessful division could be reduced by automation. Other consultants had already suggested that automation would provide needed additional production capacity, rapidly compensating for the investment in capital equipment. However, the organizational response and associated psychosocial attitudes prevented this division from acting on this information.

In summary

Organizational responses significantly influenced how CTDs were prevented and managed at each facility. The successful organization's response was based on the work of a strong project leader with management and labor support, who cultivated effective worker involvement. This successful division displayed flexibility, changing from old work practices and relationships to adapt to a new, corporate culture. Goals have been clearly communicated between management and workers, with the necessary commitment of resources. Finally, the injury management program seems to directly benefit from the team-building and flexible thinking of the successful problem-solving process.

DISCUSSION

The concept of organizational response as a key factor in determining a variety of outcomes is not new. In the business literature, the relation between this response and product costs, time to market, and quality have been thoroughly reviewed. Organizational issues have recently been a focus of the safety literature, especially in the context of TQM approaches to safety organizations, and analysis of the limitations of traditional safety programs in addressing injury rates (Sukay, 1993). Here, the organizational response model is focused on a specific industrial safety problem, that of CTDs. However, any sort of analysis relating an organization's response to CTDs is uncommon in the medical literature. Perhaps this deficiency explains the impotence of the medical model in addressing occupational CTDs. For us, this departure from a traditional medical approach has provided our analyses with a greater depth of understanding, as well as an ability to explore fully all barriers to resolving CTD problems.

For clarity of illustration, our discussion and case examples have provided a somewhat isolated focus on the organizational response and its relation to outcomes. In practice, we find that this response originates from an environment of business and psychosocial factors, and that these factors continue to determine how the organizational response evolves. Our illustrations of positive and negative organizational responses occur in the settings of organizations that, in themselves, may be viewed as positive or negative. Several conceptual models have been developed to characterize the nature of the organization, in ways that are directly relevant to the range of responses to a problem that might be expected. McGregor's theory X and theory Y and Ouchi's theory Z organizational models contrast flexible and progressive organizations (theory Y or Z), versus those that are highly structured and regressive (theory X) (Ouchi and Johnson, 1978). Obviously, theory X organizations will have much more difficulty in positively responding to CTD problems. In contrast, lower levels of formal structure, flexible distribution of authority, and responsiveness to change are some of the characteristics of theory Y or Z organizations that enhance ability to achieve success with CTD problems. The ongoing, iterative nature of an organizational response is only briefly addressed here, but a continued willingness and ability to change are characteristics of the successful response.

Several new trends will certainly impact organizational responses. The Americans with Disabilities Act will motivate companies to examine accommodations and job modifications, in the interest of accommodating workers who have had CTDs. These accommodations are likely to require collective effort to maintain productivity and prevent reinjury; the benefit will ultimately be jobs that will have less risk of causing CTDs.

REFERENCES

Adams, E. 1993 Second stage: Using macro-ergonomics to 'design out' cumulative trauma risk, *Occupational Health and Safety*, **62**, 40–5.

Loss Control Programs: The 10 Most Significant Flaws 1993 *Risk Management*, **40**, 79–84.

Bers, J. 1992 Social ergonomics: Interesting spin on human factors issues, *Facilities Design Management*, **11**, 44–7.

BRAZIER, I. 1993 The ergonomic office – Fad or fiction: The facts, *Facilities*, **11**, 20–3.

HADDON, K. I. and HADDON, M. L. 1987 Identifying corporate strategies, ch. 19 in *Strategic Management*, Englewood Cliffs, NJ: Prentice-Hall.

HADLER, N. M. 1992 Arm pain in the workplace: A small area analysis, *Journal of Occupational Medicine*, **34**, 113–19.

HAYES, E. C. 1993 Value analysis and total quality management: A comparison, *Industrial Engineering*, **25**, 18–19.

KADEFORSE, R., ENGSTROM, T., JOHANNSON, J., JOHANSSON, M., KLINGENSTIERNA, U., LINDSTROM, I. and RUBENOWITZ, R. 1992 Musculoskeletal complaints, ergonomic aspects and psychosocial factors in two different truck assembly concepts, *Arbete Och Halsa*, **17**, 145–6.

KARASEK, R. A. 1979 Job demands, job decision latitude, and mental strain: Implications for job redesign, *Administrative Science Quarterly*, **24**, 285–309.

KOHN, J. P. and FRIEND, M. A. 1993 Quality and ergonomics: The team approach to the occupational people factor, *Professional Safety*, **38**, 39–42.

LAABS, J. J. 1993 Steelcase slashes workers' comp costs, *Personnel Journal*, **72**, 72–8.

LAWLER, E. E. and MOHRMAN, S. 1987 Quality circles after the honeymoon, *Organizational Dynamics*, **1**, 42–54.

LINTON, S. J. and KAMWENDO, K. 1989 Risk factors in the psychosocial work environment for neck and shoulder pain in secretaries, *Journal of Occupational Medicine*, **31**, 609–13.

MAHONE, D. B. 1993 Quick-fix solutions to ergonomic hazards: Watch out, *Industrial Engineering*, **25**, 23–6.

MARASH-STANLEY, A. 1993 The key to TQM and world-class competitiveness, Part II, *Quality*, **32**, 43–6.

MILLAR, J. D. 1993 Valuing, empowering employees vital to quality health & safety management, *Occupational Health and Safety*, **62**, 100–1.

MYKLETUN, R. J., BERGE, W. T., BRU, E., SITTER, A. and LINDOE, P. 1992 Organizational interventions to reduce musculoskeletal pain of female hospital staff, *Arbete Oche Halsa*, **17**, 245–7.

OUCHI, W. and JOHNSON, J. B. 1978 Types of organizational control and their relationship to emotional well-being, *Administrative Science Quarterly*, **23**, 293–317.

OXENBURGH, M. S., ROWE, S. A. and DOUGLAS, D. B. 1985 Repetition strain injury in keyboard operators, *Journal of Occupational Health and Safety* (*Australia/New Zealand*), **1**, 106–12.

PIPINICH, R. E. 1993, Ergonomics: A high priority at Lockheed Fort Worth facility, *Industrial Engineering*, **25**, 20–2.

PORTIS, B. and HILL, N. 1989 Improving organization effectiveness through employee involvement, *Business Quarterly*, **53**, 58–60.

RIGDON, J. E. 1992 How a plant handles occupational hazard with common sense, *Wall Street Journal*, September 28, A7.

ROUGHTON, J. 1993a Cumulative trauma disorders: The newest business liability, *Professional Safety*, **38**, 29–35.

ROUGHTON, J. 1993b Integrating quality into safety and health management, *Industrial Engineering*, **25**, 35–40.

RUNDCRANTZ, B. L., JOHNSSON, B., MORITZ, U. and ROXENDAL, G. 1991 Occupational cervico-branchia disorders among dentists, *Scandinavian Journal of Social Medicine*, **19**, 174–80.

SILVERSTEIN, B. A. 1990 Evaluation of interventions for control of cumulative trauma disorders, ch. 7 in *Ergonomic Interventions to Prevent Musculoskeletal Injuries in Industry*, Chelsea, MI: Lewis Publishers.

SNYDER, T. B., HIMMELSTEIN, J., PRANSKY, G. and BEAVERS, J. D. 1991 Business analysis in occupational health and safety consultations, *Journal of Occupational Medicine*, **33**, 1040–5.

SOLOMON, B. 1993 Using managed care to control workers' compensation costs, *Compensation & Benefits Review*, **25**, 59–65.

SUKAY, L. D. 1993 Safety programs alone don't work in reducing workers' compensation costs, *Risk Management*, **49**, 43–50.

TERBOURG, J. R. 1988 Organizational context, in JOHNSON, K., LAROSE, J. H., SCHEIRER, C. J. and WOLLE, J. M. (Eds), *Proceedings: Methodological Issues in Worksite Research*, pp. 21–34, Washington, DC: US Department of Health and Human Services, US Public Health Service.

URSIN, H., ENDRESEN, I. M. and URSIN, G. 1988 Psychological factors and self-reports of muscle pain, *European Journal of Applied Physiology*, **57**, 282–90.

WESTGAARD, R. H., JENSEN, C. and HANSEN, K. 1993 Individual and work-related risk factors associated with symptoms of musculoskeletal complaints, *International Archive of Occupational and Environmental Health*, **64**, 405–13.

CHAPTER SIXTEEN

Cumulative trauma disorder research

Methodological Issues and Illustrative Findings from the Perspective of Psychosocial Epidemiology

STANISLAV V. KASL and BENJAMIN C. AMICK

INTRODUCTION

This chapter utilizes the perspective of psychosocial epidemiology to analyze and discuss research design and data analysis strategies useful for planning more effective studies of the etiology of cumulative trauma disorders (CTDs) in the work environment. The perspective of psychosocial epidemiology represents an analytic framework in which the interplay of biomedical, physical, and psychosocial/behavioral risk factors and moderators in the etiology of a physical disorder is of central importance. The complexity calls for theoretical models sufficiently rich to encompass a potentially large and diverse set of risk factors and moderators, and the possibly complicated etiological dynamics among them. In addition, however, disorders of complex etiology tend to demand stronger or more definitive research designs, which inevitably translate into prospective studies of initially healthy cohorts, and, possibly, special monitoring for intermediate outcomes as well. Furthermore, there is also a greater need to set up data analysis strategies that will be sensitive to the complexity of the theoretical models: identify exposures, adjust for confounders, search for vulnerability factors, determine possible underlying mediating processes, and so on.

It is, of course, difficult to discuss epidemiologic approaches to the study of the etiology of CTDs when the fundamental issues about how to conceptualize this disorder and how to measure it have not yet been settled (e.g. Chapter 8). Textbooks in epidemiology, which offer guidelines about etiological research, typically assume that issues regarding diagnostic criteria and operational procedures for the outcome of interest have been resolved (Kelsey *et al.*, 1986). Few, if any, textbooks offer guidelines about how to investigate the etiology of a condition or disorder, while at the same time still trying to answer fundamental empirical questions about the proper formulation of the construct.

In this chapter we assume that enough consensus exists regarding approximate CTD criteria and their measurement. Therefore it is not premature to discuss etiologic research strategies in the framework of psychosocial epidemiology. However, we also recognize that when a particular disorder has not yet been fully explicated, it is a good strategy to collect in epidemiologic studies as much separate and distinct information about the phenomenology of the disorder as possible, so that future changes in the diagnostic algorithm can be accommodated by re-analysis of existing data rather than having to conduct new studies.

Previous reviews of the epidemiology and possible etiology of CTDs, or highly related syndromes such as repetition strain injury (RSI) (e.g. Bammer and Martin, 1988, 1992; Kiesler and Finholt, 1988), have strongly suggested that the etiology of the disorder is unlikely to be fully encompassed by a narrow biomedical or biomechanical framework. Instead, it appears that we need to also consider a possibly long list of psychological, social, organizational, and cultural influences which may also play a role in the etiology, detection, manifestation, and consequences of the disorder (Kuorinka and Forcier, 1995). However, there is a difficulty, in the context of this chapter which attempts to discuss epidemiologic research strategies, in being able to strike a proper balance between (1) the need to define the phenomenon and its etiology broadly enough so that all crucial aspects of the causal dynamics have a chance of being identified, and (2) the need to circumscribe the CTD phenomenon sufficiently so as to be able to develop a manageable epidemiologic research agenda.

There are certain aspects of the CTD phenomenon that we intend to ignore or downplay in this chapter. These include: (1) international variations in the incidence and prevalence rates across groups of workers with apparently similar exposures; (2) secular trends in the incidence and prevalence rates within a single country which reveal puzzling increases and declines in rates apparently not explained by changing work exposures; and (3) influences on detection and identification of cases of CTD which may reflect a variety of possible biases and distortions, such as (a) readiness to seek medical attention for symptoms and complaints, (b) availability of medical services for diagnosis and treatment, and (c) decision processes regarding compensability of CTDs. Instead, we wish to concentrate on a 'simplified' epidemiologic paradigm which is ahistorical, insensitive to cross-cultural variations, and utilizes investigator-based outreach efforts in order to identify cases without bias (e.g. bias due to treated status, or sociopolitical and economic influences on case detection).

DESIGN AND DATA COLLECTION ISSUES IN CTD ETIOLOGIC RESEARCH

It is always easier to advocate rigorous and demanding research designs on paper, and in conferences, than it is to implement such advice in one's own work. Practical and financial constraints on observational research in the work setting can play havoc with one's a priori knowledge or intentions about good research designs. So the intent of this section is not to make abstract assertions about good epidemiologic research, but rather to analyze and discuss the benefits – in terms of added knowledge and understanding of the etiological process – that accrue from more demanding and complex designs. What also needs to be kept in mind is that the persistence of questions regarding the role of psychosocial factors in the etiology of CTDs suggests that the accumulated evidence so far, based as it is on predominantly cross-sectional surveys and surveillance efforts, has not been able to provide adequate answers regarding psychosocial factors.

The classical approach in epidemiology is a prospective design in which a cohort of individuals, initially free of the disease or disorder of interest, is assessed at baseline in order to characterize their exposure experiences (risk factors) and to assess additional variables which may act as confounders, controls, and moderators. The cohort is then monitored for initial events of disease (incidence), as these occur during a predetermined length of follow-up. Baseline data are then examined in order to identify independent, joint, and interacting risk factors for the outcome. Depending on models being tested, baseline variables may be arranged in analyses into various combinations of risk factors, antecedents to risk factors, controls or confounders, moderating influences, and so on.

The above paragraph offers only a simplified skeletal outline which can serve as a basis for raising a number of additional questions or issues about research design strategy, given the greater complexity of CTD etiology. These issues concern the composition of the cohort and the point at which follow-up should begin, the work settings represented, the type of monitoring during follow-up, the type of information to be collected, and the type of analysis to be done.

1. If the initial prevalence of cases with disorder (who are not eligible for the cohort follow-up) is fairly high (10 per cent or more), this may suggest that important etiological dynamics in that setting have already played themselves out to some extent, and that the cohort-eligible subjects who are still disorder-free may be an unrepresentative subset of less vulnerable individuals.

2. If CTDs represent a condition that develops gradually and goes through identifiable stages of symptom development and progression along severity–duration–disablement dimensions, then it may be insufficient to identify within the prospective cohort only cases that meet the 'final' diagnostic criteria for CTD. Many incident cases, especially in the early stages of follow-up, will be those making the transition from just failing to meet the diagnostic criteria to just meeting them. This may then represent a failure of the prospective intent of the study design, e.g. (a) reverse causation is not fully ruled out in that the presence of symptoms may influence the reporting of psychosocial conditions and the secure temporal ordering of study variables may be made more difficult, and (b) early stages of symptom development are not studied adequately and the identified risk factors for CTDs may turn out to be those that contribute to the progression through later stages of disorder development.

3. In planning the cohort selection, some thought must also be given to the prevalence of work-setting ergonomic exposure among the cohort subjects. While it is tempting to concentrate on high-risk work settings, because they are likely to yield a greater incidence of CTDs, it is important to understand how the etiological picture, especially with respect to psychosocial influences, may be altered by this aspect of the design. Specifically, when there is a sharp separation of workers on level of ergonomic risk, the main effect due to ergonomic exposure is well characterized and the moderating role of psychosocial variables can be estimated rather clearly. However, when there is an inadequate variation in ergonomic risk, psychosocial variables may appear in analysis as main effects, rather than as moderators, and their role may be misinterpreted or overrated.

4. In the classic epidemiological design, 'prospective' means before disease have developed. In occupational epidemiology, where risk factors of interest are often

environmental exposures (rather than characteristics of the person, such as obesity or blood pressure), the question arises whether a 'doubly prospective' design is needed, i.e. the cohort is picked up before exposure as well as disease. Pre-exposure baseline data can thus be obtained and the cohort members can be monitored as some move into exposure conditions and through possible stages of reacting to exposure and being impacted by it. Obviously, such a 'doubly prospective' design is more expensive and cumbersome, particularly if there were to be a substantial lag between onset of exposure and first appearance of clinical or subclinical manifestations. However, there are a number of advantages to such a design.

(a) It offers a better handle on the issue of self-selection into exposure conditions in that possible differences in pre-existing person characteristics can be identified and adjusted as confounders, if needed.
(b) Psychosocial influences on CTDs that represent stable characteristics of the person can be disentangled from psychosocial variables that are altered by the exposure, but precede CTD development. The former may be viewed as vulnerability factors, while the latter may be seen as psychosocial mediating processes.
(c) Cohort members can be monitored for influences on symptom progression along severity–duration–disablement dimensions so that the etiology of CTDs can be understood apart from influences on rate of progression and final level of severity of CTDs.

The above four points have dealt with design issues bearing on the nature of the cohort to be assembled and the manner in which baseline data will be collected and follow-up will be carried out. Another major design issue in such observational (nonexperimental) epidemiologic studies concerns the type of information to be collected. In the case of CTDs and its presumptively complex biopsychosocial etiology, the set of potentially relevant variables is likely to be extensive.

Within the domain of psychosocial influences, one set of variables that needs to be assessed are trait-like or dispositional characteristics that remain relatively stable and reflect the pre-exposure baseline status of individual cohort members. There are three broad, somewhat overlapping objectives that these variables are intended to help to accomplish.

1. To determine if there are self-selection biases in relation to exposure status; pre-exposure differences on characteristics that relate to the outcome (CTD) would need to be identified and controlled in analysis.
2. To assess characteristics that may influence the measurement of CTDs, primarily as influences on the self-detection (experiencing) of symptoms and on reporting such symptoms, when experienced. If such characteristics are equally distributed in the exposed and unexposed groups, then they do not represent a source of bias. However, greater precision and understanding of the etiological dynamics may still be gained by detecting such influences and controlling for them in analysis.
3. To measure vulnerability factors, i.e. those pre-existing characteristics that interact with exposure status and increase the risk of CTDs among the exposed. If such characteristics (which relate to true etiology, not just the measurement of

CTDs) are equally distributed among the exposed and unexposed groups, then they do not bias the results. The primary value in detecting such relationships is in the potential for worker selection, i.e. selecting into high-exposure jobs workers who are low on the vulnerability dimensions.

It is not possible to go into detail regarding all the trait-like or dispositional characteristics (and their measurement) which could be viewed as relevant to the three objectives outlined above. The processes that influence the symptom experience and symptom reporting appear to be quite complex (e.g. Croyle and Barger, 1993; Leventhal, 1986; Pennebaker, 1982; Vassend, 1994), and operationalization of constructs lags considerably behind theoretical formulations of possible interrelationships. Furthermore, it is important to note that the empirical literature is based on investigating a variety of symptoms, often 'psychophysiological' ones, and it is not clear how well findings apply specifically to musculoskeletal symptoms. What follows is more an illustrative discussion of a limited number of traits.

One important dimension to consider is neuroticism (e.g. McCrae and Costa, 1990). The argument is that this is a trait of considerable stability across the adult life span, which represents a predisposition or vulnerability to experiencing symptoms of physical and emotional distress. Ego strength or ego resilience (Block, 1965) may be viewed as the opposite end of high neuroticism, but this concept is much less frequently utilized in the literature. However, the notion of predisposition (i.e. a 'true' influence on etiology) is only part of the discussion surrounding this concept. Two methodological areas of concern have been raised as well. One is that neuroticism may be a powerful undetected confounder in associations between life experience or psychosocial exposures and indicators of health and well-being. For example, a relationship between low social support and high levels of symptoms of distress could reflect the underlying role of neuroticism: those high on the trait are unable to enlist social support and are also higher on symptoms. Similarly, the association between exposure to a high number of stressful life events and high levels of symptoms of distress could again reflect the fact that those high on neuroticism experience more such events, as well as more symptoms. A second concern is along the lines of confounding in measurement itself. Those high on neuroticism have a lower threshold for detecting and reporting negative perceptions, affect, and symptoms, and to the extent that two separate measures (e.g. work stress and depression) are both influenced by this lower threshold, the true association between these is overestimated. The significance of the concept of neuroticism for the study of CTDs is as follows:

1. There could be a confounding association between exposure status and neuroticism.
2. There could be a true vulnerability effect, leading to higher rates of CTDs among those with high neuroticism and high exposure.
3. Neuroticism could be influencing an association between subjective perceptions of the job setting (e.g. job demands, job satisfaction) and CTDs.
4. When objective measures of work exposure are linked to higher rates of CTDs, measurement confounding should not be an issue.

Another formulation that is relevant to the present discussion (but overlaps with the issues raised above concerning neuroticism) deals with the dimensions of negative affectivity (NA) and positive affectivity (PA), two broad influences on self-report measures of a variety of moods and affective states (Tellegen, 1985; Watson and Clark, 1984; Watson and Pennebaker, 1989). The basic interpretation is that NA is a general factor of subjective distress, while PA reflects the level of pleasurable engagement with the environment. The evidence suggests that NA is an important influence on the perception and reporting of somatic complaints (especially those that are diffuse and widespread), but does not appear related to long-term disease outcomes; the role of PA is less clear. Thus some measure of NA would seem to be appropriate for inclusion in a study of CTDs in order to control for the possible influence of this dispositional characteristic. Negative affectivity has been found to predict neck and shoulder musculoskeletal symptoms in Swedish office workers (Bergqvist, 1993). However, it is not clear (1) whether NA adds sufficiently new information to a study which has already included a measure of neuroticism, (2) what the best measure of NA might be, since all indicators are indirect or inferred measures (e.g. the Taylor Manifest Anxiety Scale, Taylor, 1953), and (3) whether the influence of NA is also on musculoskeletal symptoms (versus the more diffuse symptoms only) and is sufficiently strong to warrant concern.

Another stable characteristic that can influence symptom reporting is social desirability. Most often the scale that has been used is the Crowne and Marlowe (1964) measure of the 'need for approval,' an index that is not dependent on measuring symptoms of psychopathology or dysphoria. Because the conceptualization and operationalization of this dimension are quite different from neuroticism or NA, it is likely that social desirability can make an independent contribution to out understanding of the influences on symptom reporting. Statistical adjustments for this dimension might be particularly useful when CTDs are being linked to subjective work environment dimensions such as job satisfaction or work demands.

There are other constructs that would seem useful in gaining a better understanding of additional influences on symptom recognition and symptom reporting. For example, Hansell and Mechanic (1986) discuss the role of introspectiveness in illness behavior: the formulation is that highly introspective individuals focus attention inward and habitually monitor self-related thoughts, feelings, and bodily states. Such inward-oriented monitoring can also be influenced by external circumstances; stressful life events, for example, could increase introspection. More intense monitoring of bodily states is likely to lower the threshold for detecting symptoms and, perhaps, for rating them as severe and/or painful. Another potentially relevant concept is somatization, the tendency to express emotional conflict and dysphoria in somatic symptoms. Somatization thus could represent a vulnerability factor among those in high-exposure groups, particularly if such exposure is also associated with negative perceptions or reactions to the work setting. Unfortunately, measures of somatization (e.g. Derogatis *et al.*, 1973) are simply symptom checklists reflecting actual symptoms reported, rather than measuring the 'tendency to somatize,' independently of the presence of actual symptoms.

In addition to measuring presumptively stable traits or characteristics, an investigation of the psychosocial influences on CTDs also needs to include measures of concepts that are intended to represent various subjective evaluations, perceptions, and reactions (states rather than traits) of the individual to his or her life and work circumstances. The primary objectives of including these state-like measures are (1) to determine whether they are altered by ergonomic exposures, prior to any development of musculoskeletal symptoms, (2) to determine whether they increase the vulnerability to CTD development among the exposed, and (3) to examine the possibility that they are influenced by CTDs but do not play a prior etiological role in CTD development.

Within the domain of the work environment, a plethora of measures is available to assess a wide range of psychosocial (nonergonomic) work dimensions and reactions to the work setting (Kasl, 1991). The relevant ones may be grouped as follows:

1. Temporal aspects of the work day and work itself:
   (a) shift work, particularly rotating shift;
   (b) overtime, unwanted, or 'excessive' hours;
   (c) two jobs;
   (d) piece work versus hourly pay (pay mechanism influencing pace);
   (e) fast pace of work, particularly in the presence of high vigilance demands;
   (f) not enough time to complete work deadlines;
   (g) scheduling of work and rest cycles;
   (h) variation in work load; and
   (i) interruptions.
2. Work content (other than temporal aspects):
   (a) fractionated, repetitive, monotonous work having low task/skill variety;
   (b) autonomy, independence, influence, control;
   (c) utilization of existing skills;
   (d) opportunity to learn new skills;
   (e) mental alertness and concentration;
   (f) unclear tasks or demands;
   (g) conflicting tasks or demands;
   (h) insufficient resources, given work demands or responsibilities (e.g. skills, machinery, organizational structure).
3. Interpersonal – work group:
   (a) opportunity to interact with co-workers (during work, during breaks, after work);
   (b) size, cohesiveness of primary work group;
   (c) recognition for work performance;
   (d) social support;
   (e) instrumental support;
   (f) equitable work load;
   (g) harassment.
4. Interpersonal – supervision:
   (a) participation in decision-making;
   (b) receiving feedback and recognition from supervisor;
   (c) providing supervisor with feedback;
   (d) closeness of supervision;
   (e) social support;
   (f) instrumental support;
   (g) unclear, conflicting demands;
   (h) harassment.

5. Organizational conditions:
   (a) size;
   (b) structure (e.g. 'flat' structure with relatively few levels in the organization);
   (c) having a staff position (versus line position);
   (d) working on the boundary of the organization;
   (e) relative prestige of the job;
   (f) unclear organizational structure (lines of responsibility, organizational basis for role conflict and ambiguity);
   (g) organizational (administrative) red tape and cumbersome (irrational) procedures;
   (h) discriminatory policies (e.g. hiring, promotion).

In addition to the above psychosocial work dimensions, it is important to consider the role of job satisfaction. While in principle it might be argued that in assessing the above-listed dimensions, one would be accounting for a large segment of the influences on job satisfaction, it would seem that job satisfaction (and its various components or dimensions) is worth monitoring in its own right. Job satisfaction reflects one type of an accommodation to the job and it need not parallel closely the evaluations and perceptions provided by other measures. In particular, it would be interesting to contrast two groups of workers: those who are satisfied, even though their perceptions are rather negative, and those who are dissatisfied, even though their perceptions and evaluations are rather positive. These two groups could experience and report on musculoskeletal symptoms in different ways.

While this chapter emphasizes psychosocial etiology and does not deal explicitly with 'objective' work environment characteristics that define the basic exposure factors, it needs to be emphasized that the above psychosocial dimensions are seen as possible moderators and/or mediators of the basic exposure–CTD association, not as independent risk factors. Among the objective, ergonomic factors that help to define exposure, the following are important to consider:

1. The biomechanical aspects of tasks that need to be performed (Keyserling *et al.*, 1991; Stock, 1991):
   (a) rapid repetitive movements and less frequent, more forceful exertions;
   (b) static muscle loading;
   (c) awkward work postures and extreme joint position;
   (d) localized contact stresses; and
   (e) whole-body or segmental vibrations.
2. The temporal distribution of these tasks, including total percentage of time and scheduling of rest periods.
3. Biomedical characteristics of individuals that represent special musculoskeletal strengths and/or vulnerabilities.
4. Aspects of the ambient physical environment, such as noise, temperature extremes, dust, and so on.

In addition to the perceptions and evaluations that focus on the work environment, it would seem that some monitoring of the nonwork setting and of its impact is needed. These nonwork influences may represent (1) buffers, such as high levels of social–emotional support from spouse, and (2) vulnerabilities, such as recent experiences of stressful life events, or chronic financial distress. Unfortunately, the choice of measures in this area is enormous (Cohen *et al.*, 1995), and yet these variables are secondary in the overall study of psychosocial influences on CTDs. As a drastic compromise, the following indicators could be recommended for inclusion in repeated assessments of the cohort as it is followed for development of musculoskeletal problems: (1) a general screening measure of distress, such as the demoralization scale (Dohrenwend *et al.*, 1986), in order to monitor fluctuations in mental health and well-being; (2) a general measure of subjective stress exposure, such as the perceived stress scale (Cohen *et al.*, 1983) in order to monitor changes in global subjective exposures; (3) an abbreviated checklist of stressful life events (Turner and Wheaton, 1995); (4) some brief index of marital role stressors (Lepore, 1995); and (5) some monitoring of lifestyle habits (e.g. smoking, alcohol consumption, physical activity) and social–leisure activities. It should be noted that the first two measures listed will be quite highly correlated with each other (and with neuroticism and NA) in cross-sectional analyses, but over time, their fluctuations should be less correlated and should provide useful independent information on changes in stress and distress.

Our final comments on data collection concern company records which can provide additional useful information. For example, data on work absences can reveal different patterns of relationships with musculoskeletal symptoms, such as individual differences in duration or intensity thresholds for triggering absences, or the use of absences to gain temporary relief from symptoms. Many of the psychosocial variables discussed above may help to explain such differential dynamics. Similarly, medical-care information, including the use of medication, may detect individuals who have a high use of services or medication for a relatively low level of severity of symptoms; rate of progression to CTD and ultimate severity level of CTD may be affected by such differences. Or, differences between workers with CTDs of comparable severity who do versus those who do not seek workers' compensation may again be partly explained by the psychosocial data collected. However, it should be emphasized that any and all of the associations with absences, medical-care variables, and workers' compensation claims filing may remain ambiguous: on the one hand, such associations may serve to 'verify' or 'legitimize' the musculoskeletal complaints, or, on the other hand, they may represent exaggerated responses, secondary gain seeking, or 'malingering.'

In the last section we want to offer brief comments on data analysis strategies and the conceptual/theoretical model which may be most appropriate to guide such analyses. We believe that the *sine qua non* of the analysis, the basic first step, is to establish the association between objective descriptors of the work environment – the objectively characterized biomechanical and ergonomic factors which represent the exposure variable that is the fundamental risk factor – and the progression of musculoskeletal symptoms up to meeting the criteria for CTD diagnosis. The second step in analysis should be to add precision and refinement to understanding the basic association between exposure and CTDs: (1) examine the role of length of exposure; (2) daily proportion of exposure episodes; (3) scheduling of rest periods or breaks or periods of exercise; (4) workstation ergonomic factors; (5) posture; (6) musculoskeletal strengths and weaknesses of individual workers. These two steps are intended to characterize the 'basic' relationship at the biomedical/biomechanical level before psychosocial factors are entered in analysis. Subsequent steps in analysis can then examine the ways in which psychosocial variables alter our understanding of the 'basic' relationship. There would seem to be two primary ways in which this happens:

1. Psychosocial variables can be causally antecedent to variables that increase CTD risk: for example, nonsupportive supervisors could result in workers taking fewer rest breaks, or workers in psychologically demanding jobs that allow very little discretion in carrying out the tasks could have poor posture and more muscle tension.
2. Psychosocial variables can moderate the effect of exposure so that for some levels of the psychosocial variable exposure has a strong effect on CTDs, while for other levels it has a weaker effect (but the mechanism of this moderating influence is unknown and does not appear to involve the basic biomechanical dynamics).

Two additional types of associations between psychosocial variables and CTDs may be observed: (1) CTDs increase the level of a variable, such as general distress, but the variable plays no role in the etiology of CTDs; (2) a psychosocial variable is an independent risk factor for CTDs (a main effect) even when the multivariate analysis adjusts for all the variables that define high-risk exposure. The last association may be difficult to interpret. It could represent a measurement influence (self-detection and/or reporting of musculoskeletal symptoms), it could indicate a non-ergonomic, nonwork-related risk factor for CTDs, or it could point to a subset of (unexposed) workers who do not have 'true' CTDs. In the absence of a definite golden standard for assessing CTDs, we will not be able to choose among these interpretations.

PRELIMINARY RESULTS REGARDING POSSIBLE PSYCHOSOCIAL INFLUENCES ON CTDs AMONG OFFICE WORKERS

In this section of the paper, we present some preliminary cross-sectional evidence on the role of psychosocial factors in the epidemiology of CTDs. The data come from the 'Ergonomics and Your Health Project.' The project originated in 1991, when the authors were approached by the Director of Occupational Safety and Health for a large aerospace manufacturing company to help to develop an approach to managing ergonomic-related health problems in the workforce. The request was motivated by company staff estimates that ergonomic factors in the work environment were the root cause of 50 per cent of the injuries and workers' compensation costs. In collaboration with labor and management, the 'Ergonomics and Your Health Project' was designed to: (1) identify health problems before they result in functional disabilities, reporting injuries, and expensive workers' compensation claims; (2) prioritize ergonomic interventions to direct capital expenditures into the jobs with the most significant health problems; and (3) carry out a follow-up survey to assess the effectiveness of interventions.

From September, 1991 to May, 1992 we collaborated with workers to develop and pilot-test a survey. Thirty-eight workers participated in the pilot project. Significant changes resulted from the pilot testing: (1) drinking questions were dropped from the survey based on strong comments from workers; (2) more questions were added to assess the 'work relatedness' of musculoskeletal symptoms; and (3) a large number of questions were added to assess psychosocial stressors in the work environment. The finding that workers felt that more questions were needed to identify whether the CTD was work related provided a unique opportunity to extend the typical National Institute for Occupational Safety and Health (NIOSH) CTD symptom-reporting question battery.

Prior to distributing the survey, a letter went out from the president of the company and the president of the union local in support of the project. The sample was established jointly by members of business units within the company and the occupational safety and health staff. Jobs were identified where there was a high likelihood of musculoskeletal injury and presumably a need for ergonomic intervention and a group of comparable jobs that were viewed as low risk. The company approved workers completing the survey on company time. The survey was distributed within the company during October, 1992–February, 1993. The overall response rate for the survey was 64 per cent – 1779 workers completed the survey. In the following analyses, we report on cross-sectional data collected from 805 salaried (office) workers who had an overall participation rate of 65 per cent. The sample of office workers was composed of 282 women and 523 men.

While visual, cardiovascular, and respiratory symptoms were also measured, we report here only on musculoskeletal CTDs of the hand–wrist. Following NIOSH (1992), a work-related CTD was defined as: symptoms present in the previous year; symptoms occurred with a frequency of once per week or symptoms had a duration of one month or more. The symptom must be reported as being work related and beginning on the current job. Finally, people were excluded if they reported a previous accident or trauma to the hand–wrist region that may have caused the symptoms. Appendix 1 contains the section of the questionnaire that questioned workers about symptoms in the hand/wrist. Because workers were asked to assess symptoms over the past year, all estimates are one year period prevalence estimates.

While a large amount of the survey is devoted to identifying musculoskeletal problems in the neck–shoulder, elbows, hand–wrist, back, and lower extremities, we also attempted to measure a variety of psychosocial factors. A major concern of the company was that individual differences in perceiving and reporting symptoms would be more important determinants of the prevalence of CTDs rather than the work environment. To answer these concerns we included measures of neuroticism and social desirability. Neuroticism was measured using the NEO 48-item measure developed by Costa and McCrae (1992). This measure has been shown to be a relatively stable trait in adult life. People who are neurotic tend to report more symptoms than nonneurotics. To measure a possible response bias, we used the 13-item social desirability scale derived from the original Crowne–Marlowe measure of social desirability (Reynolds, 1982). The higher the score, the more likely it is that individuals seek to present themselves in a favorable light and report fewer symptoms. Both measures were recoded as indicator variables with 1 representing a higher score.

Worker reports of the importance of psychosocial stressors and growing evidence in the literature that psychosocial conditions of work predict CTDs (Kuorinka and Forcier, 1995) led us to include a range of measures of psychosocial work environment factors. The job-strain model developed by Karasek and Theorell (1990) predicts that workers in jobs with little job-decision latitude and heavy psychological demands experience job strain. We measured both psychological job demands and job-decision latitude with measures from the Karasek Job Content Survey (Karasek, 1991). The higher the score on the five-item psychological demands scale, the more the demands. Job-decision latitude is the sum of two scales – a six-item measure of skill discretion and a three-item measure of decision authority. In analyses reported here, we use these scales rather than creating the job-strain measure. Because several parts of the company were reorganizing from an assembly-line production system to a cell-based production system, we hypothesized that roles may change to create ambiguity or conflict. We used measures developed by Kahn and colleagues to assess role conflict and role ambiguity (Caplan *et al.*, 1975). We reverse-scored the four-item role ambiguity scale so that it measures role clarity. The higher the score, the more clarity and less ambiguity. However, the higher the score on the four-item role conflict measure, the greater the conflict. Because of the economic problems in the aerospace industry we measured job insecurity. One additional item was added to the three-item job insecurity measure in the Karasek instrument (Karasek, 1991). This item asked workers if their security was completely tied to the future of the company. Finally, we included an 18-item measure of cognitive demands. This experimental measure is under development by Dr Naomi Swanson at NIOSH (used with permission). The measure was designed to assess information-processing demands in office workers. The index is composed of six subscales (short-term memory, long-term memory, divided attention, focused attention, decision-making and overall task difficulty). In these analyses, we present results for the overall task difficulty scale. The higher the score, the more task difficulty experienced.

Social relationships at work may buffer the affect of demanding work conditions on health (House, 1981). We measured support from the supervisor, co-workers, and spouse using measures developed by House (1992). The higher the score on each of these four-item measures, the greater the level of combined instrumental and emotional support.

Satisfied workers may interpret their job differently or report symptoms differently compared to those who are dissatisfied (Spector, 1992). We measured the satisfaction of the worker with a range of work conditions, for example, pay, boss, co-workers, use of skills, chances for promotion, job security, workstation, and tool use. We summed responses to 10 items to create an overall satisfaction scale. Finally, individual psychological functioning may influence (and be influenced by) the reporting of work conditions and CTDs. We used a well-validated 27-item measure of global demoralization developed by Dohrenwend and colleagues (1986). The higher the score, the more nonspecific psychological distress the individual experiences.

To protect the confidentiality of workers as well as for purposes of analysis, we used a standard occupational coding system developed by the company Human Resources Department to group manufacturing jobs. Jobs were grouped if they required similar types of biomechanical actions and would likely require similar types of ergonomic interventions. The grouping was done by company engineers trained in ergonomic assessment and the health and safety staff of the company.

To group salaried jobs, we asked members of each business unit to group jobs by the amount of video display terminal (VDT) use. These groupings were reviewed by occupational safety and health staff responsible for office ergonomics in the company and familiar with the jobs. Any questionable groupings were reviewed by both business unit personnel and occupational safety and health staff. The final groupings were 0–29, 30–49, 50–79, 80–100 per cent, and 'variable' VDT usage. The variable category represents workers initially classified as using VDTs at least 50 per cent of the time, but it was difficult to place these people precisely in either the 50–79 per cent or 80 per cent and above categories. Furthermore, these workers were more often professionals whose use of the VDT varied because they were either in their office or on the shop floor solving a problem. We present results in this chapter for workers using the VDT 49 per cent or less of the time (low exposure) and those using it 50 per cent or more of the time (high exposure).

One problem that a cross-sectional design will not allow us to untangle is self-selection into jobs. We examined whether workers classified as high exposure differed from workers classified as low exposure for three health questions: measures of neuroticism, social desirability, and demoralization. We found no differences for the three individual states and traits and for self-reported health (poor to excellent), perceived effect of job on health (no effect to caused health problems), or perceived control that the individual has over his/her health (no control to complete control). We also considered whether the psychosocial work conditions varied by VDT use and surprisingly found no differences in measures of social support, skill discretion, decision authority, psychological job demands, and role clarity. Given that these data are cross-sectional, some associations would have been ambiguous, but the absence of an association is not (unless one assumes selective attrition which took place prior to data collection).

Table 16.1 shows the prevalence of hand–wrist CTDs by levels of VDT use. Women office workers have a higher prevalence for all levels of VDT use. These prevalence rates can be compared to hourly (manufacturing) workers. For example, assemblers had a prevalence of hand–wrist CTDs of 29.4 per cent, equipment metal-forming workers 33.3 per cent, and hand-finishing workers 28.0 per cent. Some hourly jobs had low rates, such as fusion welding 0 per cent, and inspection 5.2 per cent.

Table 16.2 shows the odds ratios for the classification used in Table 16.1. The inclusion of workers with 'variable' VDT exposure adds more professional women and men (engineers) into the high-risk category. While it increases the odds ratio for men, the risk remains nonsignificant; however, the significant risk for women becomes marginally significant. The significant risk is likely due to the large number of data-entry type jobs that women hold in the company (known to be high-risk

Table 16.1 Prevalence of hand–wrist CTDs by level of VDT use stratified by gender.

	Level of VDT use			
	<50%	≥50%	Variable	Total
All (%)	5.7	10.4	9.4	8.5
Women (%)	8.2	17.2	12.1	14.3
Men (%)	4.9	4.8	8.3	5.4

Table 16.2 Odds ratios for the risk of hand–wrist CTDs with and without variable VDT use stratified by gender

	Level of VDT use	
	<50% vs. ≥50% (excludes variable exposure)	<50% vs. ≥50% (includes variable exposure)
All (%)	1.92 (1.17–3.13)	1.87 (1.06–3.28)
Women (%)	2.33 (1.09–4.97)	2.19 (0.90–5.32)
Men (%)	0.97 (0.47–2.00)	1.19 (0.55–2.54)

jobs), which becomes less significant when the professional women are included. These differences were not changed when adjusted for age.

In Tables 16.3 and 16.4 we begin to examine the NIOSH definition of CTDs. Table 16.3 shows the risk for four components of the definition and three additional

Table 16.3 Odds ratios for components of hand–wrist CTD diagnosis.

	Level of VDT use	
	<50% vs. ≥50% (excludes variable exposure)	<50% vs. ≥50% (includes variable exposure)
Symptoms past year	1.47	1.38
Symptoms at least 1 per week	1.56	1.45 (ns)
Symptoms last at least 1 month	1.27 (ns)	1.33 (ns)
Pain intensity at least 'moderate'	1.41 (ns)	1.33 (ns)
Work makes symptoms worse	1.76	1.75
Vacation makes symptoms better	1.68	1.64
Symptoms started in current job (vs. other job, or not job related, among those with symptoms)	2.29 (70.7% vs. 51.3%)	2.19 (67.7% vs. 51.3%)

Table 16.4 Comparison of percent reporting onset of symptoms on current job to all others among those office workers with symptoms.

Hand–Wrist Symptoms				
		Males (%)	Females (%)	Total (%)
How often (frequently or almost always)	Current	42.0	45.2	43.4
	Others	41.9	50.0	44.9
How long (>1–2 weeks or longer)	Current	20.1	24.0	21.8
	Others	22.6	26.5	24.1
Intensity (moderate or worse)	Current	52.9	67.7	59.1
	Others	47.3	74.8	57.7
Last 7 days (experience a problem)	Current	49.8	51.6	50.6
	Others	49.7	61.2	54.0
Effect of work (makes worse)	Current	42.4	47.0	44.4
	Others	22.0	34.0	26.6
Effect of vacation (makes better)	Current	47.1	51.6	49.0
	Others	16.8	33.3	23.0
Exercise to relieve problem	Current	30.6	39.1	34.2
	Others	25.9	29.1	27.1
Onset (gradual)	Current	78.5	80.4	79.3
	Others	52.7	71.8	59.9

items (working makes the symptoms worse, vacation makes the symptoms better, intensity of symptoms). Compared to the overall risk of 1.92 when using the NIOSH CTD case definition, only 'whether the symptoms started on the current job' has a significantly higher risk for those in the high-exposure category. The table also shows, again, that inclusion of the 'variable' exposure category does not substantially change the findings, but the odds ratios are slightly lower in most comparisons. This would be expected since workers in the 'variable' exposure category would have a less continuous exposure to VDT work and would be exposed for periods of shorter duration, both contributing to a lower frequency. Additionally, it appears that questions of symptom intensity rated by 'pain' and symptom duration of at least a month do not significantly differ across the exposure levels. Yet, whether work and vacation influence symptoms does significantly differentiate high- from low-exposure categories. If this is a cumulative work-related injury, then we would expect the symptoms to be worse at work compared to nonwork and to get better on vacation. If the symptoms have progressed to a pathological state (such as carpal tunnel syndrome), we might not expect these items to differentiate exposure. However, the significance of these items in a general office worker population points to their potential utility in an active surveillance program to identify the high-risk jobs. These findings suggest the need to monitor symptoms in the early stages of CTD development, as well as using additional sensitive items not part of the NIOSH CTD case definition such as work and vacation effect on symptoms.

Table 16.4 considers whether those who report that 'the symptoms are related to their current job' differ from those who report that symptoms were related to either another job or not work related. This table only reports on those workers who responded yes to the symptom-screener question shown in the appendix. The three notable findings are: the effect of work, the effect of vacation, and the gradual onset. These findings reinforce the results of Table 16.3 which pointed to the importance of the work and vacation items for monitoring early stages of CTD.

Table 16.5 broadly summarizes the effects of several psychosocial factors on the components of CTDs and on the additional item measuring whether work makes the symptoms worse. The lack of an effect for social desirability is reassuring.

Table 16.5 Summary of psychosocial influences on components of CTD.

	Effect of neuroticism	Effect of demoralization	Effect of social desirability
How often in the past year	0	0	0
How long does problem usually last	0	0	0
Describe intensity of problem (pain)	0	+	0
Job attribution: started on present job	++	++	0
Effect of regular work activities: makes it worse	++	++	0

However, we found a moderately strong effect for neuroticism. The findings suggest that neuroticism may operate as a possible bias by influencing attribution of symptoms to the job and the judgment that work makes symptoms worse. The effects of demoralization appear similar to those of neuroticism, in part, because the two scales are well correlated cross-sectionally. The fact that pain intensity relates to demoralization only, suggests that pain influences demoralization rather than that demoralization represents a reporting bias. The differential role of neuroticism versus demoralization awaits prospective, longitudinal data for more definitive interpretation.

In Table 16.6, we consider the effect of adjustment and stratification on the risk of CTDs comparing office workers in high-risk jobs (50 per cent or more time at VDT) to low-risk jobs. Adjustments for a range of factors do not significantly alter the overall unadjusted relationship between VDT use and CTDs, represented by the odds ratio of 1.87. The only exception to this is spouse support. This finding suggests that spouse support is acting as a negative confounder. Respondents who are low on spouse support (where the effect of VDT exposure is much stronger) are more likely to be found in the low VDT exposure groups.

The stratification results in Table 16.6 are far more revealing. Notably, the findings suggest a stronger effect within one of the levels of several psychosocial vari-

Table 16.6 Influences on odds ratio comparing high to low VDT exposure.

All subjects	1.87 (1.06–3.28) Adjustments	Stratified analysis	
Sex	1.58 (0.88–2.83)	Women	2.19 (0.90–5.32)
		Men	1.19 (0.55–2.54)
Age	1.87 (1.06–3.30)	≤35	2.00 (0.90–4.43)
		≥36	1.75 (0.80–3.80)
Education	1.74 (0.98–3.09)	<College	2.14 (0.98–4.68)
		≥College	1.34 (0.59–3.04)
Neuroticism	1.87 (1.06–3.30)	Low	1.96 (0.95–4.06)
		High	1.86 (0.72–4.81)
Demoralization	1.88 (1.06–3.31)	Low	1.42 (0.62–3.25)
		High	2.31 (1.09–4.92)
Overall job satisfaction	1.90 (1.07–3.38)	Low	1.58 (0.77–3.26)
		High	2.43 (1.00–5.89)
Social support supervisor	1.92 (1.08–3.40)	Low	2.13 (0.95–4.77)
		High	1.65 (0.76–3.56)
Co-worker support	1.84 (1.04–3.25)	Low	1.52 (0.72–3.23)
		High	2.32 (1.00–5.37)
Spouse support	2.55 (1.24–5.23)	Low	4.46 (1.29–5.40)
		High	1.29 (0.67–2.48)
Skill discretion	1.85 (1.04–3.26)	Low	2.51 (1.08–5.80)
		High	1.39 (0.65–2.96)
Psychological job demands	1.83 (1.03–3.23)	Low	0.84 (0.35–2.00)
		High	2.99 (1.38–6.47)
Role conflict	1.86 (1.05–3.29)	Low	1.61 (0.58–4.46)
		High	1.97 (1.01–3.85)

Note: Includes the variable exposure group.

ables: gender, education, demoralization, job satisfaction, supervisor and co-worker support, skill discretion, and psychological job demands. Not all findings fit an expected vulnerability relationship, suggesting that other dynamics may be contributing to the distribution of CTDs among office workers. High levels of co-worker support and of job satisfaction increase the risk of CTDs when working at a VDT. The contrast between supervisor support and co-worker support is particularly interesting. The risk estimates may reflect, in part, the influences on measurement of CTDs in a survey instrument, but without a 'gold standard' to assess true prevalence this type of effect must be cautiously interpreted. Finally, the skill discretion, job demand effects suggest that the combined impact, as hypothesized by Karasek to be 'true' job strain, may produce an even more substantial odds ratio. Overall, these findings support the assertion by workers in the company that psychosocial factors are important in the etiology of CTDs.

In Table 16.7, we adjust for the role of VDT use and consider how the variables in the table influence (or are influenced by) CTDs. The results reveal several significant relationships. Some psychosocial variables appear to increase the risk of CTDs such as demoralization, role conflict, and psychological job demands. The psychological job demand risk is highest for workers in the high VDT use group. However, other factors such as job satisfaction, skill discretion, and task difficulty protect the worker from developing CTDs. Given that these are cross-sectional data, we cannot disentangle the underlying explanation for the observed relationship. For example, workers who develop CTDs may become demoralized rather than demoralization producing CTDs. A job may be more psychologically demanding as a consequence of the presence of CTDs rather than the job demands producing the condition.

However, an alternative, yet equally plausible explanation is that these psychosocial work environment measures create a picture of high-risk jobs. These jobs would have little skill discretion, conflict would exist about the role of the person and there

Table 16.7 Some correlates of hand–wrist CTDs adjusted for VDT use.

	OR (confidence limits)
Neuroticism	1.54 (0.93–2.55)
Demoralization	1.65 (1.00–2.73)
Overall job satisfaction	0.50 (0.30–0.84)
Job insecurity	1.10 (0.67–1.83)
Supervisor support	0.94 (0.87–1.01)
Co-worker support	0.91 (0.82–1.01)
Spouse support	1.01 (0.90–1.14)
Skill discretion	0.58 (0.35–0.95)
Decision authority	0.71 (0.43–1.17)
Role conflict	1.97 (1.13–3.45)
Task difficulty	0.57 (0.36–0.97)
Psychological job demands	1.93 (1.13–3.31)
– Within low VDT use	0.79 (0.31–2.05)
– Within high VDT use	2.82 (1.45–5.47)

Note: Includes the variable exposure group.

Table 16.8 The role of social desirability in hand–wrist CTDs

Continuous scoring	1.19 (0.35–4.07)
Dichotomous scoring	1.00 (0.60–1.66)
By level of VDT use	
– Low	0.61 (0.24–1.58)
– High	1.18 (0.65–2.14)
Association of VDT use with CTDs	1.87 (1.06–3.28)
– Low social desirability	1.30 (0.57–2.93)
– High social desirability	2.50 (1.14–5.43)

Note: Includes the variable exposure group.

would be heavy job demands. This type of job represents the job of workers in companies where there have been layoffs, workers have been asked to perform more and often to take on supervisory responsibilities. We might expect that jobs with more overall task difficulty would place workers at greater risk, but in the company that we studied, jobs with task difficulty have more skill discretion commensurate with the difficulty. These jobs are more likely to be the engineering jobs that comprise a substantial proportion of the 'variable' exposure category. As suggestive as the evidence in Table 16.7 is, the cross-sectional design precludes any definitive conclusion.

Table 16.8 examines the role of social desirability in CTDs. The unexpected result of this table is that workers in high-exposure jobs who are more likely to respond in a socially desirable way are at greater risk. We are uncertain at this point how best to interpret this finding, since all other analyses found no relationship between level of social desirability and symptoms of CTD.

In summary, we have presented results from a study confirming people who use VDTs for more than 50 per cent of the time are at greater risk of hand–wrist CTDs, using a NIOSH self-report definition of CTD. In concert with a range of studies we have found women office workers to be at greater risk. We have suggested a potential moderating role for a range of psychosocial variables including job demands and skill discretion. Further suggestive evidence indicates that psychosocial variables may have either an independent influence on the development of CTDs or influence the reporting of CTDs. These findings await confirmation with longitudinal data.

SUMMARY

In this chapter, we have discussed the psychosocial epidemiological perspective as one research paradigm to use to investigate the etiology of CTDs. We highlighted several major conceptual, design, and analytic issues to consider when planning to conduct a study of the role of psychosocial factors in the etiology of CTDs. Then, we presented cross-sectional evidence from our study of CTDs in a large aerospace manufacturing company. Results suggested several plausible contributions of psychosocial variables to the process of CTD development and identification. Definitive interpretation of the results requires prospective evidence.

APPENDIX 1: SURVEY QUESTIONNAIRE FOR 'ERGONOMICS AND YOUR HEALTH' PROJECT (HAND/WRIST SYMPTOMS)

We would like to ask you some questions about how you feel in the HAND/WRIST areas shown in the four diagrams below.

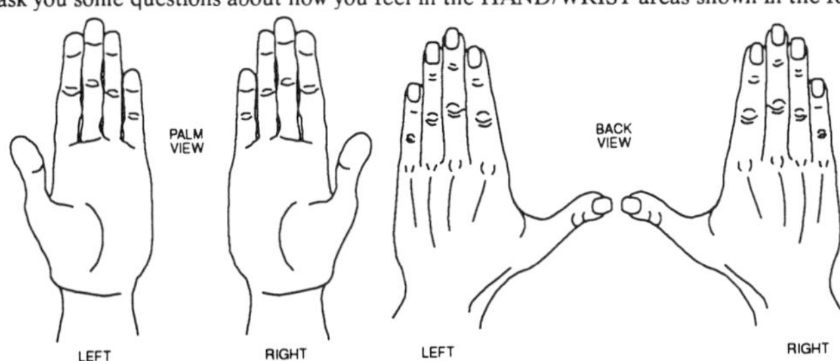

6. In the PAST YEAR, have you had pain, aching, stiffness, burning, numbness, or tingling in the area shown in the diagrams?
   Yes ☐ 1
   No ☐ 2 ☞ IF NO, please go to Question 6zz on page 19

6a. Which hand bothers you most? Right ☐ 1 Left ☐ 2 Both ☐ 3

6b. **HOW OFTEN** have you had this HAND/WRIST problem in the PAST YEAR?
   Almost never (every 6 months or less) ☐ 1
   Rarely (every 2–3 months) ☐ 2
   Sometimes (once a month) ☐ 3
   Frequently (once a week) ☐ 4
   Almost always (daily) ☐ 5

6c. **HOW LONG** does this HAND/WRIST problem usually last?
   Less than one hour (< 1 hour) ☐ 0
   1 hour to one day (< 24 hours) ☐ 1
   More than 1 day to 1 week ☐ 2
   More than 1 week to 2 weeks ☐ 3
   More than 2 weeks to 4 weeks ☐ 4
   More than 1 month to 3 months ☐ 5
   More than 3 months ☐ 6

6d. On average, describe the **INTENSITY** of this HAND/WRIST problem using the scale below: (Check ✓ the best answer)

0	1	2	3	4
(no pain)	(mild)	(moderate)	(severe)	(worst pain ever in life)
☐	☐	☐	☐	☐

6e. Have you had this HAND/WRIST problem in the past 7 days?
   Yes ☐ 1 No ☐ 2

6f. Are you taking any medication for this HAND/WRIST problem?
   Yes ☐ 1 No ☐ 2

6g. Which statement most accurately describes when this HAND/WRIST problem first started?
   Before the past year ☐ 1
   During the past year ☐ 2

6h. When you first experienced this HAND/WRIST problem, was it the result of:
   A sudden action with clear beginning to problem ☐ 1
   Gradual buildup with no clear beginning to problem ☐ 2 ☞ **IF GRADUAL**, please go to Question 6j

6i. If this was a sudden action, was the first time you experienced this HAND/WRIST problem:
   Related to a work activity ☐ 1
   Related to an activity at home ☐ 2
   Related to a sporting activity ☐ 3
   Related to a motor vehicle accident ☐ 4
   Other ☐ 5 Please describe ____________________

Please go to Question 6k

6j. If gradual buildup, what activity (or activities) do you associate with this HAND/WRIST problem?
   A specific activity or task at work ☐ 1
   My work in general ☐ 2
   Not related to my work ☐ 3
   Don't know ☐ 4

6k. Going back to when you first experienced this HAND/WRIST problem, what job were you in?

My problem is not job related	❑ 1
I was on my current job at Hamilton Standard	❑ 2
I was on a previous job at Hamilton Standard	❑ 3 Please describe job ____________
I was on a previous job outside the company	❑ 4 Please describe job ____________

6l. Since you first experienced this HAND/WRIST problem, has it changed in any way?

No change	❑ 1
Has gotten better	❑ 2
Has gotten worse	❑ 3

6m. Does this HAND/WRIST problem usually wake you from sleep? Yes ❑ 1 No ❑ 2

6n. Does shaking your hands in the air make this HAND/WRIST problem:

Better ❑ 1 Worse ❑ 2 No change ❑ 3

6o. On a day-to-day basis, do regular work activities make this HAND/WRIST problem:

Better ❑ 1 Worse ❑ 2 No change ❑ 3

6p. When on vacation, does this HAND/WRIST problem get:

Better ❑ 1 Worse ❑ 2 No change ❑ 3

6q. In the PAST YEAR, has this HAND/WRIST problem resulted in your:

	No	1–5 times	More than 5 times
a. Seeing a Physician, nurse, physician assistant, nurse practitioner	❑ 1	❑ 2	❑ 3
b. Seeing a Chiropractor	❑ 1	❑ 2	❑ 3
c. Seeing a Physical therapist	❑ 1	❑ 2	❑ 3
d. Seeing a Therapeutic masseuse	❑ 1	❑ 2	❑ 3
e. Missing work	❑ 1	❑ 2	❑ 3
f. Wearing a splint	❑ 1	❑ 2	❑ 3
g. Assigned temporarily to light duty	❑ 1	❑ 2	❑ 3
h. Assigned to another job	No ❑ 1	Yes ❑ 2	
i. Getting injections	No ❑ 1	Yes ❑ 2	

6r. Which word or set of words would you use to describe the pattern of this HAND/WRIST problem? (Please check ✓ the one best answer)

❑ 1	❑ 2	❑ 3
Continuous	Rhythmic	Brief
Steady	Periodic	Momentary
Constant	Intermittent	Transient

6s. Do you do exercises to relieve this HAND/WRIST problem?

Yes ❑ 1 No ❑ 2 ☞ IF NO, please go to Question 6u

6t. If yes, during an average work day, how many times do you stop to do exercises?

1 time a day	❑ 1
2–3 times a day	❑ 2
4–5 times a day	❑ 3
6–8 times a day	❑ 4
More than 8	❑ 5 How many? ________

6u. Has your physician ever recommended surgery for problems in your HANDS/WRISTS?

Yes ❑ 1 No ❑ 2 ☞ IF NO, please go to Question 6z

6v. Have you ever had surgery for problems in your HANDS/WRISTS?

Yes ❑ 1 No ❑ 2 ☞ IF NO, please go to Question 6z

6w. If yes, please describe the surgery and the year you had it:

Surgery	Year
____________________	19______
____________________	19______
____________________	19______
____________________	19______
____________________	19______

6x. Has any of the surgery described above been for <u>your current HAND/WRIST problem</u>?

Yes ❑ 1 No ❑ 2 ☞ **<u>IF NO,</u>** please go to Question 6z

6y. If yes, did this make your current HAND/WRIST problem:

Better ❑ 1 Worse ❑ 2 No change ❑ 3

6z. Have you ever had an accident or sudden injury to your HANDS/WRISTS, such as a sports injury, a motor vehicle injury, the loss of a hand or a digit, a laceration requiring stitches, or a tendon tear <u>not related to your current hand/wrist problems</u> you have been describing?

Yes ❑ 1 No ❑ 2

Please go to Question 7 on page 19

REFERENCES

BAMMER, G. and MARTIN, B. 1988 The arguments about RSI: An examination, *Community Health Studies*, **12**, 348–58.

BAMMER, G. and MARTIN, B. 1992 Repetition strain injury in Australia: Medical knowledge, social movement and de facto partisanship, *Social Problems*, **39**, 219–37.

BERGQVIST, U. 1993 *Health Problems During Work with Visual Display Terminals*, Stockholm: Institute for Environmental Medicine, Karolinska Institute, Series No. 28.

BLOCK, J. 1965 *The Challenge of Response Sets*, New York: Appleton-Century-Crofts.

CAPLAN, R., COBB, S., FRENCH, J. R., VAN HARRISON, R. and PINNEAU, S. 1975 *Job Demands and Worker Health*, USDHEW (NIOSH) 75–160, Washington, DC: US Government Printing Office.

COHEN, S., KAMARCK, T. and MERMELSTEIN, R. 1983 A global measure of perceived stress, *Journal of Health and Social Behavior*, **24**, 385–96.

COHEN, S., KESSLER, R. C. and GORDON, L. U. (Eds) 1995 *Measuring Stress*, New York: Oxford University Press.

COSTA, P. and MCCRAE, R. 1992 *NEO PI-R Professional Manual*, Odessa, FL: PAR.

CROWNE, D. P. and MARLOWE, C. 1964 *The Approval Motive: Studies in Evaluative Dependence*, New York: Wiley.

CROYLE, R. T. and BARGER, S. D. 1993 Illness cognition, in MAES, S., LEVENTHAL, H. and JOHNSTON, M. (Eds), *International Review of Health Psychology*, Vol. 2, pp. 29–49, Chichester: John Wiley.

DEROGATIS, L. R., LIPMAN, R. S. and COVI, L. 1973 SCL-90: An outpatient psychiatric scale: Preliminary report, *Psychopharmacology Bulletin*, **9**, 13–27.

DOHRENWEND, B. P., LEVAV, I. and SHROUT, P. E. 1986 Screening scales from the Psychiatric Epidemiology Research Interview (PERI), in WEISSMAN, M. M., MYERS, J. K. and ROSS, C. E. (Eds), *Community Surveys of Psychiatric Disorders*, pp. 349–75, New Brunswick: Rutgers University Press.

HANSELL, S. and MECHANIC, D. 1986 The socialization of introspection and illness behavior, in MCHUGH, S. and VALLIS, T. M. (Eds), *Illness Behavior: A Multidisciplinary Model*, pp. 253–60, New York: Plenum Press.

HOUSE, J. 1981 *Work Stress and Social Support*, Reading, MA: Addison-Wesley.

HOUSE, J. 1992 *The America's Changing Lives Survey*, Ann Arbor, MI: ISR, University of Michigan.

KARASEK, R. 1991 *The Job Content Questionnaire User's Guide*, Lowell, MA: Department of Work Environment, University of Massachusetts.

KARASEK, R. A. and THEORELL, T. 1990 *Healthy Work: Stress, Productivity, and the Reconstruction of Working Life*, New York: Basic Books.

KASL, S. V. 1991 Assessing health risk in the work setting, in SCHROEDER, H. E. (Ed.), *New Directions in Health Psychology Assessment*, pp. 95–125, New York: Hemisphere Publishing.

KELSEY, J. L., THOMPSON, W. D. and EVANS, A. S. 1986 *Methods in Observational Epidemiology*, New York, NY: Oxford University Press.

KEYSERLING, W. M., ARMSTRONG, T. J. and PUNNETT, L. 1991 Ergonomic job analysis: A structured approach for identifying risk factors associated with overexertion injuries and disorders, *Applied Occupational and Environmental Hygiene*, **6**, 353–63.

KIESLER, S. and FINHOLT, T. 1988 The mystery of RSI, *American Psychologist*, **43**, 1004–15.

KUORINKA, I. and FORCIER, L. (Eds) 1995 *Work Related Musculoskeletal Disorders (WMSDs): A Reference Book for Prevention*, London: Taylor & Francis.

LEPORE, S. J. 1995 Measurement of chronic stressors, in COHEN, S., KESSLER, R. C. and GORDON, L. U. (Eds), *Measuring Stress*, pp. 102–20, New York: Oxford University.

LEVENTHAL, H. 1986 Symptom reporting: A focus on process, in MCHUGH, S. and VALLIS, T. M. (Eds), *Illness Behavior: A Multidisciplinary Model*, pp. 219–37, New York: Plenum Press.

MCCRAE, R. R. and COSTA, P. T., JR. 1990 *Personality in Adulthood*, New York: Guilford Press.

NIOSH 1992 *US West Communications, Health Hazard Evaluation Report, HETA 89-299-2230*, Atlanta: National Institute for Occupational Safety and Health.

PENNEBAKER, J. 1982 *The Psychology of Physical Symptoms*, New York: Springer Verlag.

REYNOLDS, W. 1982 Development of reliable and valid short forms of the Marlowe–Crowne social desirability scale, *Journal of Clinical Psychology*, **38**, 119–25.

SPECTOR, P. 1992 A consideration of the validity and meaning of self-report measures of job conditions, *International Review of Industrial and Organizational Psychology*, **7**, 123–51.

STOCK, S. R. 1991 Workplace ergonomic factors and the development of musculoskeletal disorders of the neck and upper limbs: A meta-analysis, *American Journal of Industrial Medicine*, **19**, 87–107.

TAYLOR, J. A. 1953 A personality scale of manifest anxiety, *Journal of Abnormal and Social Psychology*, **48**, 285–90.

TELLEGEN, A. 1985 Structure of mood and personality and their relevance for assessing anxiety, with an emphasis on self-report, in TUMA, A. H. and MASER, J. D. (Eds), *Anxiety and the Anxiety Disorders*, pp. 681–706, Hillsdale, NJ: Erlbaum.

TURNER, R. J. and WHEATON, B. 1995 Checklist measurement of stressful life events in COHEN, S., KESSLER, R. C. and GORDON, L. U. (Eds), *Measuring Stress*, pp. 29–53, New York: Oxford University Press.

VASSEND, I. 1994 Negative affectivity, subjective somatic complaints and objective health indicators: Mind and body still separated?, in MAES, S., LEVENTHAL, H. and JOHNSTON, M. (Eds), *International Review of Health Psychology*, Vol. 3, pp. 97–118, Chichester: John Wiley.

WATSON, C. and CLARK, L. A. 1984 Negative affectivity: The disposition to experience aversive emotional states, *Psychological Bulletin*, **96**, 465–90.

WATSON, D. and PENNEBAKER, J. 1989 Health complaints, stress, and distress: Exploring the central role of negative affectivity, *Psychological Review*, **96**, 234–54.

PART THREE

Commentaries

CHAPTER SEVENTEEN

Work disability in an economic context

LESLIE I. BODEN

Work disability is a reduction in earnings or earning capacity caused by functional limitations. When workplace injury causes disability, workers become entitled to receive workers' compensation benefits. Longer recovery periods and more severe impairments lead to higher benefit payments. Frequently, employers prefer to pay less than workers would like to receive, and conflict ensues.

Unfortunately, the terms of discussion in this area often have focused on the worker, and the discussion has been conducted in pejorative terms: malingering, fraud, and so on. These refer to attempts by workers to stay off work while collecting benefits although they are fit. In recent years, several television shows have videotaped workers engaged in strenuous physical activities, workers who had fraudulently declared themselves disabled.[1]

While the media have paid attention to assertions of fraud and malingering by workers (for example, Dateline USA, 1995; Kerr, 1991), no credible evidence suggests substantial levels of this behavior. Thoughtful observers involved in disability evaluation and management have concluded that fraud and malingering by workers are quite rare (Foley *et al.*, 1987; see Chapter 8 of this volume). Studies do show that workers report more injuries and stay off work longer when workers' compensation benefit levels rise (Boden, 1995; Gardner, 1989). Yet these studies do not necessarily demonstrate malingering. They may simply mean that higher benefits lead to workers' reporting additional legitimate injuries and recuperating for appropriate, if longer, periods.

Picture, for a moment, injured workers arrayed on a continuum. At one end are workers like those videotaped for the television shows. They clearly have engaged in fraudulent behavior. On the other end are workers who, though badly injured and in much pain, come to work. Other injured workers fall between. In the middle of this continuum, an outside observer could not be certain whether a worker returned to work at just the right time, too soon, or too late.

Nobody knows the proportion of injured workers in each group. I would guess that, at most, 3 per cent of injured workers fall into the fraud category and that injured workers usually return to work after a reasonable time. Still, for many injuries, reasonable people can disagree about the appropriate recovery period.

Given the subjected nature of disability and the different incentives faced by workers and employers, disability determination engenders a great deal of dispute and mistrust between workers and employers. The popular view of this issue focuses on the morals (or lack thereof) of the people involved. Because worker fraud occurs only in small proportion of cases, this focus distracts us from a fuller understanding of the important physical, psychosocial, and economic factors that affect disability.

This chapter describes the system of economic factors affecting workers *and* employers and their possible effects. It also addresses the workplace system within which both injuries and workers' compensation claims occur. In doing so, I hope to shed some light on the causes of observed behavior. We can explain this behavior, recognizing that most of us are ethical individuals whose decisions are affected by the incentives we face.

This chapter focuses on four issues. First, it presents a job-mismatch model of injuries and disability, one that provides a labor-market context that is consistent with ergonomic and psychosocial models discussed elsewhere in this volume. Second, it describes how general employment conditions interact with physical limitations to cause unemployment or reduced wages among injured workers. Next, it shows how incentives inherent in workers' compensation affect the behavior of workers, employers and insurers, and medical-care providers. Finally, this chapter discusses perceptions of disability-related behavior of workers and how those perceptions can influence the actions of employers, physicians, and workers. In each of these cases, conflicts can develop, conflicts that interfere with medical treatment and with return to work.

JOB MATCH AND INJURY RATES

Many features of the employment situation can contribute to high injury rates, poor recovery, and extended time lost from work. Other papers in this volume discuss job stress, the organizational environment, job control, and other factors that can influence disability besides the physical stresses leading to cumulative trauma disorders (CTDs).

One cause of injuries and disability is a mismatch between the capabilities and needs of workers and the characteristics of their jobs. This includes the physiological match between the worker and job demands, the focus of ergonomics. Indeed, if the term were not already taken, I would choose ergonomics to describe the broader concept of job match, including psychosocial demands, pay, stress, security, the organizational environment, job control, and so on. Generally speaking, if a worker and a job are ill suited to each other, we expect the risk of injury and disability to be higher than otherwise. Note that a bad match could occur between a 'good' worker (a worker who would do well in other jobs) and a 'good' job (one that would suit other workers well).

At the time of hire, workers have acquired limited information about the job, and employers have similarly limited information about the worker. Over time, this information improves. As it does, workers and employers may find that the fit between the worker and the job is worse than they initially believed. This newly acquired information may lead to the worker's leaving or the employer's discharging the worker. This phenomenon partially explains the relatively high turnover of recently hired workers. But, while the parties are learning, and until the workers find new jobs or are fired, short-tenure workers may be employed in jobs that do not suit them. (See Viscusi, 1983, ch. 4.)

A bad fit between a worker and the job (caused by incomplete labor-market information during the search process) can cause poor productivity, increased risk of accidents, and low job satisfaction. Workers who are less productive and more dissatisfied are more likely to be disciplined and fired. Dissatisfied workers are more likely to quit. Also, as workers gain experience on the job, they discover the mismatch and may revise their initial estimate of the value of the job and quit; or employers may see accidents as a signal of a bad job fit and look to replace them. Finally, some injuries worsen the match between worker and job because the worker experiences disability.

This is one reason that studies have found that recently hired workers are more likely to be injured than workers with longer tenure (Hale and Hale, 1982). It is also consistent with results reported by Gardner and Butler in Chapter 14 of this volume. They show that workers receiving disciplinary notices more frequently file disability claims. They suggest that unit managers and problem workers collude to use disability insurance to foster removal of these workers. An alternate explanation is that disciplinary notices are signs of job mismatch and that mismatch increases the odds of injury or illness. Also, unit managers may not believe worker's assertions that they cannot work because of chronic illness or injury (especially for largely subjective complaints). This may lead them to issue disciplinary notices in such cases.

THE IMPACT OF EMPLOYMENT CONDITIONS ON DISABILITY

Disability – the loss of earnings or earning capacity caused by functional limitations – can change even when the worker's job match, impairment, skills, motivation, and so on, do not. It changes with a worker's access to employment opportunities.

Consider two equally skilled and motivated construction workers, one of whom has developed chronic lower back pain, while the other has not. Each typically moves from job to job and among various employers. When construction is booming and the labor market is tight, both may find new jobs quickly after current construction projects are completed. But, during a recession, unemployment among construction workers may be 20 per cent or greater. If employers preferentially hire healthy workers (despite the provisions of the Americans with Disabilities Act), workers with no health problems will find work more easily than those with lower back pain.

Joint causation of unemployment by economic conditions, impairment, and other factors can make it difficult to know whether to attribute a worker's income losses to a workplace injury. It creates a gray zone in entitlement to benefits. If a worker becomes unemployed but was not injured, that worker may be entitled to receive unemployment insurance benefits, at least until they expire. In addition, a disabled worker has access to workers' compensation benefits. Thus, workers and employers can disagree about the ambiguous impact of impairment on unemployment. Of course, workers will prefer to receive the more generous benefit. Research shows that the relative attractiveness of unemployment and workers' compensation benefits affects how frequently workers use the two systems (Fortin and Lanoie, 1992).

This can complicate compensation decisions, leading to uncertainty and litigation. In Florida, workers' compensation pays a proportion of the difference between current wages and pre-injury wages for workers with long-term disabilities. There are called wage-loss benefits. When an injured worker becomes unemployed or takes a low-paying job, that worker may apply for wage-loss benefits. The employer (or a workers' compensation judge) must then decide whether the income loss resulted from the injury or would have occurred in the absence of injury. Disagreements over the cause of income losses have led to substantial litigation and widespread concern and about resolving this problem (Berkowitz and Burton, 1987; Brainerd, 1990).

ECONOMIC INCENTIVES IN WORKERS' COMPENSATION

Let us turn to another example, that of a construction laborer in Illinois with a severe back strain who earns $900 per week. While he remains off work on workers' compensation, his medical care is fully paid and he receives $600 per week in tax-free workers' compensation benefits, perhaps more than his after-tax wages (Beck, 1993; Workers' Compensation Research Institute, 1993). Transport this construction laborer to neighboring Indiana, where the maximum temporary total disability benefit in 1994 is $394. In Indiana, he loses about $200 in after-tax income for every week that he stays home recuperating. Further, in Indiana the waiting period for workers' compensation benefits is seven days: in Illinois it is only three days. So, for injuries that might last between four days and a week, workers may receive over $100 a day in Illinois, but nothing in Indiana. Not surprisingly, most workers with equivalent injuries will return to work more quickly in Indiana. Indeed, some injured workers who would miss no work if injured in Indiana might stay home from work if they were injured in Illinois.

Workers in Indiana may not be more honest, have a stronger work ethic, or be more stoical than workers in Illinois, despite reporting fewer injuries and returning to work more quickly. The disparity is reported disability is caused by the greater economic pressures faced by injured workers in Indiana. Further, we cannot say whether the recuperation time of workers in Illinois or Indiana is closer to some 'medically appropriate' time way from work. Workers in Indiana might, on average, return to work too soon, may work in pain, and may be reinjured more often; or workers in Illinois might typically take longer than necessary to return.

Workers' compensation income benefits uncouple workers' incomes from work; in doing so, workers' compensation reduces incentives to return to work. Economists and insurance professionals call this *moral hazard*. This type of moral hazard changes disability behavior. As their benefits increase, covered workers will choose to recuperate longer (lose more work) after injury. Observed disability thus increases with income benefits.

This is only one example of moral hazard, which is a very widespread phenomenon. Wherever insurance buffers people from the costs associated with their behavior, it invites more of that behavior. Moral hazard is virtually a necessary consequence of insurance. Moral hazard can be reduced by limiting insurance (through, say, copayments and deductibles) or by monitoring behavior – which can be expensive, ineffective, or both.

Health-care insurance, for example, reduces the costs of individuals of the health-care services that they purchase. It thus leads them to purchase more than they otherwise would. This increases the costs of health care for us all. Still, the insurance provides access to preventive and curative care that otherwise would go unused.

Gardner and Butler (Chapter 14 of this volume) show that providers in health-maintenance organizations (HMOs) can have incentives to misclassify non-occupational injuries as compensable under workers' compensation or, at least, to classify cases of unclear etiology as compensable. HMOs typically receive a flat amount per covered employee, not per treatment or condition. However, they receive additional fees when they treat injuries covered by workers' compensation. This extra income distorts financial incentives to diagnose injuries and illnesses as work related.[2] It is most likely to affect physician behavior for occupational diseases and CTDs, where cause and effect are not simultaneous.

Employers are not immune from distorted incentives under workers' compensation. The premiums of small insured employers do not change with their injury experience (Russell, 1974). Small employers with high injury rates pay the same premiums as safer employers. Insurance uncouples their costs from workplace safety. This form of moral hazard leads small employers to underinvest in safety. In effect, they 'buy' more accidents by investing their capital in production rather than safety.

On the other hand, larger employers may have incentives to discourage claim filing, to reject worker's compensation claims, and to compel workers to return to work before they are ready. These incentives can be particularly great if the employer lacks group health and disability insurance plans or if these plans are not self-insured or experience-rated. If the additional workers' compensation costs of injuries are high compared with sick leave and group medical costs, the employer will prefer to see injuries classified as nonoccupational.

One study reported that two community colleges more aggressively challenged the compensability of claims after switching to self-insurance (Chelius and Kavanaugh, 1988). Self-insurance increased the impact of injuries on worker's compensation costs, leading employers to report fewer injuries. Spieler (1994) notes that, if employers initiate aggressive loss-control programs, injured workers may fear retaliation and avoid filing injury claims. Rising costs may also cause employers to institute safety contests with group rewards for injury-free periods. Pressure from fellow workers may then decrease reporting by injured workers. Other studies have also found that financial incentives affect employer reporting of injuries (Ruser and Smith, 1988) and hazardous conditions (Boden and Gold, 1984).

Higher benefits increase the potential for dispute between injured workers and their employers and insurers. The latitude for dispute is greatest where objective measures of impairment apply the least and where reported pain and discomfort are primary criteria. This description applies partially well to musculoskeletal injuries for two reasons. First, objective verifiable diagnostic criteria frequently do not exist. Second, physicians may find the relationship between such criteria and the injured worker's perception of disability tenuous and confounded by other factors which they do not understand. For musculoskeletal injuries, employers may be suspicious that injured workers exaggerate their symptoms and take advantage of worker's compensation benefits. Workers, on their side, may feel unjustly accused by malingering; they may be angry with their employers, who do not validate their symptoms, do not trust them, and try to compel them to return to work before they are ready.

MORAL HAZARD AND THE PERCEPTION OF DISABILITY

Less tactful circles may label behavior affected by moral hazard as fraud or malingering. In the United States, folk wisdom and media reports suggest that workers commonly file workers' compensation claims fraudulently. Musculoskeletal injuries, where diagnosis often relies primarily on workers' reports of symptoms, are thought to be particularly prone to fraud and malingering. This perception itself often leads to counterproductive behavior by both employers and injured workers.

Some years ago in Massachusetts, it was common in cases involving permanent impairment for employers to refuse to settle a claim without a written agreement from the injured worker to look elsewhere for employment. Some employers believed that the workers, upon receipt of a large settlement, would appear the following day at work, driving a new car bought with workers' compensation proceeds and completely 'cured.' The employers were fearful that other workers would attempt to duplicate this presumed windfall, and an epidemic of 'injuries' would follow.

Physicians also may mistrust patients presenting with symptoms of musculoskeletal injury. Such suspicions may have been bred from past instances where they believed they had been misled. But patients perceive these attitudes and mistrust the physician in turn. This makes successful treatment less likely than otherwise.

On the other hand, patients faced with mistrust and disbelief can view their duty as convincing physicians and employers of the validity of their illness (Reid *et al.*, 1991). This may lead to their exaggerating and prolonging symptoms, particularly if compensation (which they believe is due them) depends on this.

Stern (1989) tried to measure whether people who were not employed were likely to exaggerate their disabilities using data from the 1979 Health Interview Survey. In this survey, respondents were considered disabled if they reported that their health limited the amount or kind of work that they could do. This survey also contained physician-diagnosed health conditions among respondents and information about whether workers were employed. Stern tested statistically whether people's employment status affected their reporting of disability, given their observed health conditions. He found no evidence that being out of work led people to exaggerate their disability.

In many states, we find a typical pattern of behavior for injuries involving permanent disability. Employers and insurers hire physicians to assess impairment. These physicians, often suspicious of workers' motivations, rarely find impairment and, when they do, find little. Injured workers, in response, hire attorneys who find physicians who are much more generous in their approach to assessing impairment. Thus begins a pattern of litigation that absorbs about one-third of income benefits, increases animosity between workers and employers, and imposes impediments to reemployment (Boden, 1988, 1992).

CONCLUSION

Economic conditions affect the behaviour of injured workers, employers and insurers, and medical-care providers. Because the ability to work is not an objective, easily measured phenomenon, divergent incentives often result in conflict. Employers deny claims for compensation. Workers and their physicians mistrust each other. Workers believe that they are not getting benefits that they deserve and that employers are forcing them to return to work too early. Employers feel that workers are malingering.

These conflicts carry their own negative consequences. Injured workers are not rehired, or they quit. Workers and their employers become embroiled in litigation that thwarts medical treatment and reemployment. Physicians and their patients become entangled in a web of mistrust that undermines effective treatment.

Each of these issues is part of a *system* of employment, wages, and disability compensation. Attributing base motivation does not advance a primary goal of both medical treatment and worker's compensation: returning workers to productive and gainful employment. We can achieve this goal only by recognizing the psychosocial and economic conditions that affect disability and altering those features of the employment, medical, and disability systems that stand in its way.

NOTES

1 Employers and providers also engage in fraud, although most evidence also is anecdotal. Massachusetts recently indicted an employee leasing firm for underreporting the number of workers on its payroll, thus paying $600 000 instead of $5 million in annual premiums (Bureau of National Affairs, 1995). Similarly, medical-care providers may overbill, charge for services they did not provide, or solicit workers to file claims even when they were not injured at work (Kerr, 1991; Silverstein, 1992; Boden, 1994).

2 Still, another recent study found lower workers' compensation medical payments and somewhat lower income benefits among HMO enrollees (Zwerling *et al.*, 1991).

REFERENCES

BECK, M. 1993 *Income Replacement in Pennsylvania*, Workers Compensation Research Institute Research Brief 9(3S), Cambridge, MA: Workers Compensation Research Institute.

BERKOWITZ, M. and BURTON, J. F., Jr. 1987 *Permanent Disability Benefits in Workers' Compensation*, Kalamazoo, MI: W.E. Upjohn Institute for Employment Research.

BODEN, L. I. 1988 *Reducing Litigation: Evidence from Wisconsin*, Cambridge, MA: Workers' Compensation Research Institute.

BODEN, L. I. 1992 Dispute resolution in workers' compensation, *Review of Economics and Statistics*, **74**, 493–502.

BODEN, L. I. 1994 *Medicolegal Fees in California: An Assessment*, Cambridge, MA: Workers Compensation Research Institute.

BODEN, L. I. 1985 Workers' compensation in the United States: High costs, low benefits, *Annual Review of Public Health*, **16**, 189–216.

BODEN, L. I. and GOLD, M. 1984 The accuracy of self-reported regulatory data: The case of coal mine dust, *American Journal of Industrial Medicine*, **6**, 427–40.

BRAINERD, S. J. 1990 Déjà vu in Tallahassee: Florida tries again, *John Burton's Workers' Compensation Monitor*, **3**(4), 3–10.

BUREAU OF NATIONAL AFFAIRS 1985 Employee leasing company, owner charged with workers' comp fraud, *BNA Workers' Compensation Report*, **6**(1), 3.

CHELIUS, J. R. and KAVANAUGH, K. 1988 Workers' compensation and the level of occupational injuries, *Journal of Risk and Insurance*, **55**, 315–23.

COMMISSION ON THE EVALUATION OF PAIN 1987 *Report*, Washington, DC: Social Security Administration.

DATELINE USA 1995 You pay the bill, NBC, January 10.

FORTIN, B. and LANOIE, P. 1992 Substitution between unemployment insurance and workers' compensation: An analysis applied to the risk of workplace accidents, *Journal of Public Economics*, **49**, 287–312.

GARDNER, J. 1989 *Return-to-Work Incentives: Lessons for Policymakers from Economic Studies*, Cambridge, MA: Workers' Compensation Research Institute.

HALE, A. R. and HALE, M. 1982 *A Review of the Industrial Accident Research Literature by the National Institute of Industrial Psychology*, London: HMSO.

KERR, P. 1991 Vast amount of fraud discovered in workers' compensation system, *New York Times*, **141**(48, 829), 1, 14.

REID, J., EWAN, C. and LOWY, E. 1991 Pilgrimage of pain: The illness experiences of women with repetition strain injury and the search for credibility, *Social Science and Medicine*, **32**, 601–12.

RUSER, J. W. and SMITH, R. S. 1988 The effect of OSHA records-check inspections on reported occupational injuries in manufacturing establishments, *Journal of Risk and Uncertainty*, **1**, 415–35.

RUSSELL, L. B. 1974 Safety incentives in workmen's compensation, *Journal of Human Resources*, **9**, 361–75.

SILVERSTEIN, S. 1992 Fraud disables state's workers' compensation program, *Los Angeles Times*, August 23, D1 + .

SPIELER, E. A. 1994 Perpetuating risk? Workers' compensation and the persistence of occupational injuries, *Houston Law Review*, **31**, 119–264.

STERN, S. 1989 Measuring the effect of disability on labor force participation, *Journal of Human Resources*, **24**, 361–95.

VISCUSI, W. K. 1983 *Risk by Choice*, Cambridge, MA: Harvard University Press.

WORKERS COMPENSATION RESEARCH INSTITUTE 1993 Income replacement in Minnesota, *WCRI Research Brief* 9(5S), Cambridge, MA: Workers Compensation Research Institute.

ZWERLING, C., RYAN, J. and ORAV, J. 1991 Workers' compensation cost shifting: An empirical study, *American Journal of Industrial Medicine*, **19**, 317–25.

CHAPTER EIGHTEEN

Musculoskeletal disorders in office work

The Need to Consider Both Physical and Psychosocial Factors

LAWRENCE J. FINE

MAGNITUDE OF WORK-RELATED MUSCULOSKELETAL DISORDERS

Overall in the United States, the magnitude of the work-related musculoskeletal disorders of the upper extremity (WRMUE) is increasing. From 1982 to 1992 the number of illness cases of disorders associated with repeated trauma (the category that includes most musculoskeletal disorders of the upper extremity) increased from 22,600 to 282,000 cases (USDL, 1993). This trend is not some generalized phenomena related to the reporting of all workplace disorders or injuries, since other disorders such as work-related skin disorders have not shown an increase of similar magnitude. The reasons for this increase are not clear, but the suggestion is that workplace and societal factors can influence both the incidence of symptoms and physical signs of WRMUE, and whether workers decide to report these disorders to their employers and seek workers' compensation for these disorders.

WRMUE are commonly associated with office work involving video display terminals (VDTs). Surveys of individual workplaces both in the United States and other countries have found high rates in some office workplaces and specific jobs. For example, 22 per cent of telecommunication and 41 per cent of newspaper employees using VDTs had WRMUEs in recent NIOSH studies (Bernard *et al.*, 1993; Hales *et al.*, 1994). While most of these disorders were not associated with work disability, approximately one-third of the workers with WRMUE have sought health care. Nevertheless, most national and state-based surveillance data suggest that the incidence of these disorders is less in VDT-associated work than in manufacturing industries. The variation in the rates of WRMUE across industries with different technologies argues strongly for the etiological importance of specific psychosocial and physical workplace factors in both the development and reporting of WRMUE. One of the reasons that the etiology of these WRMUE in the office setting are controversial is that the specific anatomical cause of the upper-limb pain in these office workers is often not clear in contrast to the WRMUEs associated with highly repetitive and forceful tasks often found in some other risk industries such as meat packing (NIOSH, 1989).

PROPOSED EXPLANATIONS FOR WORK-RELATED DISORDERS

Individual, workplace psychosocial and physical, and societal factors have been postulated as causes of WRMUE and the increased incidence of these disorders (Bongers *et al.*, 1993). Most recent models that have been proposed to explain the etiology of WRMUE directly identify the importance of individual and workplace factors while indirectly addressing the role of societal factors (Armstrong *et al.*, 1993; Bongers *et al.*, 1993; Chapter 1 of this volume). The causal role of individual factors such as overall mental health or personality traits is not clear based on the results of longitudinal studies of WRMUE (Bongers *et al.*, 1993). The definition of individual causal factors in each study tends to be different. The individual factors seem unlikely to explain the recent increase in the incidence of WRMUE since, over a decade, it is unlikely that the distribution of individual factors such as personality traits is rapidly changing.

The workplace factors are both physical and psychosocial working conditions. In the office setting the separation of physical from psychosocial factors is not always clear. For example, is working under deadline as a newspaper reporter primarily a psychosocial or physical stressor? That is, does it cause one to type faster or does it increase muscle tension independent of the speed of keying? Individual factors in these models do influence the relationship between workplace factors and the development of adverse health outcomes. However, the study of individual factors seems most useful as confounders or effect modifiers.

From an epidemiological perspective, it is difficult to investigate societal factors postulated in several of the chapters in this volume. Such studies would need either to measure societal changes in compensation systems, overall ergonomic conditions, medical practice, and other social processes over time in the same society, or compare different societies on both exposure and health outcome variables. While these types of ecological studies have provided important support for hypotheses related to cancer and cardiovascular disease, they have not been feasible in occupational epidemiology.

IMPORTANCE OF PHYSICAL AND PSYCHOSOCIAL WORK FACTORS

Given the postulated stability of individual attributes over the last decade and the difficulty in studying societal factors, it seems most practical to focus epidemiological or field studies on physical and psychosocial workplace factors. In contrast to job tasks in some manufacturing jobs that involve exposure to repetitive work and which require forceful exertions of the muscles of the forearm and shoulder girdle, VDT-related job tasks generally do not require forceful exertions to the same extent. This is an additional reason that it is important to investigate more closely the role of physical and psychosocial occupational factors in the office workplace. Another reason that studying these two distinct classes of exposure variables is important arises from the need to understand the likely complex interactions between them. Finally, studying the role of workplace factors in WRMUE could also help to explain the development of substantial impairment or disability in a minority of those who are affected.

One of the critical steps in studying physical and psychosocial factors is to decide how to study each set of factors most efficiently since including both is likely to require substantial resources. Theoretical models that help the investigator to identify the most important exposure factors in specific workplaces are therefore useful. While difficult, the development of exposure assessment strategies that incorporate the investigation of both physical and psychosocial factors should assist in the development of effective prevention strategies and greater scientific understanding of the problem of WRMUEs associated with VDT work.

REFERENCES

ARMSTRONG, T. *et al.* 1993 A conceptual model for work-related back and upper-limb musculoskeletal disorders, *Scandinavian Journal of Work, Environment and Health*, **19**, 73–84.

BERNARD, B., SAUTER, S. L., FINE, L., PETERSEN, M. and HALES, T. 1994 Job task and psychosocial risk factors for work-related musculoskeletal disorders among newspaper reporters, *Scandinavian Journal of Work, Environment and Health*, **20**, 356–65.

BONGERS, P. M., DE WINTER, C. R., KOMPIEK, M. A. J. and HILDEBRANDT, V. H. 1993 Psychosocial factors at work and musculoskeletal disease, *Scandinavian Journal of Work, Environment and Health*, **19**, 297–312.

HALES, T. R., SAUTER, S. L., PETERSON, M. R., FINE, L. J., PUTZ-ANDERSON, V., SCHLEIFER, L. R., OCHS, T. T. and BERNARD, B. P. 1994 Musculoskeletal disorders among visual display terminal (VDT) users in a telecommunications company, *Ergonomics*, **37**(11), 1603–21.

NIOSH (NATIONAL INSTITUTE FOR OCCUPATIONAL SAFETY AND HEALTH) 1989 *HETA Report 88-180-1958*, Sioux Falls, SD: John Morrell and Co. (Cincinnati, OH: National Institute for Occupational Safety and Health).

USDL (UNITED STATES DEPARTMENT OF LABOUR) 1993 Workplace injuries and illnesses in 1992, *News*, Bureau of Labor Statistics, USDL 93-553.

CHAPTER NINETEEN

Is it time to integrate psychosocial prevention with ergonomics for cumulative trauma disorders?

LINDA M. FRAZIER, CRAIG R. STENBERG and LAWRENCE J. FINE

RELATIONSHIP BETWEEN PSYCHOSOCIAL FACTORS AND CTDs

The Durham conference and the resulting chapters in this book have explored the relationship between psychosocial factors and the development and treatment of cumulative trauma disorders (CTDs). These disorders have also been described by a wide variety of terms such as 'work-related musculoskeletal disorders.' The term 'CTD' will be used since it is the most common one, while acknowledging that it implies an oversimplified view of the causation for a diverse group of upper-limb disorders. Several presentations addressed a model by which workstyle factors and psychosocial factors could lead to upper-extremity symptoms (Chapters 1, 2, 5, and 6 of this volume). This more comprehensive model provides a more accurate description of the possible causal factors in upper-limb disorders. Some presentations explored possible societal, anthropologic, or economic explanations for when and why individuals with upper-extremity pain symptoms may report them (Chapters 3, 9, and 14). Problems in the traditional medical approach to treating pain were pointed out (Chapter 12) and alternative therapeutic constructs were proposed (Chapter 10).

Problems in existing studies of the relationship between psychosocial factors and CTDs include defining psychosocial distress and measuring it accurately, differentiating between personal psychosocial characteristics and work organization, lack of prospective designs in which psychosocial factors are measured before pain develops so as to be able to determine whether the psychosocial distress was caused by the pain or preceded it, and measuring ergonomic factors with the same degree of precision as is used to measure psychosocial factors is a given study. It will be difficult for any single study to resolve definitively the relative importance of these factors since such a study should be prospective, require intensive measurement of psychosocial and physical exposures at base line and thereafter periodically, and must involve workplaces with different combinations of low and high exposures to all major hypothesized causal factors. Despite these methodologic problems, overall current research suggests that both ergonomics (physical factors such as awkward, static postures of arms during typing tasks) and psychosocial factors are important (Chapters 9, 11, and 16).

When CTDs become a problem in a workplace, successful interventions often employ worker involvement in the design of the solution (Chapter 15). It may come as a surprise to some that successful interventions need not be exceedingly expensive. Ergonomic issues nearly always must be addressed, but work organization and communication between management and labor appear also to be important.

The traditional ergonomic paradigm may only explain part of the variance in CTD development. Clusters of CTDs may be found in one group of office workers but not in another group that has similar physical tasks and equipment. This suggests that ergonomic factors are not the only etiologic stimulus.

Increases in the number of work-related upper limb disorders have been noted in both the Bureau of Labor Statistics Annual Report and in workers' compensation systems since the early 1980s before these disorders received widespread coverage in the national media (Korrick *et al.*, 1994; US Department of Labor, 1992; Franklin *et al.*, 1991; Tanaka *et al.*, 1988). The majority of the cases of upper-limb disorders detected in these surveillance systems occurs in manufacturing industries where jobs with highly repetitive and forceful movements of the hands are common.

No research suggests that CTDs are entirely caused by psychologic pathology which the worker brings to the job. But the public may incorrectly leap to this conclusion (Chapter 13). Health professionals and ergonomists need to communicate clearly when describing the relationship between psychosocial factors and CTDs in order to avoid an invitation to blame the worker, suggesting that 'it's all in her head.' This attitude leads one to miss an opportunity to improve work organization which may very well prevent future CTDs.

PREVENTION OF CTDs

From a prevention perspective, effective strategies can be divided into three types: primary prevention directed at averting the development of the disorder; secondary prevention directed at deterring progression of a disorder from a mild state to an impairing or disabling state; and tertiary prevention preventing the impairment or disability from becoming permanent. Considering the prevention or control of CTDs from this perspective is particularly important because the causal factors that influence the initial development of the disorder might be substantially different than those that influence the development of permanent disability. The models presented during the symposium are consistent with the hypothesis that factors that initiate these disorders may sometimes be different from those that determine whether a worker, for example, files for workers' compensation. For instance, a reasonable hypothesis is that both the ability of the worker to control the pace of work and the worker's level of satisfaction with his or her job both might influence the likelihood of the worker filing for workers' compensation for a work-related carpal tunnel syndrome. Primary prevention, when feasible, is the most promising strategy because if it is successful, it can result in a permanent reduction in the numbers of disorders. It involves designing workplaces and processes to eliminate exposure to physical and adverse psychosocial factors. Particularly in the office setting, the goal of primary prevention is not the total elimination of exposure since the relationship between the level of exposure and the risk of disease may be U-shaped. Levels of exposure that are either too high or too low may be problematic. For example, the elimination of all movement may not be helpful. While not proven, preventive steps taken for the purpose of primary prevention may also improve employee morale and productivity.

Secondary and tertiary prevention are also important. Even if all primary work-related disorders could be prevented, some workers would have musculoskeletal pain or disorders which need to be accommodated during work. With some occupational health problems such as asbestos-related lung cancer, there are no practical secondary preventive actions, but with CTDs there is a substantial opportunity for secondary prevention since these disorders are often intermittent and mild. Critical to the secondary prevention is the encouragement of early reporting of symptoms and prompt evaluation of these symptoms. Evaluating the workplaces of these individuals will identify sometimes simple changes which will prevent the development of a more serious disorder. Tertiary prevention involves the rehabilitation of the seriously affected individual including reassessment of the workplace for adverse exposure.

Additional research will be very helpful in testing the efficacy of specific interventions to prevent CTDs. Controlled studies are needed of changes in work organization as well as of changes in specific ergonomic factors. But preventive efforts cannot wait until an exhaustive research base is available, especially since jobs are constantly evolving. Based on what we know now, prudent preventive interventions all of three types, primary, secondary, and tertiary, should follow several basic principles. The first step is problem definition. This allows one to tailor the intervention to the particular needs of a given workplace.

DEFINING THE PROBLEM

Surveillance data from the Occupational Safety and Health Administration (OSHA) log, workers' compensation records, or other sources can help to determine the magnitude of the problem by identifying the frequency of CTD claims, the body part affected, the specific diagnosis and the work areas that are having problems. Many companies perform injury analysis routinely. One claim is enough to conclude that further investigation is needed, at least at a basic level. This concept may be difficult to enlist others to agree with because people often believe that injuries are accidental, caused by a break in procedure or by carelessness. Incident reports and workers' compensation forms are often called 'accident reports.' This conceptualization can unfortunately make people wrongly fatalistic about the usefulness of prevention.

Ergonomic review of workstations and job tasks is ideally indicated before CTD problems develop. Certainly once musculoskeletal pain problems have surfaced, a basic ergonomic assessment is in order. This assessment should look not only for repetitive use of the upper extremity, but also for whether the repetitive motions entail significant force, significantly awkward or static posture (particularly if the task requires the application of force), significantly vibrating tools, repeated forceful direct compression of the proximal wrist, and work in refrigerated temperatures.

Input from workers can be very helpful in developing a list of job tasks that are most problematic. Informal discussions, formal surveys, and worker–management safety committees are methods of obtaining problem-identification information from workers. Employee relations issues are important to define. It is helpful at the outset to have an estimate of the budget that may be available to apply to potential solutions.

A look at work organization can help to define any problems (Peters, 1982; Oxenburgh, 1991; Kohn, 1993). Are workers able to make some decisions on how to perform job tasks, or are all policy and procedures defined in detail by management? Are workers responsible for outcomes yet unable to influence the preliminary tasks that need to be accomplished to achieve the outcome? Does machine pacing, a worker monitoring system or a piece-work incentive system influence workers to avoid taking periodic mini-pauses in muscular activity? Are worker-generated innovations in work procedures and tool design encouraged and followed up? Is there a substantive injury/disorder follow-up by workers and management to identify ways to prevent future injuries, or is the most common outcome of the 'accident' investigation 'Be more careful'?

DEVELOPING AND IMPLEMENTING AN INTERVENTION STRATEGY

Using a worker–management team approach, minor problems can be corrected at the shop-floor level. For major problems, organizational change may be needed to achieve shop-floor-level change. Define goals and a realistic budget at the outset. During tight economic times, it may not be realistic to purchase all new equipment, but some aggravating tools or work procedures could be improved with reasonable cost. Address both ergonomics and work organization, including employee relations issues. Beware of fads, both in ergonomics and work organization. Involve workers in problem identification and solution generation prior to making changes. Stepwise changes can be easier to comprehend and adjust to than sudden sweeping changes.

Above all, educate workers about the reason and manner of planned changes before implementing them. Educate supervisors about the fallacy of viewing injuries as accidents. Educate about ergonomic factors associated with CTDs, how to delegate a reasonable degree of autonomy to workers, and how to interact successfully with an unhappy or injured worker. Upper management need to look at incentive systems to ensure that they do not inadvertently encourage counterproductive behaviors such as 'every person for themselves' or skipping mini-muscle use pauses and standard breaks (Sauter *et al.*, 1985; Kohn, 1993).

CRITICAL INCIDENT DEBRIEFING WHEN CTDs OCCUR

Critical incident debriefing is an early intervention technique which is increasingly used by organizations to assist persons impacted by traumatic events such as a major accident or an episode of workplace violence. Prior to traumatic incidents, the organization is encouraged to develop a comprehensive response plan which focuses as much as possible on prevention strategies and prepares the organization to respond quickly, effectively, and compassionately if a traumatic event occurs. Following a traumatic incident, educational groups and/or individual sessions are made available by clinicians specifically trained to provide information about trauma responses and coping strategies. As facilitators, they assist the organization in processing the events that have occurred, in skills training which may help minimize longer-term negative psychological consequences, and in reviewing and revising the trauma response plan to implement additional preventative measures as needed and to improve the organization's trauma response capabilities. Importantly, the critical incident debriefing approach does not pathologize responses but, rather, helps to 'normalize' them through education about what trauma response is and by skills training which engages the individual and the organization in the recovery process. Instead of seeking help solely through professional treatment, the individual and the organization are instructed in how to be part of the recovery process. For example, supervisors and other key organizational members who sometimes do not know what to say or do and consequently do nothing (leaving the impression that the organization does not care) are given training, emphasizing the important role that they can play in sensitively listening and communicating with those most directly effected. When co-workers, managers, or others do not extend themselves in appropriate, compassionate ways, the impacted worker's recovery may be further compounded by psychosocial factors resulting from perceived criticism, rejection, and/or abandonment. As clinicians, professionals providing critical incident response services use these educational sessions as an opportunity to gather information which may lead to additional recommendations both for subsequent organizational and individual treatment interventions. They sometimes provide ongoing treatment services to symptomatic individuals and, if needed, channel them to more comprehensive services (Barnett-Queen and Bergmann, 1990; Mitchell, 1993).

While CTD cases seldom present as suddenly as many of the traumas typically addressed with critical incident debriefing, these techniques may well have utility in reducing the likelihood that a particularly difficult CTD case or small cluster of cases might develop into a more widespread epidemic (Chapter 9). Prior to the onset of CTD problems, occupational health professionals should assist the organization in developing a comprehensive prevention and early intervention response plan. Working as facilitators with upper-level management, supervisors, labor representatives, and other key parties, occupational health professionals can help to foster an organizational environment in which comprehensive prevention and early intervention programming becomes possible. After identifying a CTD incident, occupational health professionals trained in critical incident response techniques could use group and individual 'debriefing sessions' modeled after the critical incident techniques to provide education to supervisors, co-workers, and other affected parties, helping them to understand the ergonomic, work practice, and organizational factors that may have contributed to the onset of the CTD problem. While maintaining an appropriate level of confidentiality about certain specific medical details, this approach may help to 'normalize' the symptoms and reduce negative attributions which may lead to negative labeling of affected individuals. These sessions would also provide a forum within which the occupational health professional can assist supervisors and co-workers in understanding the ergonomic, work practice, and organizational factors that may foster improvement in the specific incident and which may foster a safer environment in the future.

The individual who has been labeled as having a medical problem caused by office work may experience psychological symptomatology as a result of the injury, especially fear of reinjury (Harber, 1994). These symptoms and concerns should be addressed as early as possible, again following the critical incident debriefing educational model. The patient needs a balanced explanation of causal factors (both occupational and nonoccupational) contributing to the condition, treatment options, and potential workplace interventions such as modification of job tasks and workstations. The patient should also be educated about normal psychological reactions to injury which may compound the recovery process. It is exceedingly important that the medical-care provider does not portray psychological interventions in a manner that even covertly gives the patient the message that he or she believes that the problem may be a result of psychological abnormality. Rather, psychological intervention should be presented by the physician as an opportunity to build on the coping skills already acquired by the patient so that she or he will be able to cope even more effectively with the accommodations that people have to make in order to recover most successfully. The physician should address the psychological issues at the beginning of treatment, otherwise it becomes very difficult to introduce them later without conveying the impression that after some traditional medical treatment has failed, the physician has begun to wonder if some of the problem is 'in the patient's head.' In turn, this can provoke a struggle between patient and medical-care providers and/or case managers in which the patient seeks to 'prove' that the problems are indeed real (i.e. physical), leading to frustration on both sides. Dealing with openly psychological issues from the beginning creates the opportunity for a healing partnership which does not polarize physical and psychosocial factors by dichotomizing them.

To be most effective, physicians treating CTDs need skills beyond their traditionally based medical expertise. They need both excellent individual and group 'bedside manners' which convey a sincere message of caring and confidence, thereby engaging the individual and the organization in a healing partnership. Medical education often does not provide significant training in group dynamics, group communication, or organizational consultation. Consequently, physicians working in this field would be well advised to seek additional training in these areas and/or to work in partnership with clinicians who have acquired this expertise.

To prevent CTDs, make problem assessment and solution generation part of standard operating procedure, not a one-time initiative.

CONCLUSIONS

Psychosocial factors have been correlated with musculoskeletal symptoms, without question. When these data are interpreted as indicating that personal flaws cause CTDs, it can lead to victim blaming and failure to detect problems which may be part organizational and part ergonomic. This can further lead to incorrect interventions, nonresolution of the problem, and lost productivity, both on a patient-care level and on a workplace level. When one explores the view that psychosocial factors correlate with work organization, then interventions can be designed and tested which simultaneously address ergonomic and psychosocial risk factors for CTDs. This approach makes for good science and good business.

REFERENCES

Barnett-Queen, T. and Bergmann, T. H. 1990 Response to traumatic event crucial in preventing lasting consequences, *Occupational Health and Safety*, **59**(7) 53–5.

Franklin, G. M., Haug, J., Heyer, N. Checkoway, H. and Peck, N. 1991 Occupational carpal tunnel syndrome in Washington State, 1984–1988, *American Journal of Public Health*, **81**, 741–6.

Harber, P. 1994 Impairment and disability, in Rosenstock, L. and Cullen, M. R. (Eds), *Textbook of Clinical Occupational and Environmental Medicine*, p. 94, Philadelphia, PA: W. B. Saunders.

Kohn, A. 1993 Thank God it's Monday: The roots of motivation in the workplace, in *Punished by Rewards: The Trouble with Gold Stars, Incentive Plans, A's, Praise and Other Bribes*, pp. 181–97, Boston: Houghton Mifflin.

Korrick, S. A., Rest, K. M., Davis, L. K. and Christian, D. C. 1994 Use of state workers' compensation data for occupational carpal tunnel syndrome surveillance: A feasibility study in Massachusetts, *American Journal of Industrial Medicine*, **25**, 837–50.

Mitchell, J. T. 1993 When disaster strikes: The critical incident stress debriefing process, *Annals of Emergency Medical Services*, **8**, 36–9.

Oxenburgh, M. 1991 *Increasing Productivity and Profit Through Health and Safety: Case Studies in Successful Occupational Health and Safety Practice*, Sydney: CCH International.

Peters, T. 1982 *In Search of Excellence*, New York: Harper & Row.

Sauter, S., Chapman, L. J. and Knutson, S. J. 1985 *Improving VDT Work: Causes and Control of Health Concerns in VDT Use*, Lawrence, KS: Ergosyst Associates.

Tanaka, S., Seligman, P., Halperin, W., Thom, M., Timbrook, C. L. and Meal, T. J. 1988 Use of workers' compensation claims data for surveillance of cumulative trauma disorders, *Journal of Occupational Medicine*, **30**, 488–92.

US Department of Labor, Bureau of Labor Statistics 1992 *Occupational Injuries and Illnesses in the United States by Industry, 1990*, Washington, DC: US Government Printing Office, Bulletin 2399.

Index